Patient Problems:
A Research Base for
Nursing Care

by
Jenifer Wilson-Barnett *and* **Lynn Batehup**
King's College, University of London, UK

with invited chapters from
Morva Fordham
King's College, University of London, UK

SCUTARI PRESS
London

Copyright © Scutari Press 1988

A division of Scutari Projects Ltd, the publishing company
of the Royal College of Nursing

First published 1988
Reprinted 1991, 1992

British Library Cataloguing in Publication Data

Wilson-Barnett, Jenifer
  Patient problems: a research base for
  nursing care
  1. Medicine. Nursing
  I. Title   II. Batehup, Lynn
  III. Fordham, Morva
  610.73

ISBN 1 871364 10 8

Typeset by Input Typesetting, London SW19 8DR
Printed and bound in Great Britain by
Courier International Limited, East Kilbride

Table of Contents

Preface

Although nursing is a new science there is now a substantial body of research which has implications and provides guidelines for practice. Nursing covers a wide range of clinical care and should exploit studies which explore social, psychological and physical aspects of health and illness. Reviewing, analysing and criticising research is very necessary when attempting to build up evidence for care. Yet for many aspects of care wise opinion and experience rules in the absence of systematic investigation. Despite the inadequacy of such evidence, nurses are being asked to rationalise their care and produce research justifications for nursing interventions.

This book is designed as a beginning to this process. Nursing science must cull information from other disciplines and promote its own research. So for the major challenges in patient care, these authors aim to describe the research which assists in providing assessment tools, that which explores patients' responses to health problems and those studies which evaluate interventions aimed to resolve such problems, even though they may be few in number.

Problems included in this book do not reflect a comprehensive coverage of nursing care, but they are selected as those which nurses recognise and document most frequently for patients nursed in general wards or in the community. This book is therefore written for general nurses, although many problems and interventions are relevant to other 'special' groups of patients. It is also oriented to those who are ill, in some way. However interventions aimed to alleviate problems may also at times be seen as preventive measures, in that they sometimes prevent problems occurring or worsening.

It is the wish of the authors that further books along these lines will be forthcoming, improving and integrating more research to build on knowledge relevant to practice. We hope to show that although our body of knowledge is emergent or immature it certainly covers a broad range of clinical issues. One of the most encouraging aspects in nursing is the energetic growth of research publications, more of which now tend to be relevant to nursing practice. Updating and reformulation of knowledge and ideas is therefore constantly necessary. Hence problem-oriented care is not the only process in nursing!

Chapter 1

Introduction: Nursing Knowledge, Research and Practice

Nursing knowledge is derived from many sources other than formal research. In the past decisions about the most appropriate nursing interventions were based on experience and medical orders. Although these sources are valuable the genesis and growth of nursing and related research has encouraged optimists to lay claim to a body of more formalised nursing knowledge. Exploration of such claims (and knowledge) and application by nurses should benefit all. Testing and applying such knowledge for patient care becomes a scientific challenge when choosing areas for further study and research and also requires a clear understanding of priorities in professional nursing practice. The relationship between knowledge, science, theory and research in nursing is therefore explored in this chapter. Applying proved and tested knowledge and using research as a guide to practice is essential to improve care. This book aims to demonstrate how this may be done by focusing on specific patient problems.

Nursing 'knowledge' and nursing 'science' are used interchangeably by some. Gortner (1980) (quoting other scientists) sees science as the body of codified understanding of the natural universe and of human social and individual behaviour. Thus:

> 'nursing science represents our currently limited understanding of human biology and behaviour in health and illness, including the processes by which changes in health status are brought about, the patterns of behaviour associated with normal and critical life events and the principles and laws governing life states and processes' (p. 180).

Others emphasise the difference between scientific process in research and the product or outcome which is increased knowledge (Hanson, 1975; Mulkay, 1975). Not only the facts or data of sciences are relevant but also the scientific methods of systematic empirical investigation are important. For instance McFarlane (1976) describes nursing as an applied science using the logico-deductive method, and, just as other professions do (e.g. medicine and engineering) drawing on pure sciences.

> 'In the process of application, however, the pure science is transmitted and I believe becomes part of a unique body of knowledge belonging to the practice discipline' (p. 446).

DIRECTIONS FOR NURSING RESEARCH

Application of research-based or scientific knowledge is essential for professional practice, which requires 'a commitment beyond mere understanding and describing' according to Dickoff and James (1968, p. 198) for directing care towards desirable and achievable goals. Thus both research and practice in nursing require direction and purpose. As Dickoff et al (1968a) claim, nursing is practical and 'action-oriented'. Research data only form part of what is required to improve nursing care. Theoretical ideas, which incorporate knowledge and the reality of health care, are also required. They provide focus and should stimulate further study to develop the 'scientific body of knowledge'. Reflecting the climate of thought at that time (1968a), they warn against rejection of existing knowledge which may not have been gained recently by nurses, but also against embracing procedures from other disciplines without careful scrutiny of what they have achieved for that discipline or might do for nursing. Nursing theories also provide guidelines for the methods appropriate for research as well as ideas for the subject of study. Theories should be tested through research and clearly indicate which goals are explicit for both practice and research.

Colaizzi (1975) echoes the need for a focus for research and practice exclusive to nursing, saying, 'We have not yet accomplished the initial philosophical task of identifying the proper object of nursing science' (p. 197). Nursing is consequently done

'in the interest of para-nursing technical practitioners, while the position of nursing in the health care delivery system becomes more and more attenuated' (p. 197).

Despite the more altruistic view that research should be done for the benefit of those we serve, others support the endeavour of defining a special area of focus for nursing. Colaizzi argues that nursing must combine empirical inquiry with understanding of the patients' experience or existential needs. Essentially her paper makes a plea for holism, the integration rather than separation of physical and mental processes, as centrally important to nursing. While agreeing with this, one can object to her position that only nursing-oriented research is of use to nurses. This author would maintain that several disciplines have findings and knowledge relevant to nursing practice.

Research studies which explore issues of relevance to nursing care are increasing in number each year, although their relationship to theories or theoretical concepts such as holism is less noticeable. Brown et al (1984) reviewed publications of mainly American work from four nursing research journals for over two decades. Not only the volume of such work but also the greater emphasis on clinical practice was evident in recent years from this review. Percentages of clinical practice research articles increased from 29% in 1952, to 45% in 1960, 40% in 1970 and up to 63% in 1980. Similarly, in a review of a British journal, (not exclusively a research publication) Wilson-Barnett (1986) found that the *Journal of Advanced Nursing* reflected this increasing trend for more practice-related research reports.

Parallel developments in methodological approaches were reported in both reviews. Descriptive studies tended to dominate in earlier issues but evaluative work using experimental designs have increased more recently and as Brown et al (1984) surmise this may reflect increased research sophistication. They discuss the power of certain correlational and *ex post facto* designs as well as experiments to predict and explain, suggesting the latter are seen to be superior in this. Gortner (1980) also reported a transition from descriptive to more multi-variate multi-dimensional studies. Now that statistical tests can handle such data, it seems more pertinent that more variables are studied, reflecting the complex situation of care.

In all three of these reviews, the authors recognise the failure of researchers to build a cumulative science, to follow previous leads, modify evidence in a specific area by comparing or interpreting data, and relate their findings to a body of knowledge within nursing. This may be due to a lack of conceptual sophistication (Batey, 1977), failure to locate the work within a theoretical framework (Dickoff, 1968b) or to a tradition which emphasises practical empirical work but has not, as yet, valued research evidence from which to replicate and build.

In an effort to provide more understanding and encourage more integration of theoretical ideas in research and practice a classification of the levels of nursing theories was devised by Dickoff and James (1968). Essentially they consist of a hierarchy. First level theories describe, identify and classify phenomena, thus labelled 'factor isolating', second level theories correlate or 'factor relate', third level theories predict and the higher level prescribe. Their thesis purports that practice professions must utilise all levels of theory to stimulate research and good practice, but ultimately prescriptive or situation-producing theories identify goals for activity which are situation specific. Acknowledging the complexity of professional practice, they list many factors pertinent to prescribing activities in order to achieve an explicit goal. Patient, nurse, environmental and resource implications are considered in their 'factorisation framework'. Although their ideas are somewhat difficult to understand they do provide an explicit opportunity for research to be clearly integrated with theory. Methods or designs for research also become obvious when considering the purpose of the theory and the level of evidence that is proposed.

APPROACHES TO NURSING RESEARCH

Levels or methods of research reflect previous knowledge and determine the applicability or use of findings in practice. As documented above descriptive work is still most common although more evaluative work is currently undertaken. Descriptive surveys are necessary to identify relevant factors in a given area, to report the frequency of events, and to provide maps or a matrix from which to do more work. They produce evidence which can be interpreted by the researchers or readers, certain associations may be highlighted but they cannot usually explain the effect of one variable on another. Rarely do they provide clear guidelines for practice although they may stimulate nursing action when areas of poor practice or neglect are highlighted. Such studies which aim to produce more information about a population or certain phenomenon, may classify, clarify and quantify. They cannot predict or lead to prescription.

Experimental studies are designed to test the effect of one variable on another by direct and explicit manipulation. They aim to evaluate the effects of the intervention and provide results which will allow prediction in similar situations. It is now more usual to find that more than one intervention is applied to the sample in order to control for the effectiveness or strength in moderating the dependent variable. Experiments have been held as the most powerful research studies, in that they predict and control.

However, problems of measurement, homogeneity, control and comparability across studies are well recognised (see Openshaw, 1984). In clinical settings there are so many uncontrollable variables that even large samples, randomisation and well-resourced studies fail to produce convincing results, amenable to multi-factorial analysis. Despite this, choice of interventions for care cannot always be made scientifically, even when experimental evidence exists. Evers (1985) also clearly demonstrated the artificiality of analysing outcome, without reviewing the total complex of variables affecting the pattern of care in a ward.

The logico-deductive, positivistic, classical scientific approach to building knowledge and theory is represented by descriptive and experimental studies. In descriptive work particular concepts or ideas are explored, organised and interrelated by systematic and repeated observations to provide a general picture or theory. This general picture is then tested for component relationships and association or causal connections through hypotheses for studies. Both approaches can relate to a theoretical framework or perspective (possibly created by induction, then tested and modified by deduction [McFarlane, 1976]). Perhaps this demonstrates that research is essential to theory and can be used in different ways to understand and shape nursing practice.

Many other research designs are employed by researchers who consider them more appropriate or feasible than either descriptive surveys or, at the other end of the spectrum, controlled experiments or trials. Action research for instance may serve to produce many interesting ideas and indeed be the most effective way of assessing change or innovation. It may however be more difficult to generalise from the findings, and be open to charges of subjective or biased reporting.

Other evaluative studies may employ a follow-through or longitudinal process, documenting the rationale for implementations and the outcome, which are then compared to baseline data. Changes in outcome are then associated with the intervention. For instance, in a study of diagnosis and treatment with hypertensive patients, Given et al (1979) demonstrated the value of detailed data collection at all stages. It was not the treatment regime or diagnostic exercise which effected the success of controlling the patient's condition but the patient's responses to and understanding of the interventions which were essential to the outcome. Hence the authors claim that both process and outcome variables need to be studied when evaluating care. This has obvious and clear implications for future study and for the care and ultimate self-care of patients.

Each type of research design can be utilised to produce valuable information adding to understanding about nursing care. When reviewing work relevant to patient problems it is essential that limitations and strengths of different approaches and individual studies are considered. This sort of judgement may account for the lack of application of some research in nursing practice.

APPLICATIONS OF RESEARCH TO PRACTICE

It may seem surprising to some, probably more so to non-nurses, that research has not generally been applied or explicitly used to determine care. Lelean (1982) discussed this at the European Group of Nurse Researchers conference. She pointed to the inadequacy of research evidence, to the poor dissemination of those studies with implications for nursing, and to the problem of accessibility of research findings. Despite many positive suggestions this situation has not changed substantially in the UK, that is, according to the author's anecdotal evidence from contact with clinical areas.

Implementation of nursing research in practice requires understanding of research and practice and the ability and power to evaluate research and co-ordinate practice. It would be unrealistic to expect every nurse to do this on her own. Ideally, evidence should be weighed up at every juncture where a nursing decision is made, in reality a clinical policy for each team or group of nurses should be agreed, and based, where possible, on available research. This must not be imposed, lest it become meaningless and inappropriately used. Involvement of nurses in devising a rationale for practice for an individual's care or that of a group with similar problems is necessary. Hunt (1987) claims that only through full involvement in action research will this be successful. Other models still have to be tested. For example, a research practitioner-facilitator may be equally successful, as Oberst (1985) found, constantly demonstrating how research is pertinent to practice, thus teaching and applying this within a certain clinical setting. They may then demonstrate the benefits of a scientific approach but also identify where more research is needed.

This serves as a justification for this book, which aims to discuss research related to practical problems facing patients and nurses. By reviewing work which is not only relevant to practice, but also should be used as a rationale for care, nurses can then test this research through practice, improve research ideas by suggesting further studies and become more confident of their own scientific knowledge base. This is quite ambitious given the breadth of problems in clinical practice but future work may make this beginning worth while. To provide structure for this text an overall appreciation of nursing problems or diagnoses is applied.

For both research and practice to be successful, questions and problems have to be carefully defined and specific. 'Nursing diagnosis' was first discussed as a concept by McManus (1950), since when several working groups and conferences have been held to generate, classify and validate a complete system. This activity reflects the aspirations of many theorists and researchers to create an identified field for nursing activity in practice and research. By employing a holistic framework authors in this area have been successful in differentiating patients' problems or nursing diagnoses from medical diagnoses. A medical diagnosis defines the pathological state of a patient whereas a nursing diagnosis defines altered patterns of human functioning. A nursing diagnosis must infer some independent action by the nurse although it is usually rather artificial to expect no overlap or interchange among members of a health care team.

When considering a comprehensive framework for nursing care on which to base diagnoses many have suggested Maslow's hierarchy of needs as suitably reflecting individuals as holistic beings. This includes the four systems of biophysical, psychosocial, cognitive-perceptual and cultural-spiritual. These systems in turn sustain life and the individual within the community, and create and perpetuate meaning for life for the individual and community. Within each of these categories a set of needs can be devised for which a balance must be maintained. Where a need cannot be met by the patient, and the nurse is able to meet it, a nursing diagnosis may be identified. This arises from the analysis of the unmet needs and potential nursing actions that can be taken.

In any system of diagnosis it is imperative that the classification is refined to include details of aetiology, for example anxiety *due to* lack of knowledge about surgery. This is necessary to plan for relevant care and evaluate effects of that care. (Papers on the thinking behind the nursing diagnosis development can be read in *Nursing Clinics of North America* volume 20, December, 1985.) A fuller more comprehensive account of progress is documented by Carpenito (1983) and, more recently, by Hurley (1986) in the published proceedings of the sixth Nursing Diagnosis conference.

Essentially nursing diagnoses are patient problems or statements presented by patients or their families. They are formulated as summary statements or judgements made by the nurse about the data she has gathered in her nursing assessment. Such statements should be 'relevant, complete, definite, useful, open, compatible and capable of computerisation' (Roy, 1975, p. 92). This should aid communication for nurses and others, Roy suggests and indicates to others what sort of patient problems a nurse can solve.

Once diagnoses or problems are clearly defined planning care and prescribing interventions should be possible. This obviously involves a review of relevant knowledge and evidence of best strategies pertinent to the individual. Consistent positive findings, such as providing relevant information to those who are anxious, give obvious indications for practice which is directed and justified by research. Individualising aspects of care in more complex family or social contexts from scanty or conflicting findings is much more difficult. But being aware of alternative interventions for such problems as postoperative pain may well assist a nurse to select, try out, modify, evaluate, reject and substitute interventions. Constant evaluation is necessary in order to guide practice which will alleviate problems, reduce discomfort and make general progress.

Choice of the term 'nursing diagnosis' in this context may be useful to remind nurses that it is their responsibility to treat and resolve these diagnoses, whereas 'patient problems' may infer to some that nurses do not have so much responsibility. Clarity and precision are also required with the diagnostic classification system and they could have substantial benefit for tailoring more specific interventions or care. Both terms will be used in this text, however, as they are both widely used in practice and research. Some problems are, as yet, still poorly understood and need to be explored both conceptually and empirically. Therefore chapters differ to some extent according to the specificity and recognition of problems. Whereas urinary incontinence is clearly defined and thus briefly introduced, sleep disturbance requires much more discussion and review. However, by providing a consistent format for each chapter, the authors hope to show how research evidence is relevant to each stage of the nursing process. First, assessment of a problem is vital, prior to selecting interventions. Descriptive studies have often employed measurement tools which can help to identify and measure a problem, both for an individual or a sample of subjects. These tools may be used for clinical practice to monitor progress and thereby evaluate effects of intervention. Where appropriate therefore, assessment of problems may be assisted by research. In the same way, the prevalence of a problem can only be measured using systematic criteria and measures. Prevalence should be estimated for a serious problem and when high it justifies more time by researchers, teachers and practitioners. Common problems are discussed in this book, yet even so for some the inadequacy of research to guide practice makes research-based practice impossible at present.

Once problems have been identified, or differential diagnoses made, realistic goals for outcome can be estimated. Descriptive work may indicate a likely course, but all too often prediction is a matter of nursing conjecture. However, careful deliberation and repeated practice and some research studies may help.

For each chapter it is the last major section which looks at the indications for intervention, or the research rationale for nursing care. For some problems there is sound and consistent evaluative research work. There is substantial knowledge about alleviating anxiety, urinary incontinence, pain, and wound problems, much of which has been generated by nurse researchers. However, helping with communication difficulties, confusional states, depression, mobility and breathing difficulties is hampered by inadequate knowledge. In each area therefore suggestions for more research approaches are made, some building on previous work, but many may be termed 'exploratory', laying the foundations for subsequent systematic or applied work.

This book is for all nurses and others who care for people, who need to understand how research can improve care and the state of the art and science of nursing.

REFERENCES

Batey MV (1977) Conceptualisation: knowledge and logic guiding empirical research. *Nursing Research* **26**(5), 324–329.

Brown JS, Tanner CA, Padrick KP (1984) Nursing's search for scientific knowledge. *Nursing Research* **33**(1), 26–32.

Carpenito LJ (1983) *Nursing Diagnosis: Application to Clinical Practice*. J.B. Lippincott, Philadelphia.

Colaizzi J (1975) The proper object of nursing science. *International Journal of Nursing Studies* **12**, 197–200.

Dickoff J, James P (1968) A theory of theories. A position paper. *Nursing Research* **17**(3), 197–203.

Dickoff J, James P, Weidenbach E (1968a,b) Theory in a practice discipline Part I. Practice-oriented theory. *Nursing Research* **17**(5), 415–435. Part II. Practice-oriented research. *Nursing Research* **17**(6), 545–554.

Evers H (1985) *Organisation of Work in Hospital Wards*. PhD Thesis. University of Birmingham.

Given B, Given CW, Simoni LE (1979) Relationships of processes of care to patient outcomes. *Nursing Research* **28**(2), 85–93.

Gortner SR (1980) Nursing science in transition. *Nursing Research* **29**(3), 180–183.

Hanson NR (1975) *Patterns of Discovery*. Cambridge University Press, Cambridge.

Hunt M (1987) The process of translating research findings into nursing practice. *Journal of Advanced Nursing* **12**(1), 101–110.

Hurley ME (1986) *Classification of Nursing Diagnoses*. Proceedings of 6th Conference on Nursing Diagnoses. Mosby, New York.

Lelean SR (1982) The implementation of research findings into nursing practice. *International Journal of Nursing Studies* **19**(4), 223–230.

McFarlane JK (1976) The role of research and the development of nursing theory. *Journal of Advanced Nursing* **1**, 443–451.

McManus RL (1950) Assumption of functions in nursing. In: *Regional Planning for Nurses and Nursing Education*. New York Bureau of Publications, Teachers College, Columbia University.

Mulkay MJ (1975) The models of scientific development. *Sociological Review* **23**(3), 509–526.

Oberst M (1985) Integrating research and clinical practice roles. *Topics in Clinical Nursing* **3**, 45–53.

Openshaw S (1984) Literature review: measurement of adequate care. *International Journal of Nursing Studies* **21**(4), 295–304.

Roy C (1975) A diagnostic classification system for nursing. *Nursing Outlook* **23**(2), 90–94.

Wilson-Barnett J (1986) *Research: Its Relationship to Practice and Representation in the Journal of Advanced Nursing*, pp. 53–56, King's Fund Report, London.

Chapter 2
Problems with Adjustment to Illness and Recovery

This problem is complex, somewhat nebulous and therefore difficult to define. However, failure to cope or adjust to life-threatening or chronic illness causes great suffering for patients and their families and presents an enormous challenge for nurses. To staff it may seem surprising that so many patients do learn to master discomfort and treatment regimes without abdicating other roles and sources of satisfaction. Studying their success, to gain knowledge of possible strategies for future patients, should be an important activity for nurses. Others, who initially fail to accept they have a serious condition which will limit their behaviour, may subsequently develop anxiety and depression leading to increased physical morbidity. It appears from research into coping and recovery that certain risk factors exist and these may inhibit the expected pattern of adjustment, both in the short and long term.

'Ineffective individual coping' is defined as a nursing diagnosis by Carpenito (1983, p. 144):

'A state in which the individual experiences or is at risk of experiencing an inability to manage internal or environmental stressors adequately due to inadequate resources (physical, psychological or behavioural).'

Change in one's situation, or an accumulation of change events which may induce threat, loss or challenge are potentially stressful (Lazarus, 1974), and the effects of stress may result in deterioration of health when coping is inadequate. Carpenito (1983, p. 145) lists recognisable characteristics for a person who is at risk of poor coping. She includes:

'1. Realisation of inability to cope.
2. Distortion or confusion of roles.
3. Inability to meet basic needs.
4. Inability to ask for help.
5. Destructive behaviour toward self or others.
6. Change in usual communication patterns.
7. Inappropriate use of defence mechanisms.
8. Frequent illness.
9. High rate of accidents.'

Illness itself is particularly stressful (Wilson-Barnett, 1979) for those who are fearful of its outcome, lose a great deal of self-esteem or who lack the capabilities and resources to plan for their future. Coping aimed to reduce negative emotions and solve health problems infers active participation. This may include physical or psychological coping, but without motivation and belief in one's own abilities and control this is likely to be unsuccessful.

Certain models of coping help to explain ways to facilitate the process. Craig and Edwards (1983) discuss coping with illness within Lazarus' (1974) framework. Perception of threat or appraisal of stress tends to alter as new information and resources become available. Adaptation is seen as a process of continuous appraisal and reappraisal of the situation in the light of reaching the goal. Role transition and identity change may become part of this process in chronic illness. They use Feldman's (1974) definition of adaptation as:

'coming to terms with the reality of chronic illness as a state of being, discarding false hope and destructive hopelessness, and restructuring the environment in which one now functions. Adaptation implies the reorganisation and acceptance of self so that there is a meaning and purpose to living that transcends the limitations imposed by the illness.'

So chronic or acute conditions, physical, social and psychological demands require adaptive responses. Physical discomfort or treatments need to be dealt with, incapacity or mobility restrictions may cause distress but various mechanisms and aids can reduce unwanted effects. These may include problem solving and forward planning. Psychological and social pressures include mobilising resources and 'inner strength' to avoid helplessness and isolation. Emotional defence mechanisms such as denial and projection may be adaptive at times, and cognitive aspects of information seeking and application of this for mastering of problems may be necessary for successful coping. Goals for adaptation should include absence of distressing symptoms, careful adherence to treatments, lack of emotional distress, unresolved anger or helplessness, a clear sense of self-worth, an acceptance of altered body image, and evidently satisfying pursuits. Socially, an absence of conflict at home and at work, successful alteration in roles, and appropriate levels of independence and support behaviour would reflect adequate coping. Craig and Edwards' (1983) model is clear and useful and leads logically to prescribing supportive and problem-solving behaviour from nurses and others.

Illness and adaptation may pass through transitional stages where emotional reactions and behaviours reflect distress and turmoil for patients and their spouses. For instance, Mailick (1979) has described three stages of a serious illness. Initially, during diagnosis and planning for treatment, anxiety may be observed while patients have inadequate information to realise just how much their life will be affected. At the next stage patients may learn to live with the illness and the many changes it may cause for them and their family. The final stage may be recovery or total adaptation or death. Such stages are not necessarily discrete and individuals may pass to and from each stage at various times.

Others have documented stages in reaction to acute onset of serious illness which may have chronic implications. Goldberg (1982) noted the transition from denial, through anxiety, depression, sometimes delirium and then convalescence. Most of these changes are thought to result from fear of death and loss of self-esteem. Kubler Ross's (1969) classic reactions may also be observed when diagnoses reflect loss of an optimistic future and sense of self-worth. Guilt, bargaining, denial and depression can all be observed at different times during illness.

All these reactions may be considered unproblematic if they are used intermittently and do not endanger the effects of treatments. Patients' reactions vary and coping strategies tend to be typical for that individual, frequently used in the past during stressful episodes. Lipowski (1983) identified several reactions to acute illness, some of which may be seen as coping or defensive reactions to this crisis situation:

1. Regression—dependency and clinging to the 'sick role'.
2. Manipulation for attention, control, or avoidance of responsibilities via sympathy and guilt of others.
3. Hypochondriasis or 'neuroses'.
4. Dealing with illness as a challenge.
5. Treating illness as a loss.
6. Interpreting the illness as punishment.
   'Succumbing' to the illness if guilt is great enough ('giving up').
   Seeing survival as having received 'just' punishment with resulting feelings of being given a 'second chance'.
7. Compulsive need to regain control (often annoying to others and therefore alienating them).
8. Grief reaction over loss of normal functioning—may proceed to depression.
9. Defensiveness or irritability secondary to fear.
10. Minimising or denial of the significance of the illness and behaving as if it did not exist.

All these reactions reflect the 'meaning' of the illness to the patient and tend to be determined by psychosocial factors and physical reactions. They may be considered as a normal range of responses but if persistent or used inflexibly can lead to poor outcome or inadequate long-term adjustment.

Coping behaviour, aimed to reduce anxiety or depression and to control events, can also be seen in children. Analysis of case notes by Caty et al (1984) revealed that behaviour could be categorised into information-exchange, action or inaction, and intrapsychic dimensions. Action or inaction was further divided into behaviour directed towards managing either the self or the environment. These included mastery behaviours aimed at gaining competence often through rehearsal during play controlling behaviours.

FACTORS AFFECTING POOR ADJUSTMENTS

Certain factors identified in patient groups are found to be associated with poor recovery or adjustment to illness. These have been found to be both biological and psychosocial, but vary for different conditions. Older age, obesity, poor physical fitness prior to illness and other diseases are listed under biological factors by Wilson-Barnett and Fordham (1982). Highly emotional predisposition, poor perceived level of support, poor understanding of the illness and treatment, and lack of motivation to recover have also been identified as psychosocial risks.

Beliefs about the cause of illness and treatment have also been seen to determine health and illness behaviour. Coping ability could be associated with beliefs and Lowery and Jacobson (1985) attempted to study this. A sample of 296 chronically ill patients were interviewed about their illness experiences, success and failures. They tended to attribute success to their own abilities or behaviour, and failures to other causes or people. Those who could not attribute causes easily were found to fall more frequently within the 'failure' group as those who were 'not coping'.

Patients who have had treatment once unsuccessfully and need repeated treatment may be considered 'at risk'. Although this was not demonstrated conclusively, Ronayne (1985) found that such patients in hospital for vascular surgery tended to experience less favourable perceptions of health, higher levels of uncertainty, and a lower rate of adherence to discharge instructions. However, all patients found their early experiences during the convalescent period at home were most crucial for subsequently adapting to the effects of the vascular disease.

Another risk factor found to account for both psychological and physical morbidity after surgery and throughout a chronic illness is emotionality or neurotic predisposition. Mathews and Ridgeway (1981) found this to be a consistent factor in their review of surgical recovery and, more specifically, Parker (1981) also showed this with patients requiring regular haemodialysis. On following through patients categorised as high or low on trait anxiety, she found that the former group needed more clinic appointments, suffering from more fluid overload and cramps. They also had a higher incidence of all complications, except for hypotension, than the low anxiety group.

When reviewing a range of factors likely to influence outcome from cardiac surgery, Mayou (1986) found that patients with post-operative social problems could be identified prior to surgery. Those with 'overt emotional disorder, histories of psychological consultation and passive non-tackling attitudes' were considered vulnerable. Such factors could obviously be indicative of poor coping.

Several researchers have discussed the role of perceived social support during stressful periods, but in particular at times of illness and treatment. Webb (1986) has reviewed this issue and showed that women after hysterectomy have expressed support needs and frequently feel let down by their partners or significant others, and members of the health care team. Earlier work (Webb and Wilson-Barnett, 1983) also showed that those who felt less supported suffered from more recovery problems. This concept is important as it may be more amenable to nursing interventions than some other 'risk' factors.

Even when illness and treatment is finite, coping may be required for quite lengthy periods and recovery can be prolonged, even for several months after surgery. As Gould and Wilson-Barnett (1985) found, home situation, economic circumstances, and general level of support were seen to be vital for patients. Minor symptoms were frequently reported for post-hospital convalescent patients. It was not only the severity of surgical intervention but also the person's personality, style of coping and experience of life which determined the success of coping with recovery.

PREVALENCE OF POOR ADJUSTMENT

Outcome depends on the number of 'at risk' people affected by an illness and the severity and nature of the illness. This problem is more frequently found for severe and fatal prognoses. For patients adjusting to the diagnosis of a malignant condition, psychological morbidity has been documented for as long as one year later for one-third of them (Maguire, 1985). This tends to be higher where the patients are all women. After a life-threatening event such as a heart attack, the problem of 'cardiac invalidity' is less frequent than it was. Between one-quarter and one-tenth of these subjects have been judged as coping badly on various criteria (Mayou, 1984).

ASSESSMENT OF COPING WITH ILLNESS

Full adjustment is seen in a majority of individuals. They are usually free of symptoms, take measures to alleviate physical problems when necessary, resume all physical activities of daily living (ADL) which are reasonable for them, engage in pleasurable activities, understand their illness and its implications, and have no change in their usual level of emotionality. Criteria for assessing problems may therefore be classified as cognitive, physical, social cognitive and emotional. See Tables 1 and 2.

Table 1. Assessment of Problems in Adjustment to Illness

Criteria	Methods
	For overall follow-up visits and rapid assessment use schedule as advised by Wilson-Barnett and Fordham (1983), Appendix 1.
Physical	Interview and examine, question on symptoms, medications, visits to doctor, and nursing needs. Use Specific Cancer Quality of Life Scales if necessary e.g. McCorkle and Young (1978).
Activities	Interview about independence on ADL Scale. Use Roberts' inventory (1975) (appendix 2). Ask for demonstration of activities if appropriate. For resumption of work and social activities use questions tested by researchers, e.g. Mayou (1984) and West (1987).
Cognitive	Assess level of understanding by questions which require patient's explanation and description of treatment advice and regime. Ask what patient has been told about likely progress and expectations of treatment.
Emotional	Interview on moods. Use MACL (see Chapter 3) and Derogatis (1983). Psychological Adjustment to Illness Scale.

Global judgements of 'coping potential' made by staff have been tested in prospective studies. For instance, in a study by Pinkerton et al (1985) patients identified as copers and non-copers by members of a cystic fibrosis team were compared on various parameters. They found that non-copers were admitted to hospital twice as often as copers even though their ventilatory function was better. Vocational records, and poor level of family support and knowledge of cystic fibrosis differentiated poor copers. On seven factors of the Psychological Adjustment to Illness Scale (Derogatis, 1983) non-copers scored more highly. These were anxiety, depression, hostility, guilt, worry, self-devaluation and body image distortion.

West (1987), a research nurse, also demonstrated that signs evident during conversation can be used to predict poor copers pre-operatively. The patient's general level of interest in the research and surgery, and his or her level of involvement and optimism, were found to discriminate between those who ultimately recovered and coped well and the smaller proportion (of uninterested patients) whose recovery was problematic.

Table 2. Identification of Problems of Poor Adjustment

Criteria	Indicative measures	Diagnosis
Physical	No abnormality detected (ECG, pulse and blood pressure). Exercise tolerance (step test) good. Three visits to the doctor in last two months for minor worries and symptoms	Poor acceptance of (uncomplicated) myocardial infarction after 6 months (male 54 years).
Activities	Recently returned to work (routine clerical) Has not resumed sex or social activities.	
Cognitive	Has over-pessimistic appraisal of his prognosis, clear understanding of aetiology and treatment for condition.	
Emotional	Highly anxious, morbid fears, withdrawn and depressed. Family conflict reported.	
Physical	No abnormality detected apart from weight loss and inflamed leg wound surrounding oedema.	Poor recovery and coping after coronary by-pass surgery 3 months ago (female 66 years) due to lack of knowledge.
Activities	Independent. Slower doing housework. Has help with shopping. Does not go out. Sedentary hobbies.	
Cognitive	Confused over surgery, does not remember what doctor explained, physiotherapist said to increase activities but this was 'too vague'. Patient admits 'it's best to be careful'.	
Emotional	Lonely despite good support from husband who works full time.	
Physical	Scans and X-rays show no recurrence of growth locally or systemically, was not offered prosthesis. Wound well healed, muscular pains subsided. No lymphoedema.	Poor coping after radical mastectomy and adjuvant therapy 8 months ago (female 40 years) due to fears and poor self-image.
Activities	Independent on all ADLs. Has not resumed sexual intercourse or shown scar to husband. Does not engage in sports or social events.	
Cognitive	Understands pathology and aims of treatment. Sceptical about prognosis.	
Emotional	Despite recognising good marital support depressed—18 on MACL. Poorly adjusted on Derogatis measure. Self-image is one of distortion and 'ugliness'.	

Certain criteria may be assessed repeatedly by open questioning and discussion or by physical examination, while others, such as the longer, more systematic interview schedules can reasonably only be used for initial assessment and follow-up evaluation.

Assessment can be time-consuming; a nurse needs to establish an easy rapport prior to asking certain questions and utilising interview schedules. Patients are also sometimes reluctant to discuss issues which may infer criticism of the care they have received.

The diagnoses outlined above reflect illnesses and treatments which are fairly common and very serious, and build on information and problems discussed in Chapter 6.

These problems are not atypical. Although the cardiac patients described may not be classified as psychiatrically ill, they cannot be seen as fully adjusted and socially integrated. Low level morbidity such as this is quite common and may be recognised or treated without careful assessment. Females are more susceptible than men to incomplete recovery from coronary artery by-pass grafting, often due to over-protection by relatives. Patients in this cardiac group need to accept accurately their vulnerability, yet a lack of clear understanding about the expectations of the health care team is frequently observed.

Mastectomies are now usually only performed if other forms of treatment are considered inadequate. Recovery patterns from this surgery however are fairly representative of those for other cancers requiring extensive excision and sometimes causing unsightly scars or disfigurements. Adjuvant therapy such as radiotherapy or cytotoxic drugs has also been shown to increase psychological morbidity in the medium to long term. For these patients coping with immediate aspects such as disfigurement and discomfort is necessary but they also have to live with the fear of recurrence and therefore the likelihood of a foreshortened life.

GOALS

Prevention of poor coping should be the ultimate goal. However, despite extensive measures morbidity does occur, particularly in those at risk. Anxiety and depression after myocardial infarction (at six months) should be alleviated by adequate counselling in a matter of months. (The family may also need to be involved so that this goal is seen as realistic to all.)

Loneliness after major surgery may be alleviated fairly rapidly. Follow up groups or home visitors have rapid effects. In a few weeks the patient may feel more confident and able to cope by initiating meetings with her own friends and attending usual activities involving social contacts.

Grave problems in coping with cancer and its treatment may take intensive counselling therapy, medication and several months to overcome.

COPING WITH CARDIAC DISEASE (see Table 2, sections 1 and 2)

Patients who have suffered a myocardial infarction or who have been treated with surgery to replace coronary arteries by vein grafts to relieve symptoms of angina, are adjusting to an acutely stressful episode, yet must live with the knowledge they have a life-threatening condition. Wilson-Barnett (1979) has reviewed many studies which show that about one-quarter of these patients do not adjust to this reality. They suffer from anxiety and depression, reduced social enjoyment and poor family relationships. In a prospective study Mayou (1984) attempted to identify early prognostic factors. By interviewing patients during hospitalisation after myocardial infarction and then 2 months and 1 year later, he found that neither previous history of cardiac or other conditions nor severity of the infarct affected long-term adjustment although marital status and previous good level of general social functioning predicted successful and complete recovery. In another group of patients women did not recover as well as men. Kellog et al (1979) also followed a group of 100 patients and found that, after 17 months, more discomfort, measured on a range of emotional and physical symptoms, was associated with being female, having a lower occupational position, less formal education and feeling more negative. Poor coping abilities may be associated with these problems.

A patient's need for support is found to be a central variable influencing coping and recovery, and lack of it may be considered a risk factor. Closest and most meaningful support may be forthcoming from the spouse or partner. Yet they too may lack knowledge and personal resources to cope with this life crisis. A small scale study (interviews with 40 couples) by Mayou et al (1976) was conducted to assess wives' views and experiences after their husband's coronary thrombosis. High levels of distress and concern were found, the women having little understanding of what had happened. Any advice that they received with the patient seemed inadequate, vague and sometimes conflicting. Levels of knowledge have been found to be generally low among spouses and patients (Rudy, 1980) and there are many recommendations for spouses to be included in discharge planning. Yet recent work continues to document inadequate support and preparation for spouses (Hentinen, 1983). In this Finnish study of 59 wives, one-fifth said they had received no information, while one-third said they had received support from a nurse. Advice about activity graduation at home was particularly requested. Importance of a supportive spouse for successful rehabilitation is often cited, yet Hilbert (1985) did not find that this had a positive effect on compliance with health carer's advice, which is a constant problem.

Influences on recovery after cardiac surgery are very similar to those reported after myocardial infarction. Social, practical, economic and physical factors were all found to affect patients (Wilson-Barnett, 1981). One-third of patients in this sample of 60 followed up one year after surgery were found to have rather vague enduring symptoms which were reflective of underlying mood changes. In general, patients were very satisfied with treatment but still had comments to make for improving patient preparation at the time of discharge from hospital. Results of high levels of patient satisfaction were also found by Penckofer and Holm (1984). Patients' quality of life seemed to increase as they progressed through the recovery period. However, Ramshaw and Stanley (1984) found that for patients followed up one year after surgery, one subgroup indicated change for the worse after surgery. This was accounted for by a high neuroticism score and poor pre-operative coping behaviour, and demonstrated that small 'at risk' groups can be identified pre-operatively.

Differences between men and women recovering from surgery have been found by Brown and Rawlinson (1977). However, these differences are not straightforward. Social, career and domestic pressures were said to explain the small differences. Men were found to relinquish the sick role more rapidly than women and influences encouraging return to work were different for men and women. But both men and women resumed their work roles after the same convalescent period. Women tend to be more open in reporting symptoms and feelings and this finding may account for studies which aim to explain differences for other reasons.

Interventions to promote coping and treat problems with adjustment to cardiac disease

Steinhart (1984) like many others includes the spouse in a rehabilitation plan for post-infarction patients. Components of such a programme are all aimed to facilitate coping and reduce problems in the recovery period. He includes readjustment to work, learning to deal more effectively with stressful daily events, exercise tolerance, dealing with altered family dynamics and problems of self-image and self-confidence. First and foremost the patient's and the family's anxiety must be reduced by increasing their knowledge and understanding. Early mobilisation also increases confidence and reduces other risks. Group discussion with the patient and his family is indicated to help in exchanging views and answering questions. After healing is almost complete, at about 8–12 weeks, more physical reconditioning and further education is often planned. Steinhart (1984) also asserts the importance of encouraging educated participation by the patient during rehabilitation. A summary of an educational programme is provided by Steinhart (p. 21). Although details and emphasis vary, most programmes for the education of post-infarction patients cover these topics:

1. Explain the nature of a myocardial infarction.
2. Explain hospital regulations, procedures and equipment.
3. Explain risk factors for coronary artery disease and how to deal with them.
   Review eating habits. Discuss foods to eat, those to avoid, and the importance of weight control.
   Detail the dangers of, and discourage, smoking.
4. Review life patterns (e.g. work habits, physical effort, sexual activity, leisure activity) with the patient and spouse.
5. Anticipate and introduce discussion of universal (but often unspoken) concerns of the patient and spouse—especially shifts in family dynamics and feelings the shifts may generate, sexual concerns, exercise tolerance, and physical weakness.
6. Review medications.
7. Describe community resources.

Specific studies aimed to evaluate interventions tend to incorporate a package of measures, such as that outlined above and earlier studies tended to assess levels of knowledge or compliance rather than coping with illness or recovery. For instance Owens et al (1978) evaluated an educational programme of five, 45-minute discussion sessions. A sample of 36 patients was given pre- and post-operative tests and followed up at 6 weeks and 3 months post-discharge. Knowledge increased significantly but few family members attended. A year later Linde and Janz (1979) designed a 'comprehensive' teaching programme for 48 patients who had surgery for either valve replacement or coronary artery grafting. Patients were tested pre-operatively and on discharge and then at their two post-operative visits. Knowledge scores were said to have increased and compliance scores (measured by laboratory tests, clinic visits, diet and other risk factors) were judged higher than in earlier studies. Five to six individual teaching sessions were given to patients and their spouses when possible.

A medical study by Naismith et al (1979), which evaluated the effect of a nurse counsellor on patients after a coronary thrombosis, incorporated a randomised controlled experimental design. Patients in the treatment group (n=59) were approached on the third day after hospitalisation for consent and interview and followed up after 6 months. Repeated assessment and counselling sessions were given to the patients and their spouses to encourage maximum independence. Sub-minimal effort tests were also done at 6 weeks, 12 weeks and after 6 months. Those in the control group (n=65) only received usual information. There were no group differences on return to work, physical and emotional stability and psychological rehabilitation although patients in the treatment group who scored high on the neuroticism scale were compared across experimental groups: those who received counselling were superior on a global measure of rehabilitation.

Two further studies attempted to evaluate specific interventions to promote recovery after myocardial infarction. Mayou et al (1981) compared counselling by a psychiatrist with physical rehabilitation sessions. A total of 129 men were enrolled randomly into the counselling group, the physical rehabilitation group, or a control group which received no special treatment. Outcome was evaluated at 12 weeks and 18 months by exercise testing and psychological social adjustment scales. For the first group counselling or advice was provided for couples three or four times each week, after discharge from hospital. Information, advice and discussion were such 'as might have been given by a cardiac nurse'. Topics included resumption of activity, symptoms, plans, and modification of risk factors. Exercise training consisted of eight twice weekly sessions in the gym, starting within four weeks of the infarct.

There were no differences on long-term effects from physical fitness although the exercise group attained greater fitness at three months. However, patients enjoyed these sessions more than the advisory sessions which were seen as rather pointless. At 18 months, however, significant advantages were found for the advice group on overall satisfaction with recovery, hours spent at work and frequency of sexual intercourse.

Another study by Bohachick (1984) found significant advantages for supplementing exercise therapy with relaxation training. This was considered an appropriate stress management technique for this post-coronary group to utilise in future. The special treatment group (n=18) received three weeks of relaxation training in addition to their exercise therapy. Patients were compared on two measures, one assessing state-trait anxiety and the other a symptom check-list. Relaxation (treatment) was associated with significantly lower anxiety than for exercise treatment (control) and post-test scores in the treatment group were lower for socialisation and interpersonal problems, and anxiety and depression, than controls.

Major projects evaluating the effect of nurse counsellors on post-coronary adjustment show very positive results. Frazure-Smith and Prince (1985) assessed patients over a one-year intervention ischaemic heart disease life stress monitoring programme. This programme included monthly telephone monitoring of psychological symptoms of stress on the General Health Questionnaire (GHQ) coupled with home nursing visits for those found to report high stress. Interventions were personalised to educate, support and monitor progress. This study randomly allocated a large sample of 453 patients into two groups. For the treatment group, when stress levels were rated for more than four symptoms on the GHQ, a nurse would visit and attempt to reduce this. She might refer the patient if she considered this necessary. About half the monitored patients had raised stress levels. On average each patient received 5–6 hours of home visiting. When discussing fears with the nurse, 80% of patients expressed fear and uncertainty about chest pain and fatigue. Sixty per cent had feelings of anxiety and depression. Many had concerns about work. Providing information for reassurance was said to be crucial as most patients had forgotton explanations they received in hospital. Personal concerns were often raised after teaching sessions had been given. The nurse also gave the patient 'permission' to contact another professional when they were concerned with symptoms. However, these nurses did not report spending much time during the sessions to simply encourage ventilation of feelings by active listening. This is not seen as surprising by the authors who explain that these nurses had no special counselling skills above their basic training for registration. This succeeded in reducing stress symptoms and reduced mortality rates by 50%. GHQ results were superior for monitored patients. When reviewing previous studies these authors conclude that other attempts have usually failed to demonstrate advantages because programmes have been standardised rather than individualised, and samples are inadequate.

In contrast to this individualised programme Dracup et al (1984a) report on a multi-centre group counselling service for patients after myocardial infarction with 58 couples in an out-patient cardiac rehabilitation programme. Ten weekly sessions of 90 minutes were held for experimental group 1 (17 patients and their partners), group 2 had 10 sessions for patients only (22 subjects), and controls (19) did not participate in an experimental programme. The aim of the sessions which applied symbolic interactionist role theory was to effect reduction in weight, blood presure and smoking and a gradual increase in exercise. Topics covered for both experimental groups included life changes since illness, role transition, and successful rehabilitation and sex. Findings showed significant differences for experimental group 2, where weight and blood pressure showed reductions, although experimental group 1 showed more increase in exercise taken. Thus the role of the spouse was not shown to be as influential as anticipated since group 2 developed a strongly competitive spirit which was seen to account for their results.

Dracup et al (1984a) discuss the three strategies which seem to be most successful in encouraging both compliance with medical advice and coping. Behavioural contracting aimed at cueing and reinforcement of compliant behaviour, simplification of medical regime, and involvement of family members have been found effective over conventional measures. With reference to this last aspect Dracup's work is based on the interactionist role theory which holds that roles are constantly being formulated and redefined as individuals interact. This helps to explain how roles alter within the family and how the sick role and the 'at risk' role interact for a convalescent patient. Roles should not conflict and to prevent this, family members are included in plans for rehabilitation.

Dracup et al (1984b) discuss the need for these programmes to concentrate on role transition, rather than just providing patients with a better understanding of coronary artery disease. As high percentages of emotionally distressed patients are reported at various times after return home, the concept of an 'at risk' role is introduced not only to help patients cope with the dangers of their condition but also to take positive actions to enjoy life and reduce risks. In this paper they give a detailed account of the 10 sessions evaluated. Stress management and problem-solving skills seem to be emphasised, role supplementation being seen as gaining additional skills for coping. However, patients and spouses, in a final evaluation of the programme, said the most valuable aspect was the sharing of concerns and feelings with others. Morbidity and mortality rates were found to be significantly reduced in this experimental group.

COPING WITH CANCER (see Table 2, section 3)

Most reviews of patients' psychological adjustment to cancer produce evidence of a large minority who do not cope for months or years after diagnosis, which results in serious emotional problems. The reactions to loss reported for patients suffering a myocardial infarction are also true, often to a greater extent, for those with cancer. Early denial is common, and acknowledged awareness of the diagnosis fluctuates over time, whereas coronary patients tend to use only denial initially (Polivy, 1977). However, a comparative interview study by Germino and McCorkle (1985) with 56 patients with lung cancer and 65 with a first myocardial infarction explored 'acknowledged awareness' of these two life-threatening chronic illnesses. Cancer patients at both one and two months after diagnosis reported more symptoms and distress. Yet both groups were similar in the reported awareness of their diagnosis, despite the fact that the cancer patients had not received formal education and the others had.

In a review of adjustment to breast cancer, Lewis and Bloom (1978) discuss the many misconceptions that women hold about the treatments and consequences of breast cancer. Treatment is found to have many stressful effects (as for other cancers), implications for body image and perceived desirability compounding other problems. The authors discuss emotional adjustment and cite studies which tend to agree that one-third of women seek or could benefit from psychiatric care for emotional lability and depression. Depression has been found in substantial minorities up to 2 years post-operatively. Good adjustment to cancer was seen as synonymous with the capacity to face problems, a sense of life fulfilment, and marital adjustment. This was then associated with less depression, anxiety, social withdrawal and instability. The role of social support was discussed by many others whose work was reviewed by Lewis and Bloom. This was seen to be most vital when provided by the spouse, then friends and lastly professional care givers. Patients in these studies defined support as helping and listening. Results seem to show that perceived social support can prevent some negative emotional reactions, but for severe depression as a response to the diagnosis and combined stresses, it may not be adequate. These writers conclude that fewer community programmes exist for post-mastectomy patients than for others such as stroke victims or multiple sclerosis sufferers. They also call for less prescriptive work and more evaluative research in this area. However, progress since this time has been impressive.

Coping patterns vary for different individuals within this group but as a whole cancer patients may be more vulnerable to emotional distress generally. Greer's (1979) study showed that those with malignant breast lumps as opposed to benign lumps could be diagnosed by psychological signs of suppressed anger alone. This may infer that negative emotionality is a common predisposition which possibly leads to more exaggerated emotional responses during recovery. Certainly Morris et al's (1977) study showed that those with a high neuroticism and high depression score pre-operatively remained stressed, not coping well, two years after surgery. Lloyd's (1979) review of emotional adjustment studies endorses the fact that cancer is a most feared disease, that emotional problems frequently prevent coping for about one-third of patients and that depressed mood may lead to reduced immune competence and further pathology. Poor pre-operative support, lack of contact with 'Reach for Recovery' or the Mastectomy Association were associated with many physical problems and poor quality of life by Woods and Earp (1978). Adaptation for the 49 post-mastectomy patients in this study was mainly facilitated by a supportive spouse.

Despite the obvious disfiguring effects of mastectomy, other cancers may cause more grave adjustment problems. For instance Krouse and Krouse (1982) reported that gynaecological patients had more persistent depression and a negative body image still present 2 years after treatment while patients after mastectomy and biopsy did not present in this way, having resolved their crises earlier.

Since the late 1970s much research has been done demonstrating how nurses and others can reduce morbidity, yet Maguire (1985) explains continuing problems. Patients are not helped to cope with uncertainty and often suffer a loss of support, withdrawing from their family for fear of distressing them. He estimates now that one in four patients is still found to suffer psychological morbidity with chemotherapy and radiotherapy compounding this dysphoria. In one study (Maguire, 1984), 19 out of 75 patients followed up developed an anxiety state and/or depressive illness, but only two of the 19 who required help considered this to be appropriate. Problems with providing comfort and support arise from staff's fears of not being sufficiently skilled or informed and of not wishing to encourage expression of emotions which then cannot be controlled or resolved.

These findings were confirmed in a questionnaire study by Ray et al (1984) of trained nurses' opinions and perceptions of cancer patients and their care. When discussing breast cancer the nurses saw themselves as having a key role in giving comfort but were less likely to see themselves in the role of counsellor. Many felt they had not been trained to provide psychological care at this level, specialist nurses being more able.

Nurses certainly believe that patients need information to cope with cancer, but, Lauer et al (1982) found that patients and nurses have different opinions on the aspects of information that can be useful. When nurses' and patients' responses were compared nurses ranked 20 out of 36 informational items as more important than did patients. They also considered that dealing with feelings was a problem for patients, but the latter apparently disagreed. However, when specific items of care were correlated with particular outcomes for those receiving chemotherapy by Lum et al (1978), content and quality of explanation correlated with patients' positive self-esteem and knowledge levels. Involvement in care and giving patients control over their treatments was also associated with positive ratings.

Many descriptive articles explain the importance of providing careful information, particularly for patients after mastectomy. Many other authorities subscribe to the early sight of the scar by both patient and spouse, to full acknowledgement of a changed body, and to open communication between the couple. Goals for rehabilitation should be gradual and explicit. Many advise full involvement of the spouse in teaching, and that the husband should be encouraged to see and possibly touch the scar during early recovery. These nurses (and many others now) act as experts providing counselling and prostheses for patients. However, as mastectomy becomes a less common intervention, evaluation of their role becomes less possible, although comparison of psychological morbidity rates and patients' reports attest to the advantages of such specialists.

Eardley (1986) discusses radiotherapy as a potentially frightening treatment, about which patients have many misconceptions concerning benefit, purpose and side-effects. In her small descriptive study (n=39) over one-third of patients did not anticipate side-effects of such severity. Learning rates for those undergoing radiotherapy are also reviewed by Johnson and Flaherty (1980). They mention that anxiety should be reduced by providing sessions based on a carefully structured curriculum. Topics should include the machine, length of treatment, treatment plans, irradiation of others or spread of cancer, the emotional effects of radiotherapy, symptoms, and radiation reactions. This programme is all part of a course entitled 'I can cope' summarised by Johnson and Flaherty (1980, p. 66):

' 1. The patient needs accurate and current information on the disease and treatment.
2. The patient must be helped to accept and readjust to changes in body image and self-concept.
3. The patient needs to understand how to express feelings about having the disease.
4. Readjustment of major responsibilities and goals will be necessary in the face of an uncertain future.
5. The impact that the illness will have on financial status of the family should be determined.
6. There may be a need for reinforcement of basic life philosophy, i.e. spiritual needs.
7. A sense of hope must be established and maintained.
8. Meaningful interpersonal relationships with family, friends and medical personnel should be encouraged.
9. Resources that can give assistance should be identified.
10. The myths and untruths about the disease and its treatments should be discussed.'

This sort of outline is fairly representative of other educational programmes, although only a few, run by nurses, have been systematically evaluated.

Interventions to promote coping and treat problems with adjustment to cancer

Watson's (1983) review of psychological interventions with cancer patients provides a sound analysis of experimental work aimed to promote adjustment. Most of these studies involve counsellors, social workers, or a combined team of workers. Studies which evaluate group support for patients are usually designed to help patients at the time of diagnosis and much later on in the course of the illness. Results are conflicting, some seem to help reduce anxiety but have little effect on self-esteem or feelings of control. No differences were found in studies comparing group and individual treatments. Other studies which tailor interventions to individual needs seem to benefit patients by reducing anxiety and depression but these research studies seem to suggest that longer term (several months) interventions or counselling sessions are required to reduce all negative reactions. One study, by Farash (1978), compared brief individual psychotherapy with the effects of a self-help group and failed to find many differences except that body image disturbances are reduced by individual therapy.

A recent study by Worden and Weisman (1984) produced interesting findings. Patients identified from a sample of newly diagnosed patients with cancer, as 'at risk' of emotional distress were randomly allocated into two groups. Experimental subjects (n= 59) were allocated to short-term intervention, consisting of techniques designed to lower distress and aid coping, for four weeks after diagnosis. Such topics as confrontation, collaboration and developing cognitive and problem-solving skills were included. Relaxation and peer modelling were also used in the second stage of this intervention. When compared to a control group (n=58) of at risk patients receiving no special intervention it was found that experimental patients had developed enhanced problem resolution and had lower levels of emotional distress up to 24 weeks after diagnosis. This type of sophisticated psychological care may not be adequately administered by nurses without special preparation, but it provides several important suggestions for interventions to improve adaptation.

Perhaps the best known British study is by Maguire et al (1980) and Maguire (1985). A sample of mastectomy patients were matched into two groups. The treatment group (n=75) was assigned to a specialised nurse counsellor who monitored patients' progress and provided advice and counselling. Patients were assessed at 12 and 18 months. At the first assessment there was more psychological morbidity in the treatment group; they also received more referral for psychiatric help. By the 12 and 18 month assessments morbidity was significantly reduced when compared to the control patients. This improvement could be accounted for by accurate and early recognition of psychological problems, by help from the nurse or by the benefits of psychiatric referral.

Watson (1983) concludes that there is insufficient research to support any one type of treatment as superior in aiding adjustment. However, formal support of most kinds tends to alleviate emotional distress, whereas deeper psychological adjustments or behavioural responses are less amenable to influence. Protracted treatment or support is advocated for particular patients who are presenting coping difficulties, but more research is said to be necessary before such support is routinely given.

An earlier review of nursing studies by Lindsey et al (1981) demonstrates a relative paucity of controlled evaluation of nurses as therapists in contrast to Watson's coverage of specialist interventions. They do claim that patient self-help or support groups are established with proven effects. One study incorporated a volunteer member of 'Reach for Recovery', a nurse and a social worker who all worked with patients for two months from the time of diagnosis until after surgery. In this study by Bloom et al (1978) the intervention group (n=21) was compared to a control group (n=18); the former received counselling from a nurse in hospital and post-discharge contact with a social worker, an out-reach centre, and a volunteer. Both practical details (prosthesis) and continued support were therefore provided. The intervention patients initially expressed more depression but over two months had greater feelings of self-efficacy. This study was said to give support to the role of the nurse specialist and the volunteer acting as a positive role model.

A study from the Netherlands by Van den Borne et al (1987) also demonstrated that contact between cancer sufferers during their illness helped to decrease depression, anxiety and psychological complaints and increase self-esteem. This was true especially for patients undergoing treatment for breast cancer and for those whose illness had recurred. Regular contacts also helped to reduce uncertainty, even for those who had little explanation from their doctors. Patients suffering from Hodgkin's disease however were rendered more vulnerable to uncertainty with more contacts if they had not had careful explanations from their doctors. In this situation where the signs and progress of the disease are less specific contacts were only seen as helpful to augment careful, professionally given information.

Self-help groups for ostomy patients have also been studied. One rather novel idea was explored by Trinor (1982). She investigated whether patients (n=171) who acted as volunteers could, themselves, by helping others as visitors, adjust better. Results showed that when compared to non-visitors, patients did significantly better on an acceptance of disability scale. Acceptance was also significantly related to length of time spent in the visitor's role. Active participation in such programmes is said to exploit earlier ideas about the benefit of the helper therapy principle.

IMPLICATIONS OF RESEARCH FOR NURSING PRACTICE

Supportive presence, counselling and information giving have all been incorporated in various interventions whether given by nurses or others. Stress management skills and spouse counselling have also been evaluated in most of the better studies. This contrasts with some of the conventional work which provided education programmes for patients supposedly to promote adaptation and compliance with advice and treatment. Two recent reviews by Wilson-Barnett and Oborne (1983) and McClellan (1986) found that patient education studies claimed predominantly to help patients but usually consisted of administering a package of information to increase knowledge. Without considering why patients needed to know about their disease and medication most researchers assumed more knowledge was a good thing, despite evidence that this did not necessarily affect behaviour, confidence, emotional responses or coping abilities. A typical example of such a study was carried out by Tanner and Noury (1981) with hypertensive patients. This well-designed controlled trial examined the effect of structural teaching on knowledge and blood pressure control. No significant effects on blood pressure were found but knowledge increased in the experimental group. Despite this rather common and predictable finding researchers appeared content. This approach has usually failed to change coping behaviour or physical welfare. Although a majority of nursing studies reviewed by Wilson-Barnett and Oborne in 1983 achieved positive results, only a very small number influenced mood, or physical or behavioural parameters.

Patients have varying needs for support and information, yet most studies provide standardised packages. Those which attempt to modify behaviour by rehearsal and modelling tend to be more effective. For instance a small study by Perry (1981) of a group of 20 patients with chronic bronchitis and emphysema who were trained to deal with the physical problems of their condition, showed that patients' skills increased and therefore their need for others' help was reduced.

Studies which have aimed to produce and test self-instructional materials have been more successful in helping patients to cope with illness than those which simply present and test for utilisation of the material. For instance Oermann et al (1986) tested a complete self-instructional programme for sufferers of rheumatoid arthritis by randomly dividing the group of 30 patients into the experimental self-taught group and a control group. Learning objectives were set and seven self-contained units of material were designed for patients to use at their own speed. Learning, satisfaction with teaching on health status (e.g. pain, mobility) were compared across the groups after 4–5 weeks. Although health status was not subsequently found to be different for the two groups in this study, methodological problems may be responsible, as Oermann and others review several studies that did achieve significantly positive findings. Individualised self-instruction programmes are therefore generally considered advantageous for patients whose requirements, objectives and abilities can be catered for.

Despite early models such as that described by Jenny (1978), emphasising patient participation, individualisation of instruction and facilitative rather than educative roles for nurses, many past studies adhered to a controlled, standardised or inflexible approach.

More recent studies with cardiac and cancer patients, evaluating experimental and shared support sessions where skills and plans are discussed rather than taught (often by patients not professionals), seem to reflect patients' needs for coping with illness. Problems can then be identified and families rather than just patients can be helped to adjust as necessary.

In reviewing studies evaluating the use of contracting to increase therapeutic behaviour (compliance), Snyder (1985) explains the rationale for this approach as making the patient more responsible for the outcome of care. This type of collaboration also helps to avoid conflicting aims and values for treatments by making goals and agreements explicit. Studies evaluating contracting have involved a range of subjects from hypertension to unsocial behaviour, such as smoking. Evidence of benefits from this approach include change and physical improvements such as lowered blood pressure and weight loss.

Dracup and Meleis (1982) have made a real impact on this field by introducing ideas of role adjustment and interaction which involve recognition by all family members that change has occurred but that self-concept can remain appropriately positive.

Research methods are also becoming more flexible and meaningful. For example Webb's (1986) study with patients after hysterectomy established that a conversation rather than an interview resulted not only in more research information, but also in benefits for patients who received relevant guidance for recovery plans. This was in contrast to an earlier, rather unsuccessful, experiment (Webb and Wilson-Barnett, 1983) which provided a standardised package of information for patients after hysterectomy prior to their discharge from hospital. Information was probably relevant to early recovery and confidence at home (although not shown) but this was not reflected by the more quantified evaluation instruments.

Reports of innovations in practice are also encouraging. Self-help groups where individuals support each other and share common experiences or problems are becoming more prevalent and successful in meeting needs. Professionals may be involved only peripherally. Such a group was described by Schultz (1984) for parents of chronically ill children. Purposes of such groups are defined as

'1. Providing a setting to communicate with others experiencing similar stresses, thus reducing their sense of isolation.
2. Helping parents anticipate and manage common problems.
3. Making possible the identification of psychosocial risk factors that require additional intervention.'

Redman (1985), when reviewing practice and research in the field of patient education, concluded that:

'Patient education is moving closer to the emotional, self-concept and self-management skill variables and its cognitive focus is more toward patient processing of information and away from cognitive abilities to learn such as formal education level, intelligence and reasoning ability.'

FUTURE RESEARCH

Future practice and research should reflect this trend, studies such as these being required:

1. Interview studies attempting to document coping strategies in various patient groups.
2. Studies evaluating courses promoting role supplementation and self-efficacy based therapies for nurses and on their subsequent success in applying these.
3. Interventions for those 'at risk' (high neuroticism and poorly supported patients) should be designed and evaluated for those with difficult disorders.
4. More patient and partner groups should be run by clinics and hospitals, field trials of such strategies could then be more representative.
5. Effects of patient 'model' visitors should be evaluated systematically in many settings, in hospital and in the home. Both the content and the response to such visits should be carefully documented.

APPENDIX 1. OUT-PATIENTS' QUESTIONNAIRE

1. Was anyone at home to help you when you were discharged from hospital?
   ....
2. What sort of help was necessary? ....
   ....
3. What has been the most problematic aspect of your recovery at home?   ....
   ....
   ....
4. Did anyone either (a) encourage or (b) discourage your return to previous levels of activity?
   Who? (a) .... , ...
         (b) .... , ...
5. What were the most difficult activities for you to perform during your recovery, and why?
   ....
   ....
6. (If applicable) Who made the decision that you should or should not go back to work?   ....
7. Is there anything you find particularly difficult about returning to work?   ....
   ....
   ....
8. Does your work involve long periods of standing, carrying weights or travelling?
   Standing ....
   Carrying weights ....
   Travelling ....
9. Do any activities at home or work cause pain or breathlessness?   ....
   ....
10. What percentage would you give your present level of health (compared to someone of your own age)? Please ring an appropriate number

    0   10   20   30   40   50   60   70   80   90   100%

11. Now that some time has passed since you first became ill, do you feel that life has returned to normal? ....
12. Is there anything else about your recovery you would like to mention?   ....
    ....
    ....

APPENDIX 2

Data sheet
Discharged patients'
Survey

Hospital Code:

Patient's Code:

Record Number:

Specified activity	Incapacity — Score in ONE column only						Compensatory help — Score in ONE column only — Incapacity=2					Incapacity=4					Sources of help — Check ALL that apply										
	Not applicable	Minimal or no difficulty	Partially unable/difficult	Partially disallowed	Unable/very difficult	Entirely disallowed	Satisfactory/dependable	Satisfactory/not dependable	Unsatisfactory/dependable	Unsatisfactory/not dependable	No help	Satisfactory/dependable	Satisfactory/not dependable	Unsatisfactory/dependable	Unsatisfactory/not dependable	No help	Member of household	Other relative/friend	District nurse	Home help	Meals service	Other—local authority	Other—voluntary service	Other—hospital	Mechanical aid	Any other	Not ascertained
1. Dress/undress	0	0	2	2	4	4	2	1	1	0	0	4	2	2	0	0	1	2	3	4	5	6	7	8	9	0	X
2. Shave/do hair	0	0	2	2	4	4	2	1	1	0	0	4	2	2	0	0	1	2	3	4	5	6	7	8	9	0	X
3. Bath/overall wash	0	0	2	2	4	4	2	1	1	0	0	4	2	2	0	0	1	2	3	4	5	6	7	8	9	0	X
4. Eat/drink	0	0	2	2	4	4	2	1	1	0	0	4	2	2	0	0	1	2	3	4	5	6	7	8	9	0	X
5. Lavatory/commode	0	0	2	2	4	4	2	1	1	0	0	4	2	2	0	0	1	2	3	4	5	6	7	8	9	0	X
6. Prepare meal	0	0	2	2	4	4	2	1	1	0	0	4	2	2	0	0	1	2	3	4	5	6	7	8	9	0	X
7. Maintain heating	0	0	2	2	4	4	2	1	1	0	0	4	2	2	0	0	1	2	3	4	5	6	7	8	9	0	X
8. Make bed	0	0	2	2	4	4	2	1	1	0	0	4	2	2	0	0	1	2	3	4	5	6	7	8	9	0	X
9. Clean floor	0	0	2	2	4	4	2	1	1	0	0	4	2	2	0	0	1	2	3	4	5	6	7	8	9	0	X
10. Personal laundry	0	0	2	2	4	4	2	1	1	0	0	4	2	2	0	0	1	2	3	4	5	6	7	8	9	0	X

Item	Scores
13. Child care	0 0 2 2 4 4 2 2 0 0 1 1 0 0 4 2 2 0 1 2 3 4 5 6 7 8 9 0 X
14. Dependant's care	0 0 2 2 4 4 2 2 0 0 1 1 0 0 4 2 2 0 1 2 3 4 5 6 7 8 9 0 X
15. Medication	0 0 2 2 4 4 2 2 0 0 1 1 0 0 4 2 2 0 1 2 3 4 5 6 7 8 9 0 X
16. Dressing/bandage	0 0 2 2 4 4 2 2 0 0 1 1 0 0 4 2 2 0 1 2 3 4 5 6 7 8 9 0 X
17. Injection	0 0 2 2 4 4 2 2 0 0 1 1 0 0 4 2 2 0 1 2 3 4 5 6 7 8 9 0 X
18. Drops	0 0 2 2 4 4 2 2 0 0 1 1 0 0 4 2 2 0 1 2 3 4 5 6 7 8 9 0 X
19. Special diet	0 0 2 2 4 4 2 2 0 0 1 1 0 0 4 2 2 0 1 2 3 4 5 6 7 8 9 0 X
20. Exercises	0 0 2 2 4 4 2 2 0 0 1 1 0 0 4 2 2 0 1 2 3 4 5 6 7 8 9 0 X
21. Wearing appliance	0 0 2 2 4 4 2 2 0 0 1 1 0 0 4 2 2 0 1 2 3 4 5 6 7 8 9 0 X
22. Other treatment	0 0 2 2 4 4 2 2 0 0 1 1 0 0 4 2 2 0 1 2 3 4 5 6 7 8 9 0 X

Column totals:

Grand totals:

Potential maximum incapacity score: _____
i.e. 4 (22 minus number of inapplicable items)

Percentage incapacity score: _____

Residual incapacity indicator: _____

From Roberts (1975) Reproduced with kind permission of the author and publishers.

REFERENCES

Bloom JR, Ross RD, Burnell E (1978) The effect of social support on patient adjustment after heart surgery. *Patient Counselling and Health Education* 1, 1–9.

Bohachick P (1984) Progressive relaxation training in cardiac rehabilitation: Effect on psychologic variables. *Nursing Research* 33(5), 283–287.

Brown JS, Rawlinson ME (1977) Sex differences in sick role rejection and in work performance following cardiac surgery. *Journal of Health and Social Behaviour* 18, 276–292.

Carpenito LJ (1983) *Nursing Diagnosis: Application to Clinical Practice*. J.B. Lippincott Co, Philadelphia.

Caty S, Ellerton ML, Ritchie JA (1984) Coping in hospitalised children: an analysis of published case studies. *Nursing Research* 33(5), 277–282.

Craig HM, Edwards JE (1983) Adaptation in chronic illness: an eclectic model for nurses. *Journal of Advanced Nursing* 8, 397–404.

Derogatis LR (1983) *The Psychological Adjustment to Illness Scale*. Clinical Psychometric Research, Division of Medical Psychology, Johns Hopkins School of Medicine, Baltimore.

Dracup KA, Meleis AI, Clark S, Clyburn A, Shields L, and Staley, M (1984a) Group counselling in cardiac rehabilitation: effect on patient compliance. *Patient Education and Counselling* 6(4), 169–177.

Dracup KA, Meleis AI (1982) Compliance: on interactionist approach. *Nursing Research* 31(1), 31–36.

Dracup K, Meleis A, Baker K, Edlefsen P (1984b) Family-focused cardiac rehabilitation: a role supplementation program for cardiac patients and spouses. *Nursing Clinics of North America* 19(1), 113–124.

Eardley A (1986) What do patients need to know? *Nursing Times* 16, 24–26.

Farash JL (1978) Effect of counselling on resolution of loss and body image disturbance following a mastectomy. *Dissertation Abstracts International* 39(8B), 4027.

Feldman DL (1974) Chronic disabling illness: a holistic view. *Journal of Chronic Disease* 27, 16–27.

Frazure-Smith N, Prince R (1985) The ischaemic heart disease life stress monitoring programme. Impact on mortality. *Psychosomatic Medicine* 47, 431–445.

Germino B, McCorkle R (1985) Acknowledged awareness of life threatening illness. *International Journal of Nursing Studies* 22(1), 33–44.

Goldberg RL (1982) Psychologic sequelae of myocardial infarction. *American Family Physician* 25(May), 209–213.

Gould D, Wilson-Barnett J (1985) A comparison of recovery following hysterectomy and major cardiac surgery. *Journal of Advanced Nursing* 10, 315–323.

Greer S (1979) Psychological enquiry: a contribution to cancer research. *Psychological Medicine* 9, 81–89.

Hentinen M (1983) Need for instruction and support of the wives of patients with myocardial infarction. *Journal of Advanced Nursing* 8, 519–524.

Hilbert GA (1985) Spouse support and myocardial infarction patient compliance. *Nursing Research* 34(4), 217–220.

Jenny J (1978) A strategy for patient teaching. *Journal of Advanced Nursing* 3, 341–348.

Johnson J, Flaherty M (1980) The nurse and cancer patient education. *Seminars in Oncology* 7(1), 63–70.

Kellog Speegle E, Bayer LR, Greens WA (1979) Convalescent discomfort following acute coronary events. *Nursing Research* 28(3), 132–138.

Krouse HJ, Krouse JH (1982) Cancer as crisis: the critical elements of adjustment. *Nursing Research* 31(2), 96–101.

Kubler Ross E (1969) *On Death and Dying*. Macmillan, New York.

Lauer P, Murphy SP, Powers MJ (1982) Learning needs of cancer patients: a comparison of nurse and patient perceptions. *Nursing Research* 31(1), 11–21.

Lazarus RS (1974) Psychological stress and coping in adaptation and illness. *International Journal of Psychiatry in Medicine* 5(4), 321–333.

Lewis FM, Bloom JR (1978) Psychosocial adjustment to breast cancer: a review of selected literature. *International Journal of Psychiatry in Medicine* 9(1), 1–17.

Linde BJ, Janz NM (1979) Effect of a teaching program on knowledge and compliance of cardiac patients. *Nursing Research* 28(5), 282–286.

Lindsey AM, Norbeck JS, Carrieri VC, Perry E (1981) Social support and health outcomes in post-mastectomy women: a review. *Cancer Nursing* Oct, 377–384.

Lipowski ZJ (1983) Psychosocial reactions to physical illness. *Canadian Medical Association* 128, 1069–1072.

Lloyd GG (1979) Psychological stress and coping mechanisms in patients with cancer. In: Stoll BA (ed) *Mind and Cancer Prognosis* 47–72. John Wiley and Sons Ltd, Chichester.

Lowery BJ, Jacobson BS (1985) Attributional analysis of chronic illness outcomes. *Nursing Research* 34(2), 82–88.

Lum JL, Chase M, Cole SM, Johnson A, Johnson JA, Link MR (1978) Nursing care of oncology patients receiving chemotheraphy. *Nursing Research* 27(6), 340–346.

Maguire GP, Tait A, Brooke M, Thomas C, Sellwood R (1980) The effects of monitoring on the psychiatric morbidity associated with mastectomy. *British Medical Journal* 11, 1454.

Maguire P (1984) Doctor–patient communication. In: Mathews A, Steptoe A (eds) *Care and Human Behaviour*, Academic Press, London.

Maguire P (1985) Improving the detection of psychiatric problems in cancer patients. *Social Science and Medicine* 20(8), 819–823.

Mailick M (1979) The impact of severe illness on the individual and family: an overview. *Social Work Health Care* 5, 117.

Mathews A, Ridgeway V (1981) Personality and surgical recovery: a review. *British Journal of Clinical Psychology* 20, 243–260.

Mayou R, Macmahon D, Sleight P, Florencio MJ (1981) Early rehabilitation after myocardial infarction. *Lancet* ii, 1399–1401.

Mayou R, Williamson B, Foster A (1976) Attitudes and advice after myocardial infarction. *British Medical Journal* 1, 1577–1579.

Mayou R (1984) Prediction of emotional and social outcome after a heart attack. *Journal of Psychosomatic Research* 28(1), 17–25.

Mayou R (1986) The psychiatric and social consequences of coronary artery surgery. *Journal of Psychosomatic Research* 30(3), 255–271.

McClellan W (1986) The physician and patient education: a review. *Patient Education and Counselling* 8, 151–163.

McCorkle R, Young K (1978) Development of a symptom distress scale. *Cancer Nursing* Oct, 373–378.

Morris T, Greer HS, White P (1977) Psychological and social adjustment to mastectomy: a two year follow up study. *Cancer* 40, 2381–2387.

Naismith LD, Robinson JF, Shaw GB, MacIntyre MM (1979) Psychological rehabilitation after myocardial infarction. *British Medical Journal* 1, 439–441.

Oermann MH, Doyle TH, Clark LR, Rivers CL, Rose VY (1986) Effectiveness of self-instruction for arthritis patient education. *Patient Education and Counselling* 8, 245–254.

Owens JF, McCann CS, Hutelmyer CM (1978) Cardiac rehabilitation: a patient education programme. *Nursing Research* 27(3), 148–150.

Parker KP (1981) Anxiety and complications in patients on haemodialysis. *Nursing Research* 30(6), 334–336.

Pay C, Grover J, Wisniewski T (1984) Nurses' perceptions of early breast cancer and mastectomy and their psychological implications, and of the role of health professionals in providing support. *Journal of Advanced Nursing* 21(2), 105–111.

Penckofer SH, Holm K (1984) Early appraisal of coronary revascularization on quality of life. *Nursing Research* 33(2), 60–63.

Perry JA (1981) Effectiveness of teaching in the rehabilitation of patients with chronic bronchitis and emphysema. *Nursing Research* 30(4), 219–222.

Pinkerton P, Trauer T, Duncan F, Hodson ME, Batten JC (1985) Cystic fibrosis in adult life: a study of coping patterns. *Lancet* ii, 761–763.

Polivy J (1977) Psychological effects of mastectomy on a woman's feminine self-concept. *Journal of Nervous and Mental Diseases* **164**(2), 77–87.

Ramshaw JE, Stanley G (1984) Psychological adjustment to coronary artery surgery. *Journal of Clinical Psychology* **23**, 101–108.

Ray C, Grover J, Wisniewski T (1984) Nurses' perceptions of early breast cancer and mastectomy and their psychological implications and of the role of health professionals in providing support. *International Journal of Nursing Studies* **21**(2), 101–111.

Redman BK (1985) Nurses as health educators: the philosophical framework. Paper read at *Health Education Conference*, Harrogate, England May 20.

Ridgeway V, Mathews A (1982) Psychological preparation for surgery: a comparison of methods. *British Journal of Clinical Psychology* **21**, 271–280.

Roberts I (1975) *Discharge from Hospital*. RCN, London.

Ronayne R (1985) Feelings and attitudes during early convalescence following vascular surgery. *Journal of Advanced Nursing* **10**, 435–441.

Rudy EB (1980) Patients' and spouses' causal explanations of a myocardial infarction. *Nursing Research* **29**(6), 352–356.

Schultz SK (1984) Use of a support group to aid parental coping with a chronically ill child. *Paedovita* **1**(1), 22–28.

Snyder M (1985) *Independent Nursing Interventions*. John Wiley and Sons, New York. pp. 153–166.

Steinhart MJ (1984) *Emotional aspects of coronary artery disease*. Current concepts series, Scope Publishers/Upjohn, Michigan.

Tanner GA, Noury DJ (1981) The effect of instruction on control of blood pressure in individuals with essential hypertension. *Journal of Advanced Nursing* **6**, 99–106.

Tarrier N (1983) A behavioural approach to the psychological problems of mastectomy. *British Journal of Clinical and Social Psychiatry* **2**, 41–43.

Trainor MA (1982) Acceptance of ostomy and the visitor role in a self-help group for ostomy patients. *Nursing Research* **31**(2), 102–106.

Van den Borne HW, Pruyn JFA, Van den Heuvel WJA (1987) Effects of contacts between cancer patients and their psychosocial problems. *Patient Education and Counselling* **9**, 33–51.

Watson M (1983) Psychosocial intervention with cancer patients: a review. *Psychological Medicine* **13**, 839–846.

Webb C, Wilson-Barnett J (1983) Hysterectomy: a study in coping with recovery. *Journal of Advanced Nursing* **8**, 311–319.

Webb C, Wilson-Barnett J (1983) Hysterectomy: dispelling the myths. *Nursing Times*: Occasional Papers. **79**(30), 52–54.

Webb C (1986) Professional and lay social support for hysterectomy patients. *Journal of Advanced Nursing* **11**, 167–177.

West S (1987) *Recovery from Coronary Artery Bypass Surgery*. Unpublished PhD Thesis, King's College, University of London.

Wilson-Barnett J (1979) A review of research into the experience of patients suffering from coronary thrombosis. *International Journal of Nursing Studies* **16**, 183–198.

Wilson-Barnett J (1981) Assessment of recovery: with special reference to a study with post-operation cardiac patients. *Journal of Advanced Nursing* **6**, 435–445.

Wilson-Barnett J, Fordham M (1983) *Recovery from Illness*. John Wiley and Sons, Chichester.

Wilson-Barnett J, Oborne J (1983) Studies evaluating patient teaching: implications for practice. *International Journal of Nursing Studies* **20**(1), 33–44.

Woods NF, Earp JA (1978) Woman with cured breast cancer. *Nursing Research* **27**(5), 279–285.

Worden JW, Weisman AD (1984) Preventive psychosocial intervention with newly diagnosed cancer patients. *General Hospital Psychiatry* **6**, 243–249.

Chapter 3
Anxiety

Dysphoria, negative moods or affects, are experienced by most people at some time in their lives, but if they are judged to be more pronounced than usual or more prolonged, they can be seen as a problem requiring interventions from nurses to reduce them and prevent major psychiatric illness. There are also complex and important relationships between moods and physical states which holistic models of care emphasise. Physical illness is often associated with and influenced adversely by negative moods, and continuous anxiety and depression may well lead to physical problems.

DEFINITION

Carpenito's (1983) book on nursing diagnosis defines anxiety thus:

> 'A state in which the individual experiences feelings of uneasiness (apprehension) and activation of the autonomic nervous system in response to a vague, non-specific threat.' (p. 78)

Anxiety is often used interchangeably with fear or stress, yet this blurs the unique feature of a disproportionate response to a non-specific or unknown threat which might occur in the future. Fear is usually exhibited in the face of an identified threat and stress is a blanket term used in the face of increased demand for the subject to adjust to changes in his or her life or environment. Anxiety may be a temporary response to a situation which is new and possibly unclear or it may be a chronic disposition in which a person frequently responds to events with anxiety. Anxiety only becomes a problem when it is judged to interfere with other activities, or inhibit coping.

Although mechanisms by which persistent or strong anxiety causes physical symptoms and illness were poorly understood (and to some extent still are), this relationship was documented and studied in the days of Hippocrates and Aristotle. The origin of the term is even earlier, the Latin derivation being *anxietas* meaning troubled in mind.

Spielberger (1972, p. 24) defines anxiety as:

> 'a palpable but transitory emotional state or condition characterised by feelings of tension and apprehension and heightened autonomic nervous system activity.'

This is obviously closely related to the derivation from '*anxietas*' and '*angor*' meaning a sense of constriction. A threat of the unknown is often said to be the cause of anxiety. For example Lazarus and Averill (1972) explain that this feeling results from an insufficient understanding of an event, and Rycroft (1968) also points to a vague threat in the future against which there is no action. May's (1950, p. 191) definition integrates most of these elements; he describes anxiety as:

> 'a diffuse apprehension which is unspecific, vague and objectless. It is associated with feelings of uncertainty and helplessness resulting from a threat to the core or essence of the personality.'

When differentiating anxiety from fear Hoch and Zubin (1950) point to disproportionate reactions: whereas in fear these are related to directive action, in anxiety the subject lacks power to act and the threat assumes disproportionate dimensions. Failure to be able to ward off a threat results in the complex emotion of anxiety which Rycroft (1968) recognises as a combination of hope, fear, despondency and despair. Izard (1972) endorses this idea of a complex and ranked the components as follows: interest, fear, distress, disgust, guilt, surprise, shyness, fatigue, anger, contempt and enjoyment. Similarly Cattell's (1954) sub-factors included guilt, ergic tension, poor ego strength, suspiciousness, and a poorly developed self-sentiment.

Positive interpretations of anxiety exist and although it is reviewed as an uncomfortable feeling many people seek situations which evoke anxiety and seem to function better with the heightened awareness and energy it provides. Yerkes and Dodson's (1908) 'U-shaped curve' has had an immense effect on psychological thinking, in that a low or moderate level of anxiety is found to be associated with improved performance in some situations but increased levels tend to result in disorganised behaviour. Related to this, Ray and Fitzgibbon (1982) consider that arousal rather than anxiety may be a more accurate description and constructive drive. In particular, when information processing is required by individuals in a clearly stressful situation (awaiting surgery), arousal rather than anxiety is desirable.

However, the uncomfortable nature of these feelings, in itself, may spur people on to actions to reduce the threat of future events. Revising for examinations, visiting the doctor or asking questions to gain information, may all be seen as positive actions spurred by anxiety leading to constructive behaviour. However, it is obviously the situations in which they occur, and the level and frequency of anxious feelings which determine their effect and long-term influences on the physical state of the individual.

ANXIETY — NORMAL AND PATHOLOGICAL

The question of whether or not neurotic anxiety differs in quality and quantity from 'normal' everyday anxiety has been discussed by May (1950) who argues for a clear differentiation between normal and neurotic anxiety. Normal anxiety is seen to be more proportional to the threat and subsides when the threat is removed, while neurotic anxiety is enduring and disproportionate and involves developing defence mechanisms. Freud (1936) and neo-Freudians also differentiate between neurotic anxiety as pathological and normal anxiety resulting from threats or inter-personal relationships and conflicts.

More recent views by Hamilton (1969) and Lader (1975) disagree with this distinction.

Hamilton claims that his research shows the difference between anxiety felt by dermatology patients and by psychiatric patients is only quantitative, not qualitative. He designed a test for anxiety on which neurotics scored much higher than dermatology patients. Psychiatric anxiety states are explained as a lowering of a threshold so that environmental stress which would not affect a normal person evokes anxiety in a 'neurotic'. Lader (1975) talks in terms of a cut-off point on a continuum of anxiety beyond which levels are considered abnormal. Pathological anxiety is more frequent, more severe and more persistent than usual, that is, usual in terms of the individual. He classifies terms in the diagram below:

	Normal	Pathological
Trait	Anxiousness	Anxious personality
State	Feeling anxious	Anxiety state

Lader and Marks (1971) found that 3.2% of the British urban population suffers from anxiety states whereas only 2% of the rural population do so. This condition is found more frequently in females. In a transcultural study Lynn (1971) found that a thin build, alcoholism, accident proneness, high suicide rates and a low calorific intake were correlated with higher levels of anxiety.

PHYSIOLOGICAL AND PHYSICAL EFFECTS OF ANXIETY

The effects of changes in autonomic functions in anxiety are clearly categorised in Table 1 modified from Aitken and Zealley (1970, p. 216)

Both sympathetic and parasympathetic systems are stimulated in anxiety and produce the variety of symptoms listed in Table 1. Rises in catecholamine production and higher proportions of adrenaline than noradrenaline occur in acute anxiety. Resulting physical sensations have a feedback mechanism and may cause a heightened awareness of these, then experienced as greater anxiety. Breggin (1964) discusses this as a self-perpetuating feedback loop. Recurrent attacks of anxiety may strengthen the conditioned association between anxiety and its sympathomimetic symptoms, thereby increasing the intensity of further anxiety reactions.

COPING WITH ANXIETY

It is well known that both Sigmund and Anna Freud (1939) contributed to thinking on how people defend themselves against the discomfort of anxiety. Displacement, sublimation, reaction-formation, regression, rationalisation and projection are discussed at length and psychoanalysts have refined many of these early ideas. Normal functioning or coping depends on the subject using defences appropriately, without relying on one strategy to the exclusion of others.

Table 1. Changes in Autonomic Functions in Anxiety

1	Changes in thinking	Worry, dread and apprehension Reduced concentration and field of attention Distractibility and forgetfulness Irritability and depression Insomnia and nightmares Perceptual disturbance, such as depersonalisation
2	Changes in physiological activity Motor activity:	 Muscular tension and trembling Restlessness and fidgeting Incoordination and impaired performance Startle reaction 'Freezing'
	Other somatic functions:	Sympathetic: Flushing and sweating Dry mouth and anorexia Choking feeling as if lump in throat Rapid breathing and sometimes hyperventilation Palpitations, fatigue, weakness and fainting Parasympathetic: Dyspepsia and diarrhoea Urgency and frequency of micturition Impotence Menstrual disturbance

Relief from anxiety symptoms, manifest as somatic as well as psychic malaise, can also be reduced when such conditioned responses are weakened. New response patterns have to be learned which are considered appropriate to the situation and environmental constraints. Recently greater emphasis has been put on this relearning capacity as a cognitive activity within the control of the subject rather than understanding subconscious dynamics. However, they depend on the motivation and understanding of the individual. Adjustment to potential anxiety-evoking events is the overall aim in order to reduce wasteful energy and uncoordinated responses. This aim of adjustment is even more essential for those who are more vulnerable through physical weaknesses and illness.

ANXIETY AS THE CAUSE OF ILLNESS

Prolonged or excessive anxiety with accompanying physical responses is associated with an increased metabolic rate, reduced immunity, and resistance to increased demand. It is not, therefore, surprising that anxious people feel unwell and complain of physical symptoms. Many somatic complaints have been misinterpreted by medical staff as indicators of an organic pathological process which should be carefully investigated and treated. Many patients in turn explain their symptoms as part of what they deem to be a physical disorder.

Relevant to this issue was a study (Wilson-Barnett and Trimble, 1984) comparing a patient group with neurological conditions and another with psychiatric disorders with those referred for assessment of 'hysterical' complaints. Patients in this last category had suffered fits, paralysis and disturbance of sensation or motor function. However, extensive investigations had been carried out without detecting abnormalities. When measuring affective components or emotions and personality dimensions it was found those in the 'hysterical' group were highly anxious and/or depressed; in some cases severity was similar to the 'psychiatric' group. Most understood that their problems could have been psychological but tended to have an unrealistic view of their capabilities and life problems. Masked anxiety or depression resulting in physical or somatic problems such as these can be detected in many other specialties.

This area of care is frequently mismanaged, 'psychosomatic' or 'hysterical' being used by staff as a pejorative term which does not deserve medical and nursing time. It is this ignorance that tends to be associated with unsupportive reactions from staff and a worsening of the sufferer's condition.

It is sad that the fascinating mechanisms by which psychological factors affect physical health are not studied more. They affect every person and patient and may well hold the key to ways in which they could be influenced positively by nurses. Holistic understanding has been deemed one of the unique perspectives for nursing (Wilson-Barnett, 1985).

A very anxious patient, in whatever situation, will find it difficult to rest, sleep, concentrate and recover. Alleviation of this distressing emotion has therefore to be seen as vital for humanitarian and physically therapeutic reasons.

Those who are vulnerable to the effects of sympathetic stimulation, which increase the demands on the cardiovascular, digestive and immune systems, may of course fare worse under conditions of increased stress or anxiety. Angina, seen as a response to emotional excitement, is in fact named from the German 'angst' inferring constriction. It is a classic symptom associated with anxiety, and ischaemic heart disease is thought to be more prevalent in those of an anxious disposition (Olmsted and Kennedy, 1975). Those with diabetes may also be unable to respond to the increased metabolism of cells, inadequate available insulin inhibiting the uptake of glucose. Alternatively muscle wasting may occur through catabolic processes in response to other systems' need for energy and nutrients. Likewise with reduced resistance consequent on protracted anxiety (Bartrop et al, 1977), many patients would be vulnerable particularly in a hospital situation where pathogens abound.

It is now established that high anxiety is associated with both physical morbidity and a reduced ability to tolerate further discomfort. In a temporary situation, i.e. post-operatively, increased pain and anxiety correlate (Hayward, 1975) and, more persistently, as a personality dimension neuroticism is associated with more complicated and prolonged recovery (Mathews and Ridgeway, 1981).

ANXIETY AS A RESPONSE TO ILLNESS

A feedback or circular relationship tends to exist between illness and anxiety: increased anxiety leads to illness and illness is associated with greater emotional reactions of anxiety and often depression. Deep-seated fears of death and mutilation were discussed as the fundamental root of anxiety by Freud (see Jones, 1955). Feelings of deep malaise or great pain and immobility tend to lead to morbid thoughts, feelings of dependence on others, and vulnerability. Even influenza can produce such unpleasant symptoms which may evoke fears of death. 'I felt like death' is not a totally 'light-hearted' description.

Other reasons for anxiety during illness exist. In any situation the causes are individualistic or idiosyncratic, differing aspects of life seeming challenging or threatening to different people. Leaving the family, fearing disfigurement, being unable to cope with usual responsibilities and fearing the withdrawal of those one cares for, may all evoke anxiety (Lipowski, 1975).

Seeking medical aid and advice from others may be encouraged through anxious feelings but may in turn cause further concerns. In contrast delays in seeking such help may be due to the fear of disclosing some dreaded condition, as Aitken Swan and Paterson (1955) found in their famous study of cancer patients.*

PREVALENCE

'Normal' anxiety may become a problem within specific contexts or social situations for individuals. This implies a continuous phenomenon differing in severity but not type or quality of mood. Proportions of 'sufferers' vary according to the situation and 'normal' expectations of when it will subside. 'Most' significant new situations evoke slight feelings of anxiety in 'most' individuals. Enduring feelings of anxiety can affect physical health adversely and this can be particularly injurious to those who are already ill. Anxiety amongst medical ward patients has been studied throughout their hospital stay (Wilson-Barnett and Carrigy, 1978); one-quarter of those studied suffered from 'acute' anxiety for at least one-third of their stay in hospital. These patients were shown to have a peak of anxiety on admission, which sometimes lasted as long as five days. Other studies on general ward patients confirm that 24–25% experience what can be judged as severe distress or psychological morbidity. Moffic and Paykel (1975) also showed that emotional problems were complex and sometimes difficult to classify as anxiety or depression, patients frequently exhibiting signs of both. Systematic assessment of these emotions was necessary to detect this prevalence, staff having failed to recognise these problems in approximately one-half of the cases.

Persistent or recurring anxiety of excessively high levels may be described as a neurotic predisposition. At extreme levels neurotic illness or neuroses is diagnosed (this is discussed more fully later in the chapter). This may also include other manifestations, such as hysterical symptoms, phobias, obsessions and depression. Community surveys show that about 10% of the population is affected by neurotic symptoms at any one time.

'Exact prevalence is impossible to determine as neurotic symptoms are not qualitatively different from normal experience.' (Hughes, 1981, p. 29)

Anxiety states are said to have a 5% prevalence in the population.

---

* Much of this introductory section is reprinted in the Chapter on 'Anxiety—its relevance for nursing' by J Wilson-Barnett (1988) in Julia Brooking (Ed), *A Textbook of Psychiatric Nursing*. Churchill Livingstone, Edinburgh.

ASSESSMENT

Rigorous and continued efforts to assess negative moods or affects are required. There are many ways to assess a person's feelings, but this takes time and careful attention. Because it has been a relatively neglected aspect of practice, nurses should now intentionally exploit their opportunities for observing and talking to patients. Adequate opportunity to discuss feelings and problems is always required, yet too many excuses are provided by staff for lack of time to talk. Hockey's (1976) study reports nurses as saying they would like to give more psychological care and several articles bemoan nurses' lack of communication skills (Syred, 1981; Macleod Clark, 1983). Evidence to the effects of this are found from Johnston's (1982) study where nurses were unable to provide accurate assessments of mood and pain. Although Openshaw's (1984) work provided better results, overestimates of anxiety were usual and she accounts for this, in part, by suggesting that nurses felt they ought to report some negative moods. Muhlenkamp and Joyner (1986) with a sample of 30 hospitalised patients with arthritis, and 28 nurses found quite accurate assessments on a number of dimensions, but noted that higher levels of nursing education were associated with the strongest correlations between patients and nurses' ratings of anxiety.

Yet many writers argue for the potential role of the nurse as psychological supporter, friend and counsellor and studies to be reviewed here attest to their power to alleviate anxiety. Nurses are seen to have most opportunity for contact from day to day, provide 24-hour cover and include psychological care as a vital part of major models for nursing practice and education. Indeed some psychologists have supported their role expanding towards more intense psychotherapy in the psychiatric setting, rather than just in necessary support relationships, which are less intense and maintain social balance (e.g. Anderson and Mottram, 1973). Their skills in this area are therefore sometimes recognised, yet widely under-utilised.

Criteria for assessment (see Table 2)

All emotions, anxiety included, tend to have physical as well as psychological components. In anxiety, physical signs are associated with sympathetic nervous system activity, experienced as insomnia, fatigue and weakness, flushing, a dry mouth, body aches and pains, urinary frequency, restlessness, faintness, and paraesthesiae. Subjective experiences are reported as apprehensiveness, helplessness, nervousness, fear associated with lack of self-confidence, loss of control, and tension or being 'keyed up'. Behavioural sequelae include irritability, angry outbursts, crying, a tendency to blame others, criticism of self and others, withdrawal, lack of initiative, and self-deprecation. Cognitive impairment results and anxiety may lead to an inability to concentrate, a lack of awareness of surroundings, forgetfulness, rumination, orientation to the past rather than to the present or future; and memory difficulties. Level of anxiety will obviously determine the degree of such feelings and problems; mild anxiety may only be identified by one or two signs, whereas severe anxiety or panic may result in grave incapacity (Carpenito, 1983).

Table 2. Criteria and Methods for Assessment of Anxiety

Physical criteria	Methods
Vital signs. Pulse, respirations, temperature and blood pressure.	Record and monitor regularly.
Pattern of micturition and defaecation.	Record and monitor daily.
Appearance of skin—flushing or perspiration.	Careful, regular observation.
Behavioural criteria	
Activity levels, restlessness.	Observe for change. Ask relatives.
Anorexia.	Record what is eaten.
Insomnia.	Observe sleep pattern and quantity.
Crying or angry outbursts.	Record if they occur.
Subjective criteria	
Patient report of anxious feelings.	Use scales to measure self-reports daily.
Complaints of fatigue.	
Inability to concentrate, forgetfulness.	Question patient carefully.

SCALES TO MEASURE ANXIETY

Assessment of present or current levels of anxiety may be done by an observer, such as a nurse who has been trained to note certain behaviours, or by the individuals themselves.

Observer ratings

Training and standardisation of raters is essential for obtaining useful assessments of others' emotions. Scales have been designed for professionals to rate those suffering from neurotic anxiety states. An alternative method by Gelder and Marks (1966) can be used to rate any symptom of anxiety such as that shown below from Lader and Marks (1971, p. 96).

Free-floating anxiety scale for observer rating anxious mood

Rater: take note of persistent, anxious mood, subjective tension, physical manifestation, poor concentration and motor restlessness. Base your assessment on the patient's state during the previous three days.

0	1	2	3	4	5	6	7	8
No anxiety		Mild anxiety kept under control		Moderate anxiety affects behaviour		Severe anxiety disabling at times		Very severe anxiety grossly disabling

In all these tests the rater must always establish the time dimension of the emotion, whether it is a long-term symptom or, as in the case of the linear scale above, only for three days. The same applies when requesting subjects to report their own feelings. Personality tests of how anxious or depressed a person is generally ask questions in terms of 'usually' or 'often'.

Self-report 'state' scales

State scales are usually either linear or adjective check lists, although Spielberger et al's (1983) popular state-trait measure consists of 24 items which have to be rated on a four-point scale. This scale is perhaps more appropriate for research uses or continuous daily ratings with the same patient. Clinical assessment monitoring needs a brief, easily completed instrument such as a linear scale.

Linear scales can be graduated and labelled quantitatively with such labels as 'none', 'a little', 'a moderate amount' or 'extremely' or they can extend from 'none at all' to 'maximum'. The subject merely crosses the line at the appropriate spot and the score equals the length along the line from 0, as below:

```
         A 10 centimetre line used as a linear scale
         How much anxiety do you feel at this moment?
     0  ─────────────────────────*─────────────────────10
         none                              maximum
                                           amount
              Score = 5 out of 10
```

This scale is easy to mark and quantify and subjects are not distracted by a description of the amount of anxiety.

It is essential to assess why someone is anxious. Careful questioning may detect whether this is either non-specific and free-floating or related to a specific situation or whether it is acute or chronic, in their 'normal' limits or beyond. Severity and duration of anxiety will determine when certain measures need to be made and careful 'plotting' of such signs is required. In the acute setting it is particularly difficult to assess an individual's behaviour over time in order to note changes. Relatives and friends may assist by providing information and the patients themselves may remark on such changes. It is however only through careful questioning, such as that used by Narrow (1979, p. 67–69) to elicit specific worries and repeated self-reports, that accurate measures can be made. With continuous care by the same nurse or two nurses, monitoring can be achieved and a simple scale can be used either to establish whether or not a problem exists or how it is progressing. In the acute situation where there is an identifiable event or situation evoking anxiety, it may be short-lived and daily monitoring considered unnecessary. However, when it is reported to be severe and inadequately explained, use of a simple linear scale can be invaluable.

Chronic anxiety problems can be accurately assessed by careful interviews, behavioural observations and monitoring, and more sophisticated measures such as a personal construct grid, often used in cognitive therapy. For phobic anxiety, which is a specific stimulus–fear response, reactions on the whole range of criteria may be relevant for assessing the degree of aversive reaction. Ultimately 'time exposed to' the noxious stimulus becomes critical for assessment during treatment (although this is sometimes beyond the patients' control as the therapist determines this as part of the therapy).

Processing data into usable, simple graphs is essential for everyday clinical practice. This may have therapeutic value for the patient and is essential for accurate evaluation of interventions.

PROBLEM IDENTIFICATION AND CAUSES OF ANXIETY

Differential diagnoses for this major problem area relate to the cause. Once this is assessed adequately, often over the course of several conversations, interventions can be tailored to meet the specific needs.

Anxiety may be due to pathology, situation or transition of maturational stage. New, unfamiliar events or changes in routine are often associated with anxiety. Threats to valued objects, status, possessions, loved ones and anticipation of failure are also common causes. Such causes tend to require the individual to adjust and behave differently in order to meet the challenge or threat. Perceived failure to cope well, or anticipated loss may also result in depressed reactions. Opportunity to control or cope with such situations seems to evoke anxiety, whereas lack of perceived opportunity may lead to feelings of powerlessness and depression.

Physical illness may induce several emotional responses from mild irritation to deeply psychotic moods. Biochemical alterations, enforced inactivity, pain, discomfort and uncertainty are all responsible. The meaning of the event and its consequences determines the response, as does the individual's usual response to potentially stressful events. Certain conditions such as viral infections, neoplastic or neurological disease, are also more likely to be associated with dysphoric states (see Wilson-Barnett, 1979).

Treatments and aspects of care are also shown to affect patients' emotions and as these are under direct control of nurses and doctors they should be considered carefully. Inadequate explanations, rushed communication, routinisation and lack of understanding have all been cited (Robinson, 1972; Ley, 1979; Engstrom, 1984). Without adequate information and support patients are said to feel insecure and helpless, in clinics, hospital or at home.

ANXIETY RELATED TO HOSPITALISATION (see Table 3, section 1)

This diagnosis is closely related to that defined as 'powerlessness related to hospitalisation'. Vague apprehensions, emphasising elements of the unknown (Hoch and Zubin, 1950) aptly describe the responses of patients who are admitted to hospital. Although specific aspects have been reported to worry patients, such as 'being away from home', 'seeing someone else who is very ill' or 'using a bed pan' (Wilson-Barnett, 1976) the more general atmosphere of the hospital engenders widespread apprehensiveness and unease among patients (Robinson, 1972).

Specific events associated with hospitalisation are found to evoke strong feelings of anxiety and depression. In a study of 202 medical ward patients Wilson-Barnett and Carrigy (1978) found that admission to hospital evoked significantly higher negative mood scores for the sample than they reported on average for other daily ratings. Only a small minority of patients reported a complete absence of anxiety and depression, and

Table 3. Anxiety—Identification of Problem and Cause

Relevant criteria	Measures and findings	Diagnosis
Behavioural	Observation and relatives' and patients' accounts show disturbances	Anxiety experienced over several days and related to hospitalisation
Self-report	Patients may not be able to verbalise specific anxiety Narrow's interview (Narrow, 1979) reveals areas of specific concern. Linear scale scores in mid to high range. Unable to concentrate and retain information given	
Physical	Blood pressure, pulse and respirations elevated pre-operation	Anxiety experienced prior to and related to surgery
Behavioural	Observation may show disturbed sleep and elimination patterns pre-operation	
Self-report	Linear scale shows high scores. Patient usually admits anxiety and specific concerns	
Physical	Blood pressure, pulse and respirations elevated when anticipating or actually exposed to object	Phobic anxiety (e.g. elevators, open space, aeroplane flying)
Behavioural	Serious disturbance in behaviour: tremor rigidity, crying. Reduces over time	
Self-report	Linear scale shows highest score possible!	

then only those who also had extremely low ratings on the personality dimension of neuroticism as measured by the Eysenck Personality Inventory. Hospital is unfamiliar to most, infers severe illness or major treatment methods, a total institution with many specialist staff in charge. All three elements of stress may be perceived by new patients therefore. There is a need to adjust to a more dependent role, to learn the ropes or rules of being a patient and to cope with illness and treatment (Franklin, 1974).

Other events have been singled out as particularly distressing and anxiety provoking during the hospital stay. Diagnostic investigations are often lengthy invasive procedures which cause discomfort and involve physical preparation. Patients are usually conscious with a local anaesthetic being used, as their collaboration during the test is required for appropriate positioning. Reviews of responses by Hawkins (1979) and interventions by Wilson-Barnett (1984) confirm that tests certainly are stressful, yet usual care tends to neglect patients' information and support needs. Results of tests are also not usually given to patients, often apparently because they are considered routine and unnecessary for patients to know (Reynolds, 1978).

Doctors' rounds are the focus of criticism by some patients (Wilson-Barnett 1979). Not only do doctors talk among themselves and tend not to include the patient in these conversations, but also they seem to distance themselves when accompanied by colleagues. Recently (from personal observation) this does not seem to be such an obvious behaviour pattern, but the content of discussions is rarely comprehensible to the patient and may be readily misunderstood.

Anxiety is often discussed as 'the fear of the unknown' and logic would therefore suggest that more information of relevance to individual needs should be provided. Studies indicating this need have been detailed elsewhere (see Wilson-Barnett, 1979, Chapter 3); suffice it to say that over the last two decades research findings still consistently bear witness to inadequate information sources and attention to providing open and informative communications with patients. In many American hospitals the patients' Bill of Rights includes full information and fully informed consent for treatments. However, in Great Britain the ombudsman (final arbitrator of complaints) annually reports that two-thirds of complaints from patients relate to inadequate communication and lack of information.

A more recent research report from Sweden by Engstrom (1984) mirrors the UK findings, in a study exploring patients' needs for information. One hundred and twenty patients were included in the sample, 60 of whom were interviewed twice. On diagnosis, prognosis, after-care, routines and facilities, 15–34% of patients reported getting 'no information'. Yet when interviewed on their needs, over two-thirds in each group wanted substantial information on examination results, prognosis and diagnosis, which they considered most important. On other matters, over one-third of the sample needed information on ward routines and facilities, yet the same proportion found this completely inadequate. Overall, 85% of patients considered a 'fairly large' part of their information needs had been met. Information on medical matters was given by doctors for 89% of cases whereas nurses gave information on 'after-care' for 50% of the patients and together with doctors for an additional 30%. Nurses provided information on facilities and equipment for 74%, and on ward routines for 32%.

Goal setting

Anxiety related to hospitalisation is usually short-lived. In at-risk groups such as those with a particularly nervous disposition or those with stress-related disorders or cardiovascular conditions, daily observations and a simple linear scale should be completed to ensure that scores are reduced to zero (or normal for that individual) and behaviour is normalised within three days, five days being the outer limit.

Care plans or records should carry a full account of the major reasons for anxiety, where possible. Narrow's interview schedule should provide a means to encouraging conversations about such aspects.

ANXIETY RELATED TO SURGERY (see Table 3, section 2)

Perhaps the most thoroughly researched event which patients mention with foreboding is surgery. Carnevali (1966), and several authors since, have shown that patients fear the anaesthetic, post-operative pain, 'being cut', and not being a good patient by being brave after surgery. Fantasies of what occurs during surgery and afterwards may evoke more anxiety than the reality, which indicates that clear and realistic information should be provided.

When anxiety is assessed regularly over the acute peri-operative period, it tends to peak on the pre-operative day and the day of operation. Johnston (1980) found this to be a generalised pattern for most patients, anxiety subsiding gradually as patients started to recover between the third and fifth post-operative day. Discomfort due to surgery and associated technical procedures such as dressing changes, drain shortening and changing intravenous cannulae all tend to increase feelings of anxiety about recovery. Pain and anxiety post-operatively are closely correlated (Seers, 1987) and this is certainly reported as one of the greatest fears for surgical patients. Associations between anxious feelings prior to and after such events as medical investigations and surgery have frequently been studied (Johnson et al, 1970). Those who are anxious before surgery tend to be more anxious afterwards, take longer to recover and require more analgesia. This relationship has also been demonstrated in a review of surgery studies by Mathews and Ridgeway (1981). Personality factors or predispositions to anxiety, that is a 'neurotic' personality type, tend to be associated with a more lengthy recovery period and with a more uncomfortable and complicated post-operative period.

Goal Setting

The goal for 'surgical anxiety' should be to minimise or alleviate this completely. With rapid patient throughput in hospital, it is sometimes impossible to attend to patients before they become nervous, and isolating the specific cause for their anxieties usually requires a fairly lengthy conversation or interview. The primary nurse should therefore assess the patient's needs and continue to provide necessary psychological care over the pre-operative period. Nurses should also avoid assuming patients are universally anxious, by routinely including this on the care plan.

If anxiety is high, reduction to minimal anxiety before operation should be a prime goal. 'At risk' patients with high anxiety should then be the target for selective attention, while others may receive more routine preparation. Their anxiety is unlikely to be too distressing and will subside rapidly after surgery.

Much research in the field of alleviating or preventing anxiety in relation to hospitalisation and associated events has created sound knowledge providing a rationale for care for the two related diagnoses of acute anxiety.

INTERVENTIONS FOR ANXIETY RELATED TO HOSPITALISATION AND SURGERY

Information giving about hospital and aspects of care

The process of providing explanations to patients who are anxious needs to be studied carefully. Meeting their needs requires a careful assessment of what and how much they wish to know as well as whether they wish to have this in written or spoken form. Principles for imparting information have been tested by Ley (1979), Redman (1980) and many others. All agree that information has to be clearly structured, explanations must not employ technical vocabulary and important details should be given first.

Cosper (1967) and Byrne and Edeani (1983) found that several terms commonly used by staff were unfamiliar to patients. For example, 'premedication', 'incision', 'infusion', 'drain' and 'void' were not understood. Many nurses struggle to provide information (even in the classroom) without employing such terms. Practice and role play are essential to gain these skills and are shown to be effective (Tomlinson et al, 1984).

Written information must also accord to average reader ability, and illustrations or photographs are essential when explaining aspects of anatomy or equipment as Webb and Wilson-Barnett (1983) found when interviewing patients after hysterectomy.

Interaction and lack of haste are important. Patient teaching studies have shown that patients gain more understanding and benefit more from individualised material (Wilson-Barnett and Oborne, 1983). Open communication and questions from the nurse may be called for when patients have non-specific requests 'to know about the treatment or condition'. Too much information which is irrelevant to the patient will not be helpful. As with any intervention, assessing the patient's needs constantly avoids repetition or giving conflicting information. Written records of such sessions are sometimes useful to reinforce and evaluate the effects of providing information. Careful planning to achieve continuity for such care is necessary.

The mechanism by which information reduces anxiety will be discussed after reviewing studies which test the effects of different interventions.

Studies evaluating interventions to alleviate anxiety

Substantial research evidence exists from experimental studies carried out by doctors, nurses and psychologists that specific psychological interventions can alleviate anxiety. In general hospitals, for those patients undergoing various stressful procedures, there have been significant advances in research evidence which gives clear guidelines for practice. Nurses have contributed to the science of this area and have demonstrated their therapeutic abilities by acting as therapists, whose effectiveness has been assessed.

Research in the area of hospital-evoked stress commenced over three decades ago. Janis' (1958) hypothesis that the 'work of worrying' was a necessary preparation for recovery from surgery stimulated this field. He surmised that moderate anxiety helped the patient to plan for the stressful aspects of surgery and to rehearse coping strategies. Without this awareness of what would ensue, patients may deny post-operative stress and discomfort pre-operatively and feel resentful and distressed during recovery. Likewise those who were over-anxious were considered unable to think constructively and reduce their anxieties by planning for the event. Although subsequent research has demonstrated that moderate anxiety is not necessary for an optimum recovery (Johnson et al, 1978), and that there is a linear relationship between levels of pre- and post-operative anxiety, the idea that patients need to plan ahead and possibly rehearse cognitive and behaviour coping strategies lives on.

Any review of this subject cannot be comprehensive as the volume of work is so impressive. Published reviews by Auerbach and Kilmann (1977), Mumford et al (1982), Mathews and Ridgeway (1981) and Wilson-Barnett (1984) highlight the consistent advantages of certain planned interventions, while theorising on the possible mechanisms for these benefits and pointing to some of the methodological challenges in this field.

Information giving

Procedural details

Studies which aimed to prepare patients for adjustment to hospitalisation and thereby reduce anxiety associated with this event tended to use predominantly procedural information. Chronological accounts of what will occur have been provided by interview (Skipper and Leonard, 1968), by booklet (Matthews, 1982), and by film (Melamed and Siegel, 1975). Procedures of admission, routine tests, visiting time, facilities in the hospital and the role and names of staff have been included in such interventions. For children, Matthews (1982) and Melamed and Siegel (1975) demonstrated that pictorial accounts helped understanding and that playing with equipment and showing them their ward was helpful in both adjustment to hospital and subsequent post-operative recovery. Involving parents in this session was considered to be essential by these researchers. 'Transmitted' anxiety is especially important among significant others (and deserves the sub-category in the nursing diagnosis details supplied by Carpenito, 1983).

Such information is shown to augment the details in admission booklets sometimes received prior to admission. These are shown to be generally unsatisfactory providing more details on regulations than facilities (Wilson-Barnett, 1979) and despite the aim for books to be sent to all scheduled admission patients only approximately one-half actually receive one (Royal Commission on the NHS, 1979). However, Rice and Johnson (1984) have shown that specific details on recovery from surgery can be usefully included in pre-admission booklets. Patients then require less time to learn to perform exercises and seem to undertake such activities more than those who do not receive such booklets.

Stressful events associated with hospitalisation

Innovations in the area of preparation for admission to hospital include organised puppet shows, group visits for children (Fradd, 1986) and liaison nurse pre-admission home visits (Jupp and Sims, 1986). But all interventions aim to provide relevant information for patients to alleviate anxiety. Adequate study designs, interesting instruments for monitoring moods, and control groups have been used in such work, although small samples are sometimes unavoidable (Miller, 1981; Matthews, 1982). Hypotheses on why such interventions affect subsequent adjustment are not so forthcoming in this early work. It seems to be assumed that knowing more about what will occur reduces the unknown and therefore anxiety. However, associations with pleasant or funny presentations for children and particularly warm and empathic nurse intervenors (Miller, 1981) may be equally powerful. Such associations may give a 'lasting impression' of friendliness which provides more positive expectations than those possibly anticipated. Advances with children's care in the area need to be mirrored for adults. It can be more stressful waiting for a scheduled admission than being received as an emergency for relief of acute problems (Hugh-Jones et al, 1964) although emergency patients need support as Anderson et al (1965) showed. In this last study a model for continuous nursing care was evaluated, each patient being received by and constantly attended to by one special nurse. She did not provide a standard package of information as in other studies, but individualised her care, comments, information and support in accord with what she assessed to be the patient's needs. Her support was provided from emergency room admission until the patient was fully admitted to the ward.

Early work with surgical patients and those for diagnostic tests also tended to use procedural information for the alleviation of anxiety. However, this was rarely given without some additional guidance on exercises or pain control. For instance, Egbert et al (1964), and Lindeman and Stetzer (1973) provided instructions on breathing and leg exercises as well as information on anaesthetic and operative procedures. Two studies in the 1970s with surgical patients tested 'specific' or procedural information prior to surgery. Andrew (1970) did not achieve positive results on a recovery index which included emotional responses, but this study was flawed by the lack of an adequate control group and sample. De Long (1971) achieved positive benefits for specific over general information on a recovery-based index consisting of number of post-operative days until discharge, number of pain and sleep medications, number of complaints, and negative behavioural observations. Both studies attempted to assess the interaction of individual patient characteristics with response to the interventions. Those people who characteristically used and sought out information were helped by such measures, but those who usually deny or repress details or aspects of a potentially stressful episode were distressed by the experimental intervention of specific information. The contribution of these projects is perhaps the demonstration of this relationship in providing implications for careful assessment of patients prior to selecting interventions. Persistent problems exist when patients refuse to listen to details and yet seem anxious. And a small proportion choose to forgo such explanations prior to events such as surgery. For instance Ridgeway and Mathews (1982) noted that one in seven chose to be excluded from informative interventions prior to hysterectomy. There is evidence that information may make patients more anxious if they are persuaded to receive it, so for them alternative methods of coping should be considered. Only in later studies, when the effects of other types of information were compared with procedural infor-mation, was a contamination between types of message avoided. However, in the work of Wilson-Barnett (1978), information given to patients scheduled for barium X-rays could really be considered largely procedural. The information was given by interview and leaflet the night before a barium enema and explained details of bowel preparation and the screening procedure. This reduced anxiety prior to and during the test. However, this result was not achieved for those undergoing a barium meal, subjects reporting much less anxiety over this X-ray, and although a similar trend was noted, the range of scores was inadequate to demonstrate significant effects. It is important to note that such information does reduce test anxiety, as results for surgery can be equivocal for anxiety but fairly consistent for more physical or 'objective' data.

Sensory information

Major advances were made by a nurse psychologist (Johnson, 1983). She and her team employed rigorous research methods to assess the effects of providing information prior to stress, on sensations which patients are likely to experience. Work with adults undergoing gastroscopy (Johnson et al, 1973), with children having plaster of Paris casts removed (Johnson et al, 1975), and with surgical patients (Johnson et al, 1978) has shown the advantages of sensory information over procedural details. Sensory information is chronologically structured and includes details of common sensations, of what the patient will feel, see, smell and hear.

Terms are culled from patients themselves, their vocabulary reflecting both what is experienced and familiar words. Only those descriptive terms which reflect types or quality of sensations are included. Value judgements on degree of discomfort or reaction are not repeated. 'Blown-out', 'sticking', 'dull', 'pounding', 'pushing', 'darkened', 'gurgling', are examples of sensory terms. This type of information is seen to be readily accessible to patients, comprehensible and relevant to their experience. It is also considered relevant to their needs to foresee what will occur. Johnson (1983) considers this type of information provides an imaginary map which will guide the patient through the stressful time and as a traveller reaches 'landmarks' so the patient will recognise what is being done, how long it will take and when the sensation will change. The nearer the anticipated experience is to what is actually experienced the more powerful the intervention is shown to be in reducing anxiety. Many studies done by other teams also support this.

Sensory information packages have been shown to be superior to control (attention) placebo interventions by Hayward (1975) and Boore (1978) for surgical patients. These studies mirror the results of many others testing this type of information in that patients' anxiety reports, per se, were not modified, but possibly other related indicators were reduced. Hayward showed a reduction in pain medications and length of stay while Boore showed that the hydroxycorticosteroids and infection rates were reduced in the experimental group. This raises the other important benefits of such interventions, which sometimes seem not to alleviate anxiety but do often have other physical effects. A meta-analysis by Devine and Cook (1983) showed that on average one-and-a-half days' hospital stay was saved for surgical patients receiving experimental informative intervention (whether procedural or sensory).

Physical advantages probably accrue from the psychological and behavioural consequences associated with reduced stress. For instance, high cortisone levels result from continued stress. This reduces immune responses and increases the chance of infection. Cognitive impairment associated with stress and anxiety reduces concentration and thinking ability. Information and instructions may not be understood, recalled or obeyed. Associations between anxiety and pain perceptions reviewed by Hayward (1975) may also result in increased sedation from analgesics, less mobility and independence, and a longer stay in hospital. General apprehension also usually inhibits appetite and sleep which causes fatigue and reduces well-being.

Sensory information has been particularly helpful for those undergoing noxious procedures such as endoscopy and cardiac catheterisation. Johnson et al (1973) studied 99 patients scheduled for gastroscopy. They divided them into three groups and compared sensory information with procedural information, both by taped message and the use of photographs, and a control non-intervention group. Sensory information was explicit with sounds of oral suction and descriptions of sensations during tube insertion. Despite the potential for anxiety induction at the time, this group of patients was significantly less anxious than others displaying less tension behaviour and gagging, and requiring least sedation. However, procedural information was also superior in some of these respects to the control situation.

Subsequent work has confirmed these results. Finesilver (1979) in a small scale study on patients due for cardiac catheterisation and Johansen Hartfield and Cason (1981) with barium enema subjects found anxiety alleviation significantly related to sensory information.

Prior to any main study careful work on the preparation of information is essential to gain a realistic account of sensations experienced, expressed in patients' terms. All these studies tend to include some procedural details on the course of events as well as sensory information to provide a logical account of what will happen to the patient. But it is the extra component of sensory information which has been demonstrated to help physical and psychological responses to stressful events.

Advice on physical coping

Most studies that have compared a 'package' of information with usual care or control situations, have also included instructions to enhance recovery or alleviate discomfort. Surgical studies by Egbert et al (1964) discussed breathing exercises as did Lindeman (1972), Dumas and Leonard (1963), Leigh et al (1977), Hayward (1975), and Boore (1978). Although Lindeman emphasised this particularly and accounted for the success of the project in terms of increased physical capacity post-operatively as facilitated by the teaching, it is not possible to exclude totally other components of the intervention as equally potent. Certainly many accounts of such pre-operative teaching attest to the enthusiasm with which patients rehearse exercises before and adhere to regimes afterwards.

Evidence from special tests is similar. For instance Finesilver (1979) reported that muscle group exercises taught to patients for use during cardiac catheterisation were particularly well received. Stiffness and discomfort associated with this investigation were helped by these exercises. Sensory information was also provided and must have influenced satisfaction and distress ratings. Further study by Johnson's team (Fuller et al 1978) compared sensory information with physical coping advice in a four group study with women undergoing pelvic examination. However, the only positive results on physiological and psychological indicators were due to the sensory information.

Physical exercises or coping behaviours may be more appropriate for some patients, while others respond better to more cognitive forms of coping instruction. However, this sub-group analysis within samples has yet to be done conclusively. Certain procedures would also seem to be more suited to such behaviours, particularly if they are rather long and boring for the patient. Patients may well have ideas on what type of information they would prefer prior to a stressful event. Wallace (1985) set out to test this and found that 90% of her sample welcomed some type of special information. When interviewed initially most preferred procedural to other types of information such as sensory, temporal or coping. However, after exposure to different booklets most patients chose the most comprehensive containing a mixture of information types on several aspects of hospitalisation.

Relaxation

Progressive muscle group relaxation or deep breathing relaxation has also been evaluated as a technique taught to patients prior to stressful events and employed by them during the event or afterwards throughout the recovery period. For surgery this was included in a package designed and tested by Field (1974); however outcome measures relying on surgeons' ratings of patients' nervousness and speed of recovery may have been insufficiently sensitive to yield positive results. Aiken and Henricks (1971) incorporated relaxation into an intervention which also gave opportunity for patients to talk about fears. Despite small matched groups they achieved positive results from this intervention on surgical stress factors and mood ratings.

In a carefully controlled study with 70 surgical patients, Wilson (1981) achieved superior results for a relaxation only group as compared with another information intervention group. He found relaxation was associated with a reduced hospital stay, less pain and medication and increased reports of strength and energy. No accurate reporting was available on frequency of use of relaxation, but within the group it was found to benefit less-frightened patients more than those who were very frightened.

Results for the effectiveness of relaxation for surgical patients are often contradictory. For instance Pickett and Clum (1982) found no benefit, an attention redirection approach being superior in reducing post-operative anxiety. In contrast, Scott and Clum (1984) found that by dividing a surgical sample by coping style, sensitisers were found to benefit from relaxation in reports of post-operative pain whereas deniers did much better when left alone.

For tests, Fuller et al (1978) and Finesilver's (1979) work is relevant. Finesilver incorporated relaxation in the package which included sensory information, but Fuller's team found that this was not particularly appropriate for women undergoing a gynaeco- logical examination. Cardiac catheterisation was also studied by Rice et al (1986) to assess effects of relaxation, but no significant results were produced.

There is really insufficient evidence to assess when and what type of relaxation, for whom, is indicated. One factor which pertains to the lack of many positive leaders is the learning or practice times needed to achieve skills in relaxation. Although this is not complex, rehearsal is certainly indicated prior to application during and after stress. Further work needs to be done with relaxation in the general hospital setting. For instance, children have been taught relaxation strategies in a classroom study (Lamon- tagne et al, 1985) and this may well have relevance to clinical practice. It is well to remember that the use of relaxation has been widely tested on other anxiety related situations and conditions and found to be very useful (see Snyder, 1985, p. 61).

Cognitive coping strategies

Although there are only a few studies which have employed specifically taught coping strategies, the results seem to be very encouraging for patients undergoing the stress of surgery and major investigations. Positive reappraisal has had significant results in two surgical studies. Langer et al (1975) compared three groups of 20 randomly selected and stratified patients for major surgery. Coping devices were taught to the first group and this was compared with preparatory information and no attention control patients. Coping devices were taught by a psychologist and this involved practice of positive appraisal, a somewhat complex and unusual technique. The intervener would explore worries and threatening aspects of surgery and then encourage the patient to identify the positive aspects of each concern. For example, post-operative pain can be alleviated and it does not last long. This approach was found to be superior in reducing physical and psychological distress to information intervention although both interventions were significantly better on several parameters than the control situation.

In a similar study with hysterectomy patients, Ridgeway and Mathews (1982) endorsed the findings of Langer et al (1975). Patients who employed positive reappraisal were superior on hospital measures of recovery and were more self-caring three weeks after surgery, when at home. Booklets were used for intervention and should be seen as a valuable resource for further practice. This demonstrated that positive reappraisal can be used by patients without extensive specialist instructions.

Positive results using this technique with patients undergoing cardiac catheterisation were also provided in a study by Kendall et al (1979). Cognitive strategies for patients to repeat statements to themselves during the test were encouraged. Such statements aimed to minimise the threat of the procedure and enhance feelings of control throughout. Persuasive evidence from these few studies shows that this improved co-operation and reduction of perceived stress demonstrates the applicability of such techniques in many settings. However, further research is needed, in particular by nurses who might introduce this strategy.

Applications in practice

Summary guidelines for practice are provided below using elements of interventions which have been shown to be beneficial for patients prior to stressful hospital events or surgery.

1. Sessions should be interactive but provide a chronological account of the procedure and its efforts.
2. Major queries or concerns should be explored initially.
3. All information should be given in everyday language.
4. Sessions should not be longer than 20 minutes.
5. Patients should be encouraged to ask questions and write things down if they wish.
6. A written account can be used to guide the session and left with the patient for future reference.
7. Information which relates the patient's experience and sensations is most important.
8. Advice on physical coping is particularly useful if the patient is conscious during a procedure.
9. The patient should be constantly assessed for signs of fatigue or fear.
10. If information does not appear to be relevant or acceptable to the patient a different approach should be tried, i.e. exercises or relaxation.

It may be most sensible in the clinical setting to maximise the possible benefits of different interventions by using a combined approach. This is obviously only indicated where patients accept it readily or when they are in a condition to understand and use information.

If patients are reluctant or unable to identify their particular worries initially a conversation providing them with an account of the procedure may facilitate more focused discussion on the topics as raised. As long as the member of staff is sensitive to the reactions and needs of the patient this should incorporate the benefits of a comprehensive description and an exploration of specific worries. If positive reappraisal can be employed for these worries this can be an additional strength.

Advice can be interspersed with demonstration and discussion of diagrams or pictures, to avoid loss of concentration. If the patient appears to respond positively to one type of presentation this can then be exploited fully throughout the session.

If the explanation seems to require longer than 20 minutes a short break is indicated. On the other hand when a patient is quiet and passive a return visit could be required as they may need time to think through what has been said before asking questions or expressing their views and feelings.

A summary of this more combined approach, particularly relevant to patients under-going surgery, would require five more preliminary steps before using those previously listed.

1. Discuss with the patient how he or she feels about surgery.
2. Identify specific worries.
3. Explore these worries and their perceived cause.
4. Provide realistic information about these aspects of surgery.
5. Encourage one or more positive statements on each topic.

PHOBIC ANXIETY (see Table 3, section 3)

When anxiety is excessive in degree or duration or without obvious cause, the term morbid anxiety is used. In some patients this may be only one aspect of a more serious disease such as schizophrenia or depression, in which case the disease is treated rather than the anxiety (Marks, 1975). However, when anxiety is very acute and focused on a specific object it may be termed fear or a phobia, and various forms of behaviour therapy are indicated.

The origin of a phobic anxiety may have arisen from a particularly uncomfortable experience related to the specific object or situation or may be reflective of deep-seated unresolved concerns or trauma. Exploration of the roots of phobic reaction often demonstrates that it arose after a difficult life experience. Snakes, lifts, mice, spiders, aeroplanes, open spaces or crowds may each be the focus of a phobic reaction. This may well be one of a number of other neurotic problems for which a range of treatments is needed. However, some people suffer acute phobic reactions in the face of a particular object yet report a busy and fulfilled existence. It is appropriate to describe phobic reactions here because of the irrationality and disproportionate nature of the emotional response, in common with other anxiety responses.

When exposed to the phobic object, an acute fear, terror or panic reaction is suffered. The complete range of physical, behavioural and psychological symptoms becomes manifest. Increased sympathetic activity results in a raised pulse, blood pressure and respiration rate. Rigidity and tremors may be seen and the patient reports feelings of terror. These acute levels of disturbance subside if exposure is prolonged.

Goals

It is essential when setting goals that clients are totally involved in agreeing to the plan of treatment and the intensity of the programme. Time and goals for curing a phobic reaction are set according to the time schedule for therapy, more intense schedules taking a shorter overall time to be effective. Severity of reaction, motivation of the subject and availability of the therapies all affect cure rates. Several sessions of treatment are usually necessary and adherence to homework tasks also determines the success. It may be that two intense sessions will cure an aeroplane phobic, while several short treatment sessions are necessary for an older person who is phobic of crossing a foot bridge.

Rationale for nursing intervention

Behaviour therapy is particularly successful for mono-phobias (which are relatively rare), whereas chronic neurotic or generalised morbid anxiety states may require additional cognitive and/or other psychotherapies. There is little doubt that behaviour therapy (or exposure therapy) effects substantially positive results. As there are many texts on devising programmes for different approaches to therapy, details will not be provided here.

Gray's (1982) scholarly treatise on the neuropsychology of anxiety reviews the advantages and possible mechanism for effects of behaviour therapy, discussing the apparently contradictory uses of progressive desensitisation with associated relaxation and implosion or flooding therapy. He concludes that it is the total length of time for exposure to phobic objects (even when imagined) that is really therapeutically significant rather than the staging of such exposure.

Results evaluating such treatments and therapists are generally very positive. Nurses tend to be as successful if not better in caring for such patients than others and treatment may occur in the patient's home, in outpatient clinics or at the family doctor's clinic. Nurses may treat patients individually for special phobias or in groups for other treatments such as cognitive management of anxiety (Jupp and Dudley, 1984).

Careful monitoring of specialist nurses' work has been carried out in descriptive studies by Roach and Farley (1986), which show how they can work independently with patients referred from several doctors. Evaluative studies also show that community psychiatric nurses can provide more comprehensive follow-up care for those who would be treated traditionally as psychiatric outpatients (Paykel and Griffith, 1983). In this study eight nurses cared for a group of 50 patients, classified as neurotically ill, for 18 months. The patients represented one-half of an initial sample of 99, the other half being assigned to psychiatrists for outpatient care as the control group. There were no differences among the two groups in moods or symptoms over the follow-up period but consumer satisfaction was significantly higher among those cared for by nurses, particularly with regard to easy communications and the therapeutic relationship.

Marks's (1985) study with nurse behaviour therapists also demonstrates the great potential advantages for some patient groups in being cared for by a specialist nurse. When compared with services supplied for general practitioners' patients, patients randomly assigned to the nurse therapist had benefited greatly. Controls showed few gains. There was also high agreement on diagnosis and treatment plans between the nurse and psychologist and patients appreciated being treated at home, and the cost benefits of this service were high. In addition it was pointed out that community based therapists can pick up referrals much more quickly, perhaps preventing a more grave condition.

Interventions by specialists are often gradually eventually learned by other non-specialists. Some of these advanced psychological caring skills may well be appropriate for general nurses caring for generally ill patients, whether anxious or depressed or just troubled.

FUTURE RESEARCH

Evaluative studies have produced such encouraging results in this area of psychological care so central to nursing, that more should be encouraged. Promoting more nursing skills in this area and recording changes in clients' responses could be fruitful. Allowing for continuous relationships, as with primary nursing, may permit more research on effectiveness of nurse support in the hospital setting. Team research with nurses and psychologists has produced new evidence (e.g. Johnson's work). Perhaps this could be useful in less exploited areas such as day hospitals for the elderly. There is certainly no shortage of studies on which to build, or areas that would benefit from further research. Specific suggestions would include studies such as:

1. More controlled studies to evaluate the effect of patients' chosen type of coping intervention on anxiety levels during a stressful procedure.
2. Field trials where hospital nurses are trained in specific coping teaching skills and their interventions are evaluated with many patients.
3. More studies incorporating relaxation techniques for patients to employ throughout their stay in hospital, comparing psychological and physical indicators with others who do not use this technique.
4. An analysis of patient admission booklets and a redesign of these after systematic study with those who have been hospitalised on the type of information patients require.
5. Evaluation of the primary nurse in alleviating psychological stress in hospital.
6. Evaluation of intensive counselling skill courses for groups of nurses to assess the subsequent and long-term effects on their psychosocial care with patients.

REFERENCES

Aiken LH, Henrichs TF (1971) Systematic relaxation as a nursing intervention technique with open heart surgery patients. *Nursing Research* 20, 212–217.

Aitken Swan J, Paterson R (1955) The cancer patients' delay in seeking advice. *British Medical Journal* 1, 623.

Aitken RCB, Zealley AK (1970) Measurement of moods. *British Journal of Hospital Medicine* 8, 215–224.

Anderson BJ, Martz H, Leonard RC (1965) Two experimental tests of a patient-centred admission process. *Nursing Research* 14(2), 151–157.

Anderson M, Mottram K (1973) Its our problem too! *International Journal of Nursing Studies* 10, 81–85.

Andrew J (1970) Recovery from surgery, with and without preparatory instruction for three coping styles. *Journal of Personality and Social Psychology* 15, 223–226.

Auerbach SM, Kilmann PR (1977) Crisis intervention: a review of outcome research. *Psychological Bulletin* 84(6), 1189–1217.

Bartrop RW, Lazarus L, Luckhurst E, Kiloh LG, Penny R (1977) Depressed lymphocyte function after bereavement. *Lancet* i, 834–836.

Boore J (1978) *Information a Prescription for Recovery*. Royal College of Nursing, London.

Breggin PB (1964) The psychophysiology of anxiety with a review of the literature concerning adrenaline. *Journal of Nervous and Mental Diseases* 139, 558–568.

Byrne TJ, Edeani D (1983) Knowledge of medical terminology among hospital patients. *Nursing Research* 33(3), 178–181.

Carnevali DL (1966) Pre-operative anxiety. *American Journal of Nursing* 7, 1536–1538.

Carpenito LJ (1983) *Nursing Diagnosis: Application to Clinical Practice*. JB Lippincott Co, Philadelphia.

Cattell RB (1954) *Sixteen Personality Factors*. National Foundation for Educational Research, Bucks, England, and Institute for Personality and Ability Testing, Illinois, USA.

Cosper B (1967) How well do patients understand hospital jargon? *American Journal of Nursing* **Dec**, 1932–1934.

De Long RD (1971) Individual differences in patterns of anxiety arousal, stress relevant information and recovery from surgery. PhD dissertation, University of California, LA *Dissertation Abstracts International* **32**, 554B.

Devine EC, Cook TD (1983) A meta-analytic analysis of effects of psycho-educational interventions on length of post-surgical hospital stay. *Nursing Research* **32**(5), 267–274.

Dumas RG, Leonard RC (1963) The effect of nursing on the incidence of post-operative vomiting. *Nursing Research* **12**, 12–15.

Egbert LD, Battit GE, Welch CE, Bartlett MK (1964) Reduction of post-operative pain by encouragement and instruction of patients: a study of doctor patient rapport. *New England Journal of Medicine* **270**, 822–827.

Engstrom B (1984) The patients' need for information during hospital stay. *International Journal of Nursing Studies* **21**(2), 113–130.

Field D (1974) Effects of tape recorded hypnotic preparation for surgery. *International Journal of Clinical and Experimental Hypnosis* **22**, 54–61.

Finesilver C (1979) Preparation of adult patients for cardiac catheterisation and coronary cineangiography. *International Journal of Nursing* **16**, 211–221.

Franklin BL (1974) *Patient Anxiety on Admission to Hospital*. RCN Study of Nursing Care Project, Royal College of Nursing, London.

Fradd E (1986) Learning about hospital. *Nursing Times* **83**(3), 28–30.

Freud A (1936) *The Ego and Mechanisms of Defence*. International University Press, New York.

Fuller SS, Endress MP, Johnson JE (1978) The effects of cognitive and behavioural control with an aversive health examination. *Journal of Human Stress* **4**, 18–25.

Gelder MG, Marks IM (1966) Severe agoraphobia: a controlled prospective therapeutic trial. *British Journal of Psychiatry* **112**, 309–319.

Gray JA (1982) *The Neuropsychology of Anxiety: An Enquiry into the Functions of the Septohippocampal System*. Clarendon Press, Oxford; Oxford University Press, New York.

Hamilton M (1969) Diagnosis and rating of anxiety. In: Lader M (ed) *Studies in Anxiety*. 76–79. Headly Brothers Ltd, Ashford, Kent.

Hawkins C (1979) Patients reactions to their investigations: A study of 504 patients. *British Medical Journal* **2**, 638–640.

Hayward JC (1975) *Information – A Prescription Against Pain*. RCN Study of Nursing Care Series, Royal College of Nursing, London.

Hoch PH, Zubin H (1950) *Anxiety*. Grune and Stratton Inc, New York.

Hockey L (1978) *Women in Nursing: A Descriptive Study*. Hodder and Stoughton, London.

Hughes J (1981) *An Outline of Modern Psychiatry*. John Wiley & Sons, Chichester.

Hugh-Jones P, Tanser AR, Whitby C (1964) Patients' view of admission to a London Teaching Hospital. *British Medical Journal* **2**, 660–664.

Izard C (1972) *Patterns of Emotions*. Academic Press, New York and London.

Janis IL (1958) *Psychological Stress*. John Wiley & Sons, New York.

Johansen Hartfield M, Cason CL (1981) Effects of information on emotional responses during barium enema. *Nursing Research* **30**(3), 151–155.

Johnson JE (1983) Preparing patients to cope with stress. In: Wilson-Barnett J (ed) *Patient Teaching*. Vol 6. Recent Advances in Nursing Series. Churchill Livingstone, Edinburgh.

Johnson JE, Dabbs JM, Leventhal H (1970) Psychosocial factors in the welfare of surgical patients. *Nursing Research* **19**(1), 18–29.

Johnson JE, Kirchhoff KT, Endress MP (1975) Altering children's distress behaviour during orthopaedic cast removal. *Nursing Research* **24**, 404–410.

Johnson JE, Morrissey JF, Leventhal H (1973) Psychological preparation for an endoscopic examination. *Gastrointestinal Endoscopy* **19**, 180–182.

Johnson JE, Rice VH, Fuller SS, Endress MP (1978) Sensory information, instruction in coping strategy and recovery from surgery. *Research in Nursing and Health* **1**, 4–17.

Johnston M (1980) Anxiety in surgical patients. *Psychological Medicine* **10**, 145–152.

Johnston M (1982) Recognition of patients' worries by nurses and by other patients. *British Journal of Clinical Psychology* **21**, 255–261.

Jones E (1955) *Sigmund Freud: Life and Work*. Vols 1 and 2. Hogarth Press, London.

Jupp H, Dudley M (1984) Group cognitive/anxiety management. *Journal of Advanced Nursing* **9**, 573–580.

Jupp M, Sims S (1986) Going home. *Nursing Times* **82**(40), 40–42.

Kendall PC, Williams L, Pechacek TF, Gramm LE, Shisslak C, Herzoff N (1979) Cognitive-behavioural and patient educational interventions in cardiac catheterisation procedures: The Palo Alto Medical Psychology Project. *Journal of Consulting and Clinical Psychology* **47**, 49–58.

Lader M, Marks I (1971) *Clinical Anxiety*. William Heinemann Medical Books Ltd, London.

Lader M., (1975) Discussion In: L Levi (ed) *Emotions, their Parameters and Measurement*. pp. 341–367. Raven Press, New York.

Lamontagne LL, Mason KR, Hepworth JT (1985) Effects of relaxation on anxiety in children: implications for coping with stress. *Nursing Research* **34**, 289–292.

Langer EJ, Janis IL, Wolfer JA (1975) Reduction of psychological stress in surgical patients. *Journal of Experimental Social Psychology* **11**, 155–165.

Lazarus RS, Averill JR (1972) Emotion and cognition. In: Spielberger CD (ed) *Anxiety: Current Trends in Theory and Research*, Vol. 1, Academic Press, New York.

Leigh JM, Walker J, Janaganathan P (1977) Effect of pre-operative anaesthetic visit on anxiety. *British Medical Journal* **2**, 987–989.

Ley P (1979) Improving communications: effects of altering doctor behaviour. In: Oborne DJ, Gruneberg MM, Eiser JR (eds) *Research in Psychology and Medicine*. pp. 221–229. Academic Press, London.

Lindeman CA (1972) Nursing intervention with the pre-surgical patient. *Nursing Research* **21**, 196–209.

Lindeman CA, Stetzer SL (1973) Effects of pre-operative visits by operating room nurses. *Nursing Research* **22**, 4–16.

Lipowski ZJ (1975) Physical illness, the patient and his environment: psychosocial foundations of medicine. *American Handbook of Psychiatry* **4**, 1–42.

Lynn R (1971) *National Differences in Anxiety*. The Economic and Social Research Institute, February Report, London, pp. 25–56.

Macleod Clark J (1983) Nurse–patient communication—an analysis of conversations from surgical wards. In: Wilson-Barnett J (ed) *Nursing Research: Ten Studies in Patient Care*. John Wiley & Sons, Chichester.

Marks I (1975) Modern trends in the management of morbid anxiety: coping, stress immunisation, and extinction. In: Spielberger C, Sarason IG (eds) *Stress and Anxiety*. Hemisphere Publishing Co, New York.

Marks I, (1985) *Psychiatric Nurse Therapists in Primary Care*. RCN Research Series, Royal College of Nursing, London.

Mathews A, Ridgeway V (1981) Personality and surgical recovery: a review. *British Journal of Clinical Psychology* **20**, 243–260.

Matthews A (1982) *A Study to Assess the Effectiveness of a Purpose-designed Booklet in Reducing Anxiety in Children Admitted to a Paediatric Ward for Elective Surgery*. Unpublished BSc Dissertation (Nursing). King's College, London University, London.

May R (1950) *The Meaning of Anxiety*. Roland Press, New York.

Melamed BG, Siegel LJ (1975) Reduction of anxiety in children facing hospitalisation and surgery by use of film modelling. *Journal of Counsulting and Clinical Psychology* **43**, 511–521.

Miller B (1981) *Coming into Hospital*. Unpublished BSc Dissertation (Nursing). King's College, London University, London.

Moffic HS, Paykel ES (1975) Depression in medical in-patients. *British Journal of Psychiatry* **126**, 346–353.

Muhlenkamp AF, Joyner JA (1986) Arthritis patients' self-reported affective states and their care givers' perceptions. *Nursing Research* **35**, 24–27.

Mumford E, Schlesinger HJ, Glass GV (1982) The effects of psychological intervention on recovery from surgery and heart attacks: an analysis of the literature. *American Journal of Public Health* **72**, 141–151.

Narrow B (1979) *Patient Teaching: nursing practice*. John Wiley & Sons, New York.

Olmsted RW, Kennedy DA (1975) In: Millon T (ed) *Medical Behavioural Science*. pp. 200–206. WB Saunders, London.

Openshaw S (1984) *Clinical Judgements by Nurses: Decision Strategies and Nurses' Appraisal of Patient Affect*. Unpublished PhD Thesis, King's College, University of London, London.

Paykel ES, Griffith JH (1983) *Community Psychiatric Nursing for Neurotic Patients*. RCN research Series, Royal College of Nursing, London.

Pickett C, Clum G (1982) omparative treatment strategies and their interactio ith locus of control in the redction of post-surgical pain and anxiety. *Journal of Consulting and Clinical Psychology* 50(3), 439–441.

Ray C, Fitzgibbon G (1982) Stress arousal and coping wih surgery. *Psychological Medicine*, 11, 741–746.

Redman BK (1980) *The Process of Patient Teaching in Nursing*. 4th edition. CV Mosby Co, St Louis.

Reynolds M (1978) No news is bad news: patients' views about communication in hospital. *British Medical Journal* 1, 1673–1676.

Rice VH, Caldwell M, Butler S, Robinson J (1986) Relaxation training and response to cardiac catheterisation: a pilot study. *Nursing Research* 35(1), 39–43.

Rice VH, Johnson JE (1984) Pre-admission self-instruction booklets, post-admission exercise performance and teaching time. *Nursing Research* 33(3), 147–151.

Ridgeway V, Mathews A (1982) Psychological preparation for surgery: a comparison of methods. *British Journal of Clinical Psychology* 21, 271–280.

Roach F, Farley N (1986) The behavioural management of neurosis by the psychiatric nurse therapist. In: Brooking JI (ed) *Psychiatric Nursing Research*. pp. 195–211. John Wiley & Sons, Chichester.

Robinson L (1972) *Psychological Aspects of the Care of Hospitalised Patients*. 3rd edition, Davis, Philadelphia.

Royal Commission on the National Health Service (1979) *Report No. 5*. HMSO, London.

Rycroft C (1968) *Anxiety and Neurosis*. Pelican, London.

Scott LE, Clum GA (1984) Examining the interaction effects of coping style and brief interventions in the treatment of post-surgical pain. *Pain* 20, 279–291.

Seers K (1987) *Pain, Anxiety and Recovery in Patients Undergoing Surgery*. PhD Thesis. King's College, University of London, London.

Skipper JK, Leonard RC (1968) Children, stress and hospitalisation: a field experiment. *Journal of Health and Social Behaviour* 4, 275–287.

Snyder M (1985) *Independent Nursing Intervention*. John Wiley & Sons, New York.

Spielberger CD (1972 (ed) *Anxiety, Current Trends in Theory and Research*. Vol 1. Academic Press, London.

Spielberger CD, Gorsuch RL, Lushene R, Vagg PR, Jacobs GA (1983) *Manual for the State-Trait Anxiety Inventory (Form Y) 'Self-Evaluation Questionnaire'*. Consulting Psychologists Press, California.

Syred MEJ (1981) The abdication of the role of health education by hospital nurses. *Journal of Advanced Nursing* 6, 27–33.

Tomlinson A, Macleod Clark J, Faulkner A (1984) The use of role play in nurse education. *Nursing Times* 80(38), 48–51 and 80(39), 45–47.

Wallace L (1985) Surgical patients' preferences for pre-operative information. *Patient Education and Counselling* 7, 377–387.

Webb C, Wilson-Barnett J (1983) Self-concept, social support and hysterectomy. *International Journal of Nursing Studies* 20(2), 97–107.

Wilson JF (1981) Behavioural preparation for surgery: benefit or harm? *Journal of Behavioural Medicine* 4(1), 79–102.

Wilson-Barnett J (1976) Patients' emotional reaction to hospitalisation: an exploratory study. *Journal of Advanced Nursing* 1, 351–358.

Wilson-Barnett J (1978) Patients' emotional responses to barium x-rays. *Journal of Advanced Nursing* 3(1), 37–46.

Wilson-Barnett J (1979) *Stress in Hospital: Patients' Psychological Reactions to Hospitalisation*. Churchill Livingstone, Edinburgh.

Wilson-Barnett J (1984) Alleviating stress for hospitalised patients. *International Review of Applied Psychology* 33, 493–503.

Wilson-Barnett J, Carrigy A (1978) Factors affecting patients' responses to hospitalisation. *Journal of Advanced Nursing* 3(3), 221–228.

Wilson-Barnett J, Oborne J (1983) Studies evaluating patient teaching: implications for practice. *International Journal of Nursing Studies* **20**(1), 33–44.

Wilson-Barnett J (1985) *Key Functions in Nursing*. The Winifred Raphael Lecture. Royal College of Nursing, London.

Wilson-Barnett J, Trimble M (1984) Abnormal illness behaviour: the nursing contribution. *International Journal of Nursing Studies* **21**(4), 267–278.

Yerkes RM, Dodson JD (1908) The relation of strength of stimulus to rapidity of habit formation. *Journal of Comparative Neurology and Psychology* **18**, 459–482.

Chapter 4
Depression

As for any complex phenomenon there are several definitions for, and meanings ascribed to, depression. However, there is agreement on the widespread incidence of depression in Western populations; much is mild and not recognised as an illness but even quite severe depression goes untreated in various groups (Brown, 1976). This is also recognised as a more enduring and potentially dangerous emotional state than anxiety. Viewed on a continuum (ignoring the argument about endogenous and reactive depression) which extends from normal feelings of sadness and loss to serious psychiatric disorders of melancholia, nurses are in a position to recognise signs of depression and may be able to alleviate a deepening mood by providing general psychological support.

DEFINITION

Definitions of depression point to this emotion as one of deep unhappiness with a sense of self-worthlessness and hopelessness, associated with a lack of meaning or positive value to life and the world (Brown, 1975). Mood and physical (vegetative) functions tend to be depressed, while activities and performance also are usually reduced.

Depression may only be one dimension in a complex of negative moods experienced at any one time. Differentiating anxiety and depression and deciding which is most dominant in some distressed states is, therefore, quite difficult. Although a person may be primarily anxious they may also behave aggressively and report feelings of depression. Izard (1972) found many similar statements were used to describe anxiety and depression and a severe level of neurotic illness may be manifested in both anxious and depressed behaviours (Marks, 1975). Predisposition to experience negative emotions or neuroticism may also be associated with habituation and a propensity to react in a depressed way rather than with anxiety (or vice versa) when the other emotion could be predicted.

The overlap between anxiety and depression in component feelings and in clinical manifestations has been recognised for some time. The unitary school prefer to group them as 'affective states' without distinguishing the separate emotions (see Becker, 1974, p. 24). Both emotions are described as anhedonic, associated with unpleasant events or stress, and may be triggered by failure and related to threats to the self-esteem. Becker also says:

'many clinicians conjecture that anxiety reflects a mobilisation to cope with threat whereas depression reflects a passive despair, a sense of futile inevitability about an adverse outcome. The cognitive appraisal will therefore determine the kind of threat.'

Both Becker, and Brown (1976) follow the 'social' approach which sees depression in terms of threat of such things as power, status, roles and identity. Depression is therefore a multifactorial phenomenon precipitated by problems of coping with loss and adaptation to various life events.

As with anxiety a debate has occurred over whether or not there is a qualitative difference between feelings of sadness and feelings of depression in the psychiatric illnesses. Zung (1973) and Beck (1967) maintain that there is no qualitative difference between these two situations. Zung (1973, p. 330) explains,

'Depression as an affect or feeling tone is a ubiquitous and universal condition which as a human experience extends as a continuum from normal mood swings to a pathological state. Thus depression as a word can be used to describe:

1. an affect which is a subjective feeling tone of short duration;
2. a mood which is a state sustained over a long period of time;
3. an emotion which is comprised of the feeling tones along with objective indications; or
4. a disorder which has characteristic symptom clusters, complexes or configurations.'

This continuum or exaggeration of the same feelings was accepted by Beck (1967) who claimed that 'normals' and depressed subjects had significantly different scores on his inventory. The items were applicable to both groups but depressed patients scored more highly. In contrast, Akiskal and McKinney (1975) have differentiated these emotional experiences by renaming the most severe depression as 'melancholia', an old and established term.

Kendell (1976) has reviewed the main research theories of psychiatric depressive disorders, which are generally beyond the scope of this book. One central controversy about the classification and possible aetiology of the emotion divides depressive illness into two categories, the endogenous and reactive types. Endogenous depression is thus explained by a combination of genetic and biochemical factors, whereas reactive depression is initiated or provoked by undesirable or stressful events and the depression is 'reactive' to environmental circumstances. Doubt has been expressed about the dichotomy by such researchers as Kendell (1976) and Lader (1976). After reviewing research on depressed patients the latter concludes that there is little empirical evidence for the division into two as the symptoms and aetiology are often very mixed. Research has shown a relationship between 'life events' and depression (Brown, 1972; Paykel et al, 1969), especially significant 'exit' events associated with the loss or absence of a loved one.

Separation from a 'significant other' is one factor said to lead to both anxiety and depression. Bowlby's (1973) concept of 'separation anxiety' and Kendell's (1976) recent review of depression resulting from loss or separation confirms that this sort of life event is probably significantly related to negative emotions. These ideas are akin to those of Freud (1917) in *Mourning and Melancholia* and of Klein (1948). They emphasise loss of a love object and Freud viewed depression as aggressive instincts turned inwards or dammed up aggression in response to this loss. Behaviourists see this loss in terms of reduced reinforcement for actions. For instance, Liberman (1976) and Lazarus (1968) see depression based on an altered style of cognition characterised by negative expectations. A person experiences insuperable obstacles to need fulfilment and consequently feels helpless. It follows from a reduction in positive reinforcers which weaken the behavioural repertoire.

Kendell concludes that most research in this area shows that the:

> 'majority of depressive illnesses are preceded by stressful events of one sort or another and that truly endogenous illnesses are therefore quite rare; that there is little relationship between the type or severity of the preceding stresses and the symptomatology of the illness itself, and that the aetiological role of stressful environmental changes is always one of degree rather than a simple question of presence or absence.' (p. 18)

Akiskal and McKinney (1975) also summarised the interaction effects of events and illness as:

1. The association between stress and primary depressive illness is coincidental. Stress may precipitate hospitalisation, rather than the depressive episode.
2. Primary depressive illness produces stress. Individuals predisposed to affective illness display abnormal reactivity to everyday stresses, so the precipitating stressful events actually mark the beginning of the illness. Depression said to be induced by failure of some kind, may in fact have been the reason for the failure.
3. Stress does play a role in precipitating illness, particularly in those individuals who are genetically or developmentally predisposed to such illness.

PREVALENCE

Assessment of depression, cut-off points above which normal becomes seen as abnormal or treatable depression differ, and therefore results of prevalence studies are somewhat inconsistent. The prevalence of depressive illness in the population is approximated at 4%. Life-time expectancy for being admitted to hospital for depressive symptoms is about 2% for men and 4% for women (Hughes, 1981).

More evidence of the vulnerability of women to become depressed now exists (Hirschfield, 1980). Two-thirds of those who suffer are women and sociological studies provide particularly telling data. Brown and Harris's (1978) publication revealed the extent of the problem for women in urban populations. Vulnerability factors of lower socio-economic grouping, three or more children under 14, lack of a close and confiding partner and loss of mother before the age of 11 were shown to be critical. It is stated that loss events will not precipitate depressed reactions without presence of at least one of these factors. Although there is still debate on the role of life events as causal in illness, Brown (1972) suggests that for vulnerable people events can in fact determine when depression occurs. His complex model calculating time lag from his sociological data is very convincing.

A high incidence (approximately one in four cases) of serious emotional disturbance in general wards has been found (Moffic and Paykel, 1975) and poor recognition of psychological morbidity among patients by doctors and nurses resulted in inadequate care for a high proportion of these patients. Diagnosing depression in many situations is undeniably important as part of the nurse's role, but skills necessary for exploration of feelings and providing support for those who are anxious or depressed must be carefully learned.

ASSESSMENT OF DEPRESSION (see Table 1)

As for anxiety it is essential to use conversations and observations when assessing a person's mood. Open questions and those which explore how an individual is feeling 'in themselves' usually succeed in obtaining clues to a depressed mood. However, because of the evidence suggesting that nurses and doctors in general care settings sometimes miss the signs of depression, this should be done with care for all those who might be at risk.

Table 1. Criteria and Methods of Assessment of Depression

Physical criteria	Methods
Weight	Daily weight recorded
Elimination	Record
Skin condition	Observe for signs of anaemia or malnutrition
Behavioural	
Inactivity, withdrawn, crying	Observe carefully
Sleep disturbance—early morning waking	Observe carefully
Anorexia	Record how much is eaten
Subjective	
Statements of worthlessness	Open questioning
Frequently self-blaming	Complete Beck inventory initially, and
Chooses negative descriptors of mood	mood adjectives check-list regularly

In conversation an individual may use descriptions of themselves as 'worthless', 'no good', 'tired', 'discouraged', 'blue', or 'guilty'. They tend to exhibit an unexpressive way of talking, using only a few words, apparently lacking the energy for more. Conversation tends to be inward directed and egocentric and frequently interrupted by weeping. Initially, mention of 'ending it all' should be taken very seriously and this in itself should merit psychiatric help.

Behaviour alters, tending to be withdrawn, quiet and unresponsive. They may be in bed during the day time, classically feeling much worse in the morning, unable to face the day. Often they neglect personal hygiene, usual routines and social responsibilities.

Activities such as eating and sleeping become disturbed for those who are depressed. They lose all interest in food, tending to exhibit weight loss and constipation. Sleep patterns are also disturbed. Early morning waking is usual and difficulty in getting off to sleep is frequently reported. This then leads to feelings of tiredness and sometimes weakness. Failure to eat regularly can lead to anaemia and generalised malnutrition.

Research studies have demonstrated that careful assessment of moods such as depression can be undertaken with a population who are not necessarily psychologically upset. For instance Wilson-Barnett and Carrigy (1978) used a mood adjectives check-list (see Table 2) of 24 adjectives describing moods on five dimensions of anxiety, depression, fatigue, hospitality and vigour. Patients in a general medical ward completed the form each day to describe the way they felt. Each word had to be checked, patients indicating whether they 'did not feel like this', 'a little', 'moderately', or 'extremely'. This took between 2 and 5 minutes each day and even less time to score. Out of 202 patients only one refused. It was, therefore, acceptable, many admitting that they found the exercise relevant.

Table 2. The Mood Adjectives Check-list (MACL)

| Name .... |
| Below are a number of words which describe moods. Please put a cross to indicate how much you have felt the way described today. |

	Not at all	A little	Quite a bit	Extremely
Shaky				
Sluggish				
Resentful				
Nervous				
Weary				
Vigorous				
Hopeless				
Lively				
Guilty				
Tired				
Unhappy				
Tense				
Full of pep				
Active				
Worthless				
Miserable				
Worn out				
Discouraged				
Spiteful				
Depressed				
On edge				
Angry				
Furious				
Helpless				

When it seems appropriate to assess patients' moods, either once, or to monitor them over time, this check-list is suitable. Because of the choice of adjectives it seems relevant to a wide range of subjects detecting the mixed nature of moods on several dimensions and it is particularly valid for individual comparisons over time.

When assessing a person who is depressed for the severity or depth of mood a more comprehensive instrument has been well tried and tested. Beck's (1969) inventory is a lengthy self-report test which asks for reports of subjective, behavioural and physical signs of depression. Low scores may indicate some 'normal' levels of unhappiness but above a certain cut-off point, depression is estimated to reach the level of a psychiatric illness. Webb and Wilson-Barnett (1983) used this instrument to assess for depressed mood amongst women after hysterectomy. For the majority of patients this was seen as an acceptable part of the research data collection procedure. However, a small number found it somewhat irrelevant and almost suggestive that they were expected to be distressed. In most situations where depression is suspected and because of its previous wide use it can be employed as an assessment tool providing reliable evidence of morbidity.

Any comprehensive assessment should include a series of interviews, preferably by the same member of staff. Continuity within such a relationship is essential to elicit an accurate picture of how the patient is feeling and to what they attribute their depressed state.

CAUSES OF DEPRESSION (see Table 3)

Causes of depression are less easily identified than for anxiety, onset may be gradual and even those events which are thought to be precipitative could have occurred many years ago. Loss is generally associated with depressive reactions but the severity of these reactions and the factors which predispose to a major illness are not totally understood. In hospital, those with certain disorders may suffer more from depressed moods through loneliness, loss of health or attractiveness and enforced inactivity.

DEPRESSION RELATED TO PHYSICAL ILLNESS (see Table 3, section 1)

If physical illness is likely to be resolved, it follows that depression also lifts. However, prolonged depression may retard physical recovery and should, therefore, be attended to. Those most vulnerable to a depressive reaction are those who are predisposed to neurotic illness, those with viral, neoplastic, cardiovascular or other life-threatening disorder (Moffic and Paykel, 1975); Wilson-Barnett and Carrigy, 1978). Both the condition and its treatment may be associated as the cause of depression. Medication and surgery may increase or cause depression.

It is particularly easy to miss this problem in the context of physical illness. Signs of slowed activity, poor appetite, weight loss, constipation and disturbed sleep may all be attributed to a generally poor state of health. Maguire (1985) has also shown that cues to psychological distress are often not recognised in the context of physical care.

Patients in this setting may exhibit a mixture of emotions: anxiety about their health and its impact on others, and depressed about their loss of ability, their suffering, and their spoiled self-image. Particular reasons for their depression should be elucidated and regular monitoring of moods should indicate whether psychiatric treatment is indicated or whether general adjustment and acceptance of the future means that depression has resolved.

Table 3. Depression—Identification of Problem and Cause

Relevant criteria	Measures and findings	Diagnosis
Physical	Physical signs masked by illness. Withdrawn, tearful.	Depression related to physical illness.
Behavioural	Anorexic, inactive, irritable, uncooperative, sleeping fitfully.	
Self-report	Reporting that things are hopeless, worried about recovery or continued illness. Possibly complaining about treatment. Scores high on MACL—above mid point, scores moderately on Beck—within mid-range.	
Behavioural	Unkempt appearance possibly taking alcohol more frequently. Missing appointments and obligations.	Depression due to lack of meaningful support and reward.
Self-report	Complains of feeling tired, low, useless, unappreciated and lonely. Scores low to middle on MACL. Scores low to middle on Beck.	
Physical	Weight loss. Appears pale and drawn.	Depression due to loss events (death, desertion or unwanted divorce).
Behavioural	Withdrawn, tearful at times. Unable to function. Forgetful, inattentive, self-absorbed.	
Self-report	Feels very sad, contemplates giving up. Life is meaningless. Scores high on MACL. Scores within top range of Beck.	

Children may well suffer from depression, particularly in association with physical illness and hospitalisation. Early studies by Spitz (1946) showed that children show the classic responses to separation, anxiety leading on to depression, when they realise the loss has to be endured. Lack of warm loving relationships or of enjoyable interactions makes people lonely in any setting (Francis, 1976) but this is particularly experienced during a period of stress, such as illness, even when several people are 'in attendance'.

Associated with depression (as previously discussed) is the concept of self-esteem or how we rate or value ourselves. In a comparative study by Riffee (1981) children were found to alter in their ratings of self-esteem while in hospital. Three groups of children were matched for age (6–8 years), one group consisted of those admitted for surgery, another in hospital for non-surgical treatment and a control group at school. Although the hospital stay was short, on average only three days, the surgical group showed a significant reduction in the measure of self-esteem from the day of admission to the second measure taken one month later. On other measures reflecting perceived social ratings of peers non-surgical children's scores also dropped. Interpretation of these results raises many questions. However, separation from peers obviously affects individuals at whatever age and should be assessed for longer-term influences.

Helplessness has been identified as a component in the depressed feelings, but more particularly in the elderly (Crook, 1982) and those who are institutionalised for a long time. Lack of control or rather a perceived lack of control has long been seen to result in a syndrome of helplessness (Seligman, 1975). Studies of the elderly (Chang, 1978, 1979; Ryden, 1983) show that those who perceive they have some individual power over their lives and environment report much higher ratings of morale. However, the converse was also demonstrated in that those who would like to have some control and felt this was not possible had a lower morale and lower self-esteem. Expectations are obviously important and self-esteem is dependent on judgement of others' treatment and interactions.

Goals

Once depression is recognised and the causes identified for those in a general care setting, appropriate attention is given and realistic goals for resolution should be set. For a majority of 'acute' patients substantial improvement should be expected in a week. For those who have a deeper depression with feelings of hopelessness for the future associated with a serious physical illness or long-term institutionalisation, this may take several weeks. Moods should be monitored every few days, perhaps twice weekly. Not only will this give an accurate account of what is happening, but also it will demonstrate to the patient that staff are concerned about their feelings, and trying to help. Deep depression should always be assessed psychiatrically and not go untreated. Even so progress may be slow, realistic goals may be set to try to achieve slight improvement each week.

DEPRESSION DUE TO LACK OF MEANINGFUL SUPPORT
(see Table 3, section 2)

Chronically deprived and lonely people, more often women, frequently exhibit a low but persistent level of depression. Brown and Harris' (1978) work in urban areas showed that young mothers without a close relationship or significant other were particularly likely to exhibit this picture. The cause of this unhappy, fatigued and apathetic response apparently lies in disturbed social and psychological circumstances.

For many young working class women who have children, an additional cause for depression may be overlooked. Although postnatal depression is a much researched area, over one-half of new mothers suffer from post baby blues and 10% suffer from depression. This is frequently unrecognised and untreated. Causes for this are still hypothetical although low progesterone levels may be partly responsible. Williams (1986) discusses the role of antenatal parent education on this subject and warns that fatigue and lack of support may be contributory. She also mentions that social factors (poor housing, unemployment) were found by Oakley and Chamberlain (1981) to be positively related to depression in this group. As they say, midwives must obviously be alert to these problems and recognise when counselling may be inadequate and psychiatric referral necessary.

The process by which people become vulnerable can also be seen within a behavioural (or learning) model. Lack of meaningful interaction and reward for actions, or inconsiderate treatment by others, gradually reduces self-esteem, social reinforcement being seen as necessary for healthy adjustment to life. Replacement of such recognition and added support is then said by behaviour therapists to alleviate these problems (Liberman, 1975). Related to this perspective is that of cognitive psychology. Beck (1969) conceives that lowered self-esteem is related to how one habitually views and thinks about oneself. Consistently negative self-appraisal may determine how one behaves and feels in general.

Goals

Goals for changing long-standing circumstances must be realistic; self-awareness and empowerment, behavioural and cognitive therapies take several weeks before positive results are obtained. At times it is also realistic to accept the limitations of health care staff to alter social environments, and the behaviour of partners.

DEPRESSION DUE TO LOSS EVENTS (see Table 3, section 3)

Reactions to loss, defined as bereavement, may be actual or anticipated. Anticipated loss may induce anxiety and protest, actual loss being followed by withdrawal and decreased social participation (Klerman, 1975). Losses can include such things as children leaving home, breaking a relationship or friendship or moving to another district. Only some people become depressed as a result, but failure or perceived failure to cope with these transitions is central. Accumulation of such events in the absence of a close supportive relationship tends to reduce the chance of adaptation. As with anxiety a history of successful coping provides more resources for the individual to cope in the present and future.

Classic pictures of bereavement reactions have been systematically constructed. Work by Lindeman (1944) and Parkes (1972) has confirmed that people suffer from a syndrome of both physical and psychological suffering after a major loss. Physical sensations, such as dizziness, shortness of breath and various aches and pains are not unusual. Grieving involves coming to terms with the loss but this process may take several years, during which time the lost object or person may be imagined or assumed to exist at times before the individual suddenly returns to what is said to be the 'painful' realisation once more.

Reports of increased ill health and mortality at times of loss are plentiful. Males are particularly vulnerable and their chances of fatal illness are significantly increased. Staff in the community should be alert to this potential morbidity and attempt to provide relevant support during this time of readjustment.

Goals

Once more, resolution frequently takes a very long time, and depends on the alternative sources of support from significant others or professionals. Many individuals say they never 'get over' the loss of a loved one but their state of health and ability to take interest in other activities should return within months of the loss. There is no right time period for mourning (Parkes, 1972). This may take years. Therapists should however be able to anticipate watersheds and predict when long-term adjustment will be achieved.

RATIONALE FOR NURSING INTERVENTION TO ALLEVIATE DEPRESSION DUE TO ALL THESE CAUSES

There is little research in this area of nursing care of depressed patients. Depression is potentially fatal if untreated or unresolved, but it is often a severe chronic condition which has to be treated by psychiatrists with anti-depressive medications or electroconvulsive therapy. For nurses, certain general skills are essential and for those who do not work in a psychiatric care setting, these have not to date been given a high enough priority. General counselling skills will, therefore, be discussed as they are fundamental to any psychological assessment or intervention.

REASSURANCE AND COUNSELLING FOR THOSE WHO ARE ANXIOUS AND DEPRESSED

General empathy, facilitative, caring, and supportive skills are advocated for nurses to help patients, yet rarely closely evaluated. However, studies which compare the effectiveness of nurses providing care with others are really often reflecting these behaviours in nurses.

Reassurance is a classic term, commonly used by nurses in texts and conversation but somewhat difficult to explain and put into operation. French (1979) talks about reassurance as a therapeutic skill which aims to restore the patient's confidence in himself and his treatment. It involves explanation and information about anxiety provoking situations and the future and avoids bland statements like 'there is nothing to worry about'. Reassurance seeks to help the patient cope with the unfamiliar situation and to introduce a familiar element into such a situation. He discusses touch as an important element in reassurance, where holding someone's hand during a stressful experience is an obvious example. A current British study is designed to assess the response of elderly patients to the level of touch they receive from nurses (Redfern and Le May, 1986). Even the presence of a nurse at such a time may be reassuring. French includes the ability of the nurse to control her own emotional reactions during the patient's distress as a necessary 'skill'. Counselling skills are also subsumed under the blanket of reassurance.

Counselling techniques can be seen as advanced communication skills, necessary to help distressed patients in any setting. Barry's (1984) particular expertise is in liaison psychological support given by nurses. Her section on these skills provides an excellent account aimed to alleviate anxiety and depression and prevent more serious emotional complications. Differentiating between empathy and sympathy is her first vital task. Empathy occurs when a helper borrows emotions in order to fully understand them but keeps separate from them. Sympathy may involve emotions in the helper which are not constructive. Empathy is essential to undertake a counselling role, which may not be a formally defined one, but meaningful, helpful communication. Above all nurses must realise that ultimately patients help themselves, the helper may facilitate but not determine this adjustment. So informal counselling requires a genuine feeling of warmth for the person being 'helped', a capacity really to understand how the patient is feeling and their frame of reference and to be 'genuine' and 'real'. Nurses may undertake advisory or guiding roles or merely support and explore the patient's own feelings and choices, but in counselling the nurse would serve as catalyst for the patient to air his views and solutions.

Communication skills are vital to empathic communication and counselling. Comfortable and relaxed settings are best (but a busy ward may not afford these) so that nurses may display interest and commitment to listening, summarising and interpreting what the patient is saying. It may be difficult to avoid advising someone but this is not indicated where that someone needs to decide for himself. This type of approach is useful for individual and group counselling. As with all communication skills it needs to be practised (Tomlinson et al, 1984). Anxious patients in particular are usually very willing to talk about their feelings whereas those who are depressed may need a great deal of encouragement. Active listening is important to interpret and assess whether additional interventions are necessary.

OTHER INTERVENTIONS

Given that self-esteem is so central to depression it is important to explore how nurses can encourage more positive self-esteem in patients. As with all these rather abstract concepts, describing supportive behaviours for nurses is quite challenging. However, Meisenhelder's (1985) article reviews work in this area and advocates certain principles for care. Significant others are seen as most influential to an individual's appraisal of himself by others and this paper refers to nurses as potential significant others. Positive appraisal must be explicit and perceived in order to enhance self-esteem. Praise for attempts to cope with certain problems, and identification of individual's attributes and strengths is found to be important. Non-verbal communication of affection and providing time to be with the individual also indicate their worth. Facilitating support from others who matter to the individual is vital. Lastly nurses can enhance esteem by providing relationships within groups of patients and Meisenhelder reviews work that has demonstrated the positive effect of this.

Nurses, therefore, need to exploit clinical psychological approaches as well as general counselling skills. Although nurse behaviour therapists use desensitisation approaches, designing and scheduling programmes with patients and their families, other nurses are also using cognitive therapies for those who are anxious and depressed. As described by Shaffer et al (1981) cognitive therapy may be conducted with individuals or in groups. Their study evaluated the relative effectiveness of this and showed that group therapy was as effective in reducing anxiety and depression, and in increasing assertiveness as individual therapy. Cognitive behaviour therapy consisted of progressive relaxation, cognitive restructuring and assertion training.

Cognitive therapy elicits patients' automatic thoughts and encourages rational responses to them (Beck, 1969). This therapy has been positively evaluated in outcome studies (see Persons and Burns, 1985) although the actual process by which moods are elevated is not really understood and relationships with the therapist might have a significant influence. Combined support, attention and social reward may all play a part in the success of such therapies.

More physical forms of intervention for those who are depressed have also been tried. For instance Snyder (1985, p. 80) reviews work with exercise therapy in depression. This has shown positive results, whether used as an adjunct to other therapies or in isolation. Effects relate to the intensity and duration of such exercise as jogging or swimming.

However, so many of those who suffer from loneliness and chronic depression are elderly, either living alone or in institutions. Here 'helplessness' or 'powerlessness' feelings are basic to depression.

Interventions to provide increased opportunities for 'control' have included introducing personal furniture, caring for plants, or resources such as wine to share. Also a review and study by Francis et al (1985) showed that pet visiting had very positive effects particularly when residents were treated to a weekly session with puppies!

EVALUATIVE WORK WITH NURSES AS THERAPISTS

Few examples of experimental work from which to advocate good practice exist in this field. Exceptionally Gordon's (1986) work with depressed women has made a substantial contribution. In a series of carefully controlled experiments she has demonstrated that nurses can successfully act as group facilitators who help others to utilise the principles of cognitive therapy, assertiveness training and problem solving. Groups run in the USA and the UK had positive effects. Depressed women were initially self-selecting from a public notification of the study. In London over 200 women came forward, out of which a study group (n=10) and control group (n=10) were randomly selected. All of these participants were rated as mild to moderately depressed on Beck's (1969) scale. Extensive pre- and post-study testing was undertaken in this and the previous American studies.

Group work was supervised by two trained psychiatric nurses conversant with this way of working. They had instructor's books to guide them through the process and goals for each of the 14 sessions. The women also had a manual including thir homework and further reading. Group sessions were reviewed and summarised by the nurses, but the women were encouraged to explore and record their own feelings and supportive relationships as much as possible. For many of these women the sessions provided a very necessary medium for expressing themselves and regaining their self-esteem through positive self-statements, and increasing understanding of their social situations. Assertiveness training was also much appreciated by the group (who reported some favourable consequences at home). Post-treatment ratings were significantly better on measures of self-esteem, depression and hopelessness. This study demonstrates that nurse run groups are really very effective and useful for many people—not only those who are deemed 'ill'.

PRACTICAL IMPLICATIONS FROM RESEARCH

There is obviously much less nursing research in the area of evaluating interventions to alleviate depression than anxiety. However, several encouraging leads have been provided in some studies, particularly when nurses act as independent therapists. More practice of counselling skills for assessment and treatment is required and individualisation of strategies for those recognised as depressed, is indicated. Concepts such as self-esteem are important and maintaining positive self-esteem in patients should be seen as a vital nursing responsibility, as failure to do this may lead to a far more intractable problem of depression.

FUTURE RESEARCH

This might include:

1. Studies which evaluate teaching strategies aimed to prepare nurses in assessment and cue recognition for depressed people.
2. Video feedback used systematically and evaluated as a self-learning device to assist nurses to improve their psychosocial skills.
3. In depth studies analysing nurse–patient communication and the outcome for patients' psychological state, to attempt to correlate specific counselling behaviours with patients' responses.
4. More evaluation of nurse run groups for various clients who are depressed (possibly as replication to Gordon's work) in different settings.
5. Comparative studies using behavioural techniques and cognitive therapies applied by nurses for those with depression and lowered self-esteem.
6. Many more clinically based monitoring studies, carefully detailing interventions employed by specialist nurses, with suggestions for others to employ these in different settings.
7. Evaluation of various interventions to help those in hospital to gain more control and enjoyment from their environment.

REFERENCES

Akiskal HS, McKinney WT (1975) Overview of research in depression. *Archives of General Psychiatry* **32**(March) 285–305.

Barry PD (1984) *Psychological Nursing: Assessment and Intervention.* JB Lippincott Co, Philadelphia.

Beck AT (1967) *Depression, Clinical, Experimental and Theoretical Aspects.* Hoeber Medical Division, Harper and Row, New York.

Beck AT (1969) Cognition and psychopathology. In: Beck AT (ed) *Depression: Clinical, Experimental and Theoretical Aspects* p. 253. Harper and Row, New York.

Becker J (1974) *Depression: Theory and Research.* J Wiley & Sons, London.

Bowlby J (1973) *Separation Anxiety and Anger.* Penguin Books, London.

Brown G (1976) Depression: A sociological view. *Bethlem and Maudsley Gazette* **Summer**, 9–12.

Brown GW, Harris TH (1978) *Social Origins of Depression.* Tavistock Publications, London.

Brown GW (1972) Life events and psychiatric illness: some thoughts on methodology and causality. *Journal of Psychosomatic Research* **16**, 311–320.

Chang BL (1978) Generalised expectancy, situational perception and morale among institutionalised elderly. *Nursing Research* **27**(5), 316–324.

Chang BL (1979) Locus of control, trust, situational control and morale of the elderly. *International Journal of Nursing Studies* **16**, 169–181.

Crook T (1982) Diagnosis of treatment of mixed anxiety-depression in the elderly. *Journal of Clinical Psychiatry* **43**(9), 35–43.

Francis GM (1976) Loneliness: measuring the abstract. *International Journal of Nursing Studies* **13**, 156–160.

Francis GM, Turner JT, Johnson SB (1985) Domestic animal visitation as therapy with adult home residents. *International Journal of Nursing Studies* **22**(3), 201–206.

French HP (1979) Reassurance: a nursing skill? *Journal of Advanced Nursing* **4**, 627–634.

Freud A (1936) *The Ego and Mechanisms of Defence*. International University Press, New York.

Gordon V (1986) Treatment of depressed women by nurses in Britain and the USA. In: Brooking JI (ed) *Psychiatric Nursing Research*. pp. 91–117. John Wiley & Sons, Chichester.

Hirschfield RM (1980) In: Scarf M (ed) *Unfinished Business: Pressure Points in the Lives of Women*. p. 277. Ballantine Books, New York.

Hughes J (1981) *An Outline of Modern Psychiatry*. John Wiley & Sons, Chichester.

Izard C (1972) *Patterns of Emotions*. Academic Press, New York.

Kendell RD (1976) The classification of depressions: a review of contemporary confusion. *British Journal of Psychiatry* **129**(July), 15–28.

Klein M (1948) *Contributions to Psychoanalysis 1921–1945*. Hogarth Press, London.

Klerman G (1975) Overview of depression. In: Freedman AM, Kaplan HI, Sadock BJ (eds) *Comprehensive Textbook of Psychiatry II*, second edition. Williams and Wilkins, Baltimore.

Lader M (1976) Depression. *Bethlem and Maudsley Gazette* **Summer**, 12–15.

Liberman D (1975) Depression: a behavioural view. *Bethlem and Maudsley Gazette* **Summer**, 18–23.

Lindeman E (1944) Symptomology and management of acute grief. *American Journal of Psychiatry*, **101**, 7–21.

Lindeman CA (1972) Nursing intervention with the pre-surgical patient. *Nursing Research* **21**, 196–209.

Maquire P (1985) Barriers to psychological care of the dying. *British Medical Journal* **291**, 1711–1713.

Marks I (1975) Modern trends in the management of morbid anxiety: coping, stress immunisation and extinction. In Spielberger L, Sarason LG (eds) *Stress and Anxiety*. Hemisphere, New York.

Meisenhelder JB (1985) Self esteem: a closer look at clinical interventions. *International Journal of Nursing Studies* **22**, 2, 127–135.

Moffic HS, Paykel ES (1975) Depression in medical in-patients. *British Journal of Psychiatry* **126**, 346–353.

Oakley A, Chamberlain I (1981) Medical and social factors in postpartum depression. *Journal of Obstetrics and Gynaecology* **1**, 182–187.

Parkes CM (1972) Components of the reaction to loss of a limb, spouse or home. *Journal of Psychosomatic Research* **16**, 343–349.

Paykel ES, Myers JK, Dienelt MN, Klerman GL, Lindenthal JJ, Pepper MP (1969) Life events and depression: a controlled study. *Archives of General Psychiatry* **21**, 753–760.

Persons JB, Burns DD (1985) Mechanisms of action of cognitive therapy: the relative contributions of technical and interpersonal interventions. *Cognitive Therapy and Research* **9**(5), 539–551.

Redfern S, Le May A (1986) *Ongoing Study, Nurse–Patient Touch with Elderly Patients*. King's College, University of London, London.

Riffee DM (1981) Self-esteem changes in hospitalised school-age children. *Nursing Research* **30**(2), 94–97.

Ryden MB (1983) Morale and perceived control in institutionalised elderly. *Nursing Research* **33**(3), 130–136.

Seligman ME (1975) *Helplessness*. WH Freeman, San Francisco.

Shaffer CS, Shapiro J, Sank LI, Coghlan DJ (1981) Positive changes in depression, anxiety and assertiveness following individual and group cognitive behaviour therapy intervention. *Cognitive Therapy and Research* **5**(2), 149–157.

Snyder M (1985) *Independent Nursing Intervention*. John Wiley & Sons, New York.

Spitz RA (1946) Analytic depression. *Psychoanalytic Study of a Child* **2**, 313–342.

Tomlinson A, Macleod Clark J, Faulkner A (1984) The use of role play in nurse education. *Nursing Times* **80**(35), 48–51 and **80**(39), 45–47.

Webb C, Wilson-Barnett J (1983) Self-concept, social support and hysterectomy. *International Journal of Nursing Studies* **20**(2), 97–107.

Williams J (1986) Not just the baby blues. *Nursing Times* **82**(20), 38–40.

Wilson-Barnett J, Carrigy A (1978) Factors affecting patients' responses to hospitalisation. *Journal of Advanced Nursing* **3**(3), 221–228.

Zung WWK (1973) From art to science. The diagnosis and treatment of depression. *Archives of General Psychiatry* **29**(Sept), 328–337.

Chapter 5
Communication Problems

INTRODUCTION

Clear communication is vital for any meaningful interaction between individuals. This involves the sending and receiving of a message, either verbal or non-verbal, with shared meaning. Most people take this for granted without analysing the interaction unduly but for those in the health professions this process needs to be understood and sometimes modified to promote clear understanding between patients, their relatives and others who are caring for them. It is not only problems in communication which affect patients that should be studied, despite the fact that impairment of the sensations, such as sight and hearing loss, and speech difficulties obviously affect communication abilities. But also communication difficulties are frequently cited in many situations between perfectly able and healthy individuals. In health care settings patients' needs require that staff engage in very skilful communication for explanation and reassurance, but sufficient levels of meaningful interaction are also necessary to avoid psychological distress among patients. However, there are several studies, many referred to in the previous chapter, which reveal inadequacies in staff's communication abilities. Some, for instance, (Lanceley, 1985) have interpreted poor communication skills leading to general problems in health care settings, as a mechanism for nurses to maintain control and organise the ward system into a bureaucratic, structured institution. Staff may also have additional problems in communication, many of which compound those of their patients, who have specific physical handicaps. Assessment of patients' needs and interventions by nurses inevitably depends on many of those skills which have been found sadly lacking. By focusing on the care of those with impairment it is hoped to review much that could be classified as 'good communication'.

PROBLEMS OF COMMUNICATION FOR THOSE WHO ARE PHYSICALLY ILL AND/OR ELDERLY

Difficulty in sending and receiving messages tends to become more severe with increasing age and infirmity. Those who are physically ill or elderly may well experience problems in attending to or concentrating on what is being said or what is happening in the social environment. They may also lack sufficient energy to express their thoughts and feelings. Hence their need for more rest and clear, careful communications from those attending them. Many illnesses also indirectly affect sensations, rendering individuals photophobic, hypersensitive to touch, or intolerant to noise. All these experiences need to be understood by nurses who should then moderate their styles of communication. However, evidence that nurses seem unaware of such needs is widespread, and therefore positive interventions have to be prescriptive as few research studies evaluate such specific care.

With increasing age deterioration in vision and hearing is to be expected. As so many patients in general or acute hospital areas are elderly, 'good communication' should become an especially important aspect of nursing care. Much of the nursing literature in this area prescribes good practice (e.g. Fielding, 1981) and emphasises the importance of balancing or complementing verbal and non-verbal communication. Despite this Wells (1980) and Le May and Redfern (1987) found very little evidence of explicit use of non-verbal communication; expressive touch being used very infrequently by nurses with elderly people. However Burchett (1967) showed that seriously ill elderly patients were frequently too exhausted to cope with more than the very minimum of verbal communication. Nurses may rationalise the paucity of communication of all types with the elderly by considering that their patients are too weak or tired.

Careful assessment of need, and attention to physical and environmental concerns is fundamental to promoting constructive, useful and desirable communications. Frequently, nurses need to plan to promote open communication with those who are elderly and/or physically ill. Certain factors promote this and need to be organised or manipulated. Background noise is often troublesome for those who are even slightly deaf. Poor lighting or direct lamps may also be problematic for the partially sighted. But perhaps even more of a hindrance is the absence of space or seating. Squatting by a bed or bending over a chair is uncomfortable and appears rather uncommitted. Patients may well take this cue and, wishing to prevent discomfort for others, 'release' that person from the interaction.

Given that communication with people is so central for nursing (Bridge and Macleod Clarke, 1981) those with impaired ability, however subtle, should receive more attention from nurses. Sadly, descriptive research seems to indicate that they are stigmatised (or left relatively unattended) by all, nurses included (Stockwell, 1971).

PHYSICAL PROBLEMS WHICH IMPAIR COMMUNICATION

Verbal and non-verbal communication is used to send and receive messages. These messages are, therefore, designed and sent by spoken word or gesture and then heard and interpreted or decoded. This involves thought processes or cognition, articulation and expression as well as sight and hearing. In this chapter, physically related problems of sight, hearing and speech impairment are considered, all of which increase in severity and prevalence with age.

PREVALENCE

Sight loss affects 52 adults for a population of 10,000 but for 32% (with 6/60 vision or less) this is considered severe. Major causes for blindness are cataract, macular degeneration, diabetic retinopathy, glaucoma and retinal detachment.

It has been estimated that (Royal College of Physicians, 1986) in England and Wales (which are typical of westernised countries in general) one in 10 members of the adult population has impaired *hearing*. For those over 70 years this rises to 75%, with 10% of those affected having severe impairment. This is, therefore, a very widespread disability.

Impaired *speech* is estimated to affect approximately one in 100 of the population, one-third of those affected having severe impediments. Medical diagnoses include progressive neurological disease (for one-third), stroke, cerebral palsy and head injury each accounting for roughly one-sixth, and the remainder a group of disorders including cancers.

ASSESSMENT OF COMMUNICATION PROBLEMS DUE TO PHYSICAL IMPAIRMENT (see Table 1)

This complex area of human functioning can be assessed and deemed problematic in many ways. Sophisticated models for evaluating the quality of communication exist (Macleod Clark, 1982). However, as with all nursing problems, these are defined in relation to the extent to which they impede activities of daily life. For the purpose of this chapter, communication will be divided into what is seen, (as non-verbal communication

Table 1. Assessment of Communication Problems

Criteria		*Methods*
Reception of non-verbal messages.	Awareness of people in general. Awareness of individuals attempting to communicate non-verbally (other than by touch). Response to messages (e.g. smiles). Appearance when others are near, relaxed or 'peering'.	Observe responses. Question individual and family on capacity. Optical assessment.
Reception of verbal messages.	Level of participation in conversation. Response to messages. Ease of interaction, relevance of verbal responses. Appearance during conversation while listening (tense or showing effort). Volume and tone of individual's own voice.	Test by altered volume pitch and tone of sounds and voices. Question individual and family. Audiometric testing.
Sending messages.	Level of participation in conversation. Response to messages. Quantity and nature of speech. Level of impairment: intermittent or continuous. Nature of difficulty: cognitive, emotional or muscular.	Observe conversation with staff and family. Question individual and family about difficulty. Speech therapist assessment e.g. Porch Index, Word and Picture Chart (Chest, Heart and Stroke Association, 1986).

contributes to meaning and much of the affective component), heard, and spoken or expressed. Assessment of ability to communicate relates to all these aspects. Specialists are usually available to make precise assessments in these areas, but nurses should be able to assess sight, hearing and speech, as environments and fluctuating levels of health often evoke or compound these problems.

Continuous and careful observation and purposeful conversations are essential in order to make a careful assessment of an individual's communication difficulties. By allocating the same nurse to the individual patient, the more subtle facets or influences can be noted. This takes time, but helpful observations on what helps or hinders a person's capacity may affect the future quality of life. Specialists may be able to make more accurate assessments, but nurses can report on many environmental and social influences.

IMPAIRED VISION (see Table 2, section 1)

Those who develop poor sight during their life are likely to experience more difficulties in communication than those who have been blind or seriously impaired throughout their life, and have developed compensatory mechanisms of acute hearing and more sensitivity to others' presence. In particular the elderly may be suddenly surprised by someone's voice and frequently have developed poorer hearing as well. Unaware of gestures or other visual cues to non-verbally communicated messages, they may be prone to misinterpret what is said. Those who are partially sighted or blind may also appear slow to respond appropriately, as they are possibly unaware of who is addressing them, or they are not aware of the personal context of the conversation. Also, as they have not seen who is approaching they have not had the time to prepare what they may wish to say or how to start.

Blind people may not use facial expressions or gestures as much as others. This may result in loss of the affective or expressive component of what they are saying. As they cannot see how others are using non-verbal cues, they may not then employ these themselves. For instance, some tend to smile less, have fixed expressions or frown in a rather exaggerated fashion while trying to orientate themselves.

Social isolation is obviously a great problem for those who are blind or severely handicapped and Cullinan (1986) describes how other people approach such individuals with apprehension. This is perhaps due to fear of inadequate skill in helping them appropriately or becoming involved in such commitments. Consequently social conversation may be even more difficult and those who are blind admit to providing constant reassurance and guidance for the general public and to developing reactions which will reward those who do attempt to help.

Goals

Although deterioration in the function of the eye may not be correctable, maximising opportunities for partially sighted people is a nursing responsibility. Specific objectives include obtaining appropriate spectacles and lighting, and advising those who care for

Table 2. Identification of Communication Problems

Criteria	Measures and findings	Diagnosis
Reception of non-verbal messages Observations	Statements asking for identification of others. Complaints – that faces are blurred. – that glasses are no good. – that room is too dark (or light). Requests for speaker to come nearer (or further away) and to touch them. Failure to notice those in certain visual fields (or at one side).	Impaired vision (due to general deterioration in old age).
Questions	Individual and family will report on changes in eyesight, usually gradual deterioration.	
Tests	Visual acuity poor and a full range of optical tests indicates impairment.	
Reception of verbal messages	Easier to converse if voice is louder and of lower tone.	Impaired hearing (due to deterioration, often in old age).
Observations during different speech	Familiar voices more easily heard. Frequently turns head to 'good' side.	
Questions	Family may report gradual deterioration, individual may be reluctant to admit to problem or deny it.	
Tests	Audiometric tests with hearing-aid demonstrate impairment.	
Sending messages (by speech)	Speech may be slow, poorly articulated. Recognition and naming of objects may or may not be impaired.	Impaired speech due possibly to cerebral damage.
Observation	Difficulty with certain consonants. Speech may be more difficult when the patient is upset or anxious.	
Tests	Scans and neurological assessment. Detailed speech therapist e.g. Porch Index of Communicative Ability— results may be with a wide range. Bliss symbols used—poor recognition likely at first.	

such individuals about communication. Simple measures may take a few moments, while changing others' patterns of communication to help the afflicted individual may take weeks.

Rationale for nursing interventions

Research by nurses describing communication problems and evaluating interventions with the elderly blind or partially sighted is sadly lacking. Once more nursing interventions must be based on 'accumulated wisdom'.

Nurses, therefore, need to be clearly aware of these difficulties and develop skills which will help patients, particularly in the clinic or institutional health care setting. Simple guidelines are advocated by Macleod Clark (1985, p. 56).

'1. When communicating with patients with poor vision it is essential to introduce yourself before you speak as the patient may not be aware of your presence.
2. Sit or stand in a position which suits the patient best.
3. Do not sit or stand too close. This can be uncomfortable for old people whose eyes cannot focus or accommodate to very near objects.
4. Non-verbal communication is vital, especially touch and the use of clear intonation.
5. Try to keep the patient's environment as consistent and familiar as possible.'

For the elderly it is obviously vital to assess sight carefully and supply glasses (and clean them as necessary) or other aids. Lighting preferences vary but sitting between the patient and in front of the light will cause difficulties. Positioning yourself so that the patient can also touch you is important to achieve reciprocal contact. Care to provide a sustained conversation and to describe what is going on is very important to compensate for lack of visual orientation.

Typically principles for communicating with those who are blind rely on what has been culled from experience and individuals who have experienced problems themselves rather than systematic investigation. Experts in teaching the blind also tend to be invaluable in teaching nurses. The Royal National Institute for the Blind and the Disabled Living Foundation are two British charities with such professional help.

IMPAIRED HEARING (see Table 2, section 2)

The extent of this problem has only recently been recognised and publicised and as a particular problem of the elderly this has been seen as a Cinderella service area with previously inadequate resources. Whereas specialists and schools are devoted to the young, services for older people who develop hearing problems are still relatively poorly funded. Because of this, professional and lay education and publicity which aids communication skills generally are not well developed. As a consequence 1986 was designated a special campaign year for the Royal National Institute for the Deaf on its 75th anniversary. Of the two million people in England and Wales who wear hearing-aids, about 60% are over 60 years of age. Another four million require but have not received help. This may be due to the incipient nature of the problem, so that individuals themselves do not realise what they cannot hear.

Certain facts about deafness in older age are important for skilled communication. Murphy (1986) explains that degeneration begins with the high frequencies, which include consonants ('s' and 't' which serve to differentiate word sounds). Speech, therefore, becomes a meaningless jumble of vowel sounds. Background noise affects speech differentiation, and in a large room filled with people 'noise' tends to dominate as it usually consists of low frequency sounds. Other phenomena also tend to be distressing. For instance certain sounds tend to become louder and even painful. 'Noise' such as television or radio may be intolerable. The consequences for communication are grave as meals and social gatherings become uncomfortable, lack of sound dissemination being embarrassing and the sound of cutlery and crockery may be unbearable. Withdrawal from this interaction may lead patients to become uncommunicative, antisocial or stubborn. Such effects are isolating and compound the problem.

Goals

It may take several weeks before an elderly person adjusts to using a hearing-aid, when prescribed. Helping such an individual to accept their deafness and assisting others to moderate their communication may be a long-term process. However, repeated efforts and optimistic estimates would indicate three or four weeks to effect these changes.

Rationale for nursing interventions

Little research evaluating nursing interactions or approaches has been done but evidence of the outcome of poor communication patterns with the deaf exists. For instance the quality of life amongst elderly women was examined by Magilvy (1985) by comparing early and late onset deafness and those factors most responsible for distress and isolation. Path-analysis showed that the best predictors of quality of life were the level of social hearing handicap, functional social support and perceived health. The later onset group had an overall lower perception of quality of life.

Recommendations for care are only indirectly based on research. Patients and staff should of course make every effort to deal with hearing-aids and learn special communication skills, as Murphy (1986, p. 17) says:

'Every nurse working with geriatric patients should know how to deal with hearing-aids with confidence and unobtrusive skill . . . Slow, clear speech without exaggerated lip pattern helps. Clear speech should be as unobtrusive as possible. If a patient does not understand questions, they should be rephrased. Some words and phrases are easier to lip-read than others.'

Similarly, Macleod Clark (1985, p. 57) says:

'1. Try to avoid distracting extra noises by going to a quiet room or corner.
2. Turn off the television or radio before speaking.
3. Ensure the hearing-aid, if it exists, is switched on and working.
4. Write important messages clearly on a piece of paper.
5. Repeat your message if you do not think you have been understood.
6. Give your patient time to think about what you say and respond to it.
7. Ask simple, clear questions.
8. Use short sentences.'

One useful suggestion by Drane (1986), a senior nurse in intensive care, was made in response to continued problems in understanding patients with tracheostomies, is also particularly relevant to those who are deaf. Drane attended lip-reading classes for the deaf by a speech therapist for several weeks. In her amusing and valuable article, Drane explains that females are easier to lip-read than men because they smile more when talking thus revealing their teeth and tongue. After six weeks this special diligence was rewarded by greater ability.

IMPAIRED SPEECH (see Table 2, section 3)

'Impaired verbal communication' related to 'impaired ability to speak words' and 'aphasia' (and foreign language barriers) are described as nursing diagnoses by Carpenito (1983, pp. 133–143), whose definition of impaired verbal communication is:

'That state in which the individual experiences, or could experience a decreased ability to speak appropriately or understand the meaning of words.'

Aetiology and contributing factors include cerebral impairment, that is stroke, brain damage (head injury), central nervous system depression, tumour, mental retardation or chronic hypoxia; neurological impairment of nervous system; diseases such as multiple sclerosis or myasthenia gravis or vocal cord paralysis. The most common among all these conditions is stroke.

Large numbers, that is, one-third of all patients suffering a stroke have various forms of speech impairment. Patients may suffer from dysarthria which is a problem of articulation and muscle control. This tends to be more amenable to practice and fairly simple interventions which exercise the capacity of speech. Aphasia is the complete absence of speech but more common after stroke is dysphasia which is the partial loss of speech or difficulty with speech. This can take the form of expressive dysphasia, (impaired motor function of the brain) resulting in the inability to say the correct word to imply specific meaning. Receptive dysphasia affects the auditory cortex and, therefore, understanding of what is heard, but may not affect ability to speak, although this will sound meaningless. However, the more severe the initial speech impairment or aphasia the less likely it is for recovery of normal speech (Sessler, 1981). Mental ability is usually unaffected despite severe speech impairment.

Dyslexia and agraphia also frequently accompany speech problems (Clifford-Rose, 1981) and this can be particularly devastating as it prevents use of alternative forms of communication.

Goals

Nursing goals for those with general speaking difficulties are listed as follows (Carpenito, 1983, p. 135):

'. . . the nurse will seek to:
1. Create an atmosphere conducive to communication.
2. Promote optimal communication by encouraging the person to use adaptive devices for speech and hearing if necessary (e.g. hearing-aid, artificial larynx).
3. Provide alternative methods of communicating (e.g. pad and pencil, pictures, alphabet).
4. Encourage the person to express himself in what ever way he can.'

Time for improvement of speech varies according to the extent and location of the cerebral damage. For some, muscular weakness improves in a matter of days or weeks, for others with more neurological deficit, improvement may take months.

Rationale for nursing interventions

Of the research done with patients who have speech disorders, those after stroke (affecting the left side of the brain) seem to be studied more than others. This work attempts to describe needs and services provided and evaluates attempts to restore power of speech in the acute recovery period and long term, at home. Although this may not involve nurses directly, evaluative work has much relevance to the work and potential value of nursing care.

All the evidence on care provision in the UK shows inadequate attention by and education of staff. Sawyer's (1986) study with district nurses showed their preparation and self-reported knowledge to be minimal despite the large number of stroke patients they look after for quite protracted periods of time. Not surprisingly reports from stroke patients themselves and the few studies which analyse nurse–patient communication show lack of skill.

One study by Skelly (1975) found common complaints from reports of stroke patients. These complaints were subsequently used to analyse and categorise nurse-patient, nurse-nurse and nurse-doctor conversations about stroke patients by Macleod Clark and Walton (1986). Revealing insights into the type of communications serve not only to question the quality of care but also to self-question how much one's own behaviour is recognisable. Skelly's findings included the fact that nurses did not judge patients' ability to comprehend accurately, which returned more rapidly than they supposed. They and the doctor talked too quickly with too much information or too many changes of subject to be understood. Staff were found to talk about patients without including them, because their speech was slow. They did not allow sufficient time for patients to answer, and the general noise level was far too high. Patients also complained about the lack of continuity in carers which meant they had to interact with too many new people. They also complained that their problems were not discussed with them by nurses or doctors, only with speech therapists if they visited. All this seems to point to the need for more effort to plan care much more systematically and practise communication skills with such patients. Powerful lessons can be learned from tape recordings in the real situation, to make nurses aware of the effects of their own inadequate skills.

Evaluation for improved skills for nurses has not occurred as yet but planned interventions have been designed and assessed. For instance Leutenegger (1975) claimed that early encouragement of talking results in better recovery. She designed this component of care to be included as an active part of the daily plan during the immediate post-stroke period. Speech therapists have also demonstrated that they can produce significant improvements with therapy given early on (Aronson, 1983).

Controlled trials during the later stages of stroke recovery have unfortunately been less successful in demonstrating that speech therapists are able to effect improvements. Lincoln et al (1984) found a lack of difference between 84 randomly selected patients in the treatment groups and 74 patients who did not receive treatment from 10 weeks and up to 34 weeks after stroke. Patients who received therapy had twice weekly sessions but failed to show significantly greater improvement than others. Although different strategies might have worked, the authors conclude that speech therapists should expend more energy on assessment and supporting staff and relatives by giving them skills to help others in encouraging communication.

More support for suggesting that volunteers can be helpful as long-term 'therapists' is provided by two research teams. Meikle et al (1979) conducted a small clinical trial with 31 patients. Half were treated by 3–5 weekly sessions of varying lengths with professional speech therapists. The other half of the sample who were visited at home received more sessions although these were with volunteers. Four volunteers looked after each patient who then received four visits per week as well as a group session. No differences were found between initial and final scores on the Porch Index of Communicative Ability (Porch, 1971). Many problems with this study were discussed but it certainly demonstrated that volunteers do no worse than professionals and that they can act as faithful visitors, well appreciated by patients and families. Eaton Griffith and Miller (1980) reported on a five year extension scheme of volunteer visiting for patients, and compared results on speech ability for 350 patients as rated by general practitioners, the family, speech therapist and all volunteers, after six months in the scheme. All agreed that 90–95% of patients showed great improvement and that 70% or more improved in speech.

In both these studies patients were encouraged to have more confidence by practising their speech and helped to be more stimulated and reassured that they were able to regain more speech. Simple techniques of discussing interesting topics, reading or practice with time-telling helped volunteers to visit for one hour and maintain the interaction. Isted's (1979) book provides an excellent outline for helping the lay person. Such commitment has been greatly valued by patients. It also gives families encouragement that something is being done to help. Nurses could also provide such care in many settings if they witnessed special therapy sessions and were motivated to augment the approaches and techniques employed.

More specific advice on communicating with stroke patients has not been evaluated, but authorities in this field have agreed on strategies that are useful. For instance, Macleod Clark (1985, pp. 161–162) recommends the following guidelines for communicating with stroke patients:

' 1. Ensure that you have obtained the patient's attention before speaking.
2. Ensure that the patient can see and hear you.
3. Tell the patient you are trying to help her to speak.
4. Speak directly to the patient, talking clearly and slowly but with normal intonation and phrasing.
5. Use simple sentence structure, incorporating one idea at a time.
6. Commands can be given in single words, e.g. watch, listen, wait, swallow.
7. Repeat key words, rephrase if necessary.
8. Do not shout.
9. Label important items, e.g. cup, glass, spectacles.
10. Ask simple closed questions so that the patient can answer with one word, e.g. "Would you like tea or coffee?"
11. If the patient cannot answer yes or no, try to devise a gesture or sign language for these words, e.g. thumbs up for yes and thumbs down for no.
12. Do not push your patient too hard; learn to pick up signs of distress such as perseveration (meaningless repetition of a word or act), loss of concentration, eye blinking, irritability and sweating.

13. Do not underestimate the patient's comprehension or potential capacity to communicate.
14. Avoid distractions, especially noise.
15. Give enough time for the patient to respond.
16. Find out what interests the patient (from relatives or visitors if necessary) and talk about these things.
17. Promote "ritual" communication. Familiar phrases reduce stress and improve performance.
18. Involve relatives and friends in all stages of care and teach them to help the patient communicate.
19. Use alternative methods of communication such as communication boards, written instructions, picture cards, etc. Encourage patients to use the unaffected hand for writing or drawing.'

Such advice may also be appropriate for other individuals who are suffering from speech impairment. These suggestions are echoed by other nurses such as Carpenito (1983) who advises honest communication and maximum effort by the nurse to reinforce effort and encourage attempts by the patient. Relatives may need support to interact in this same way and because they provide constant company and support often develop much more successful communication. Frustration by all should be recognised and acknowledged, but nurses must engage in conversations as an explicit component of care, seeing these as treatment sessions, planned for a time when the patient is not tired and seems willing.

IMPLICATIONS OF COMMUNICATION PROBLEMS FOR PRACTICE IN GENERAL

Simple recommendations for practice can be made. Nurses themselves need to employ more care and sensitivity to this aspect of helping their patients as what evidence there is tends to show that present communication styles probably discourage patients' attempts to practise speech rather than systematically planning to help. Practical hints are included in this chapter because there is a paucity of studies which evaluate those specially designed interventions that are needed. Social and communications skills which are tailored to meet individual needs in general must be employed for those who are partially blind or deaf and those who have speech impairment. Above and beyond this staff need to recognise that communication must be slower, that communication problems do not necessarily infer problems in cognition or mental ability in general and that patients need to feel that communicating with them is seen as important to staff. Various organisational and environmental factors require attention for those nursed in hospital. Unnecessary noise should be reduced for all patients but for those with hearing difficulties in particular, this is vital. Continuity of staff is important to reduce confusion and promote more meaningful contact for patients. One or two nurses can usually be assigned to the same patient over time if the necessity or benefit is recognised. This helps them to devise an effective plan and become familiar with the individual's abilities, problems and pronunciation.

Resources for those who care for people with communication problems need to be available and fully utilised. For instance those mentioned by the Report on Physical

Disability in the Journal of the Royal College of Physicians (1986, p. 180) included alternative communication systems; such as:

1. Sign and letter systems—e.g. Deaf alphabet, Makaton and Amarind.
2. Symbol systems—e.g. Word and picture chart (the patient points to a symbol to represent an expression).
3. Low technology aids to communication—e.g. pointing boards, pictures and word charts.
4. Medium technology aids—e.g. Canon Communicator and the Cambridge Lightwriter.
5. High technology aids for communication such as speech synthesisers and computers. They also state: 'It is clearly important that patients should not be supplied with equipment which is inappropriate. Each patient must be individually assessed and this will involve an analysis of the precise type of communication defect, physical, visual and cognitive abilities, as well as his educational background and the prognosis of the underlying disease.'

This Royal College report recommends that all patients should be assessed by a speech therapist if necessary and that equipment should be supplied quickly and that sign, letter and hospital picture boards should be available in wards and intensive care units. Nurses should ensure they are available, and be aware of helpful literature and support groups run for patients and their relatives, for example by the Royal College of Speech Therapists.

FUTURE RESEARCH

Much more descriptive and evaluative work needs to be done in this area, which is relatively deprived of systematic nursing investigation. Perhaps what is indicated, should include:

1. Descriptive study of patients' reports on communication problems in social and health related situations. This should highlight differences for those with speech and sensory deficits.
2. Staff behaviour and communication styles should be appraised by patients with communication problems, to identify 'good' communication.
3. Nursing staff should be surveyed to assess what type of further education they feel they require. Video feedback should be used to instruct nurses and other carers on their own patterns of communication and this should be evaluated with before and after records of skills.
4. Different types of speech therapy for particular problems should be taught to nurses by speech therapists and these nurses should then provide daily sessions with patients during their hospitalisation or during recovery at home. A comparison of recovery could be made for such a group with a matched or randomly selected control group, who receive attention only.
5. Nurses could rate each other as communicators, explaining why; they could then repeat this exercise after a few weeks to demonstrate any change in behaviour.
6. Pre-recorded teaching programmes need to be evaluated for use with trained staff,

on communication with those who are blind, deaf, or have speech deficits. Behaviours which are seen as good or deficient could be identified by nurses and others with these problems, to document knowledge and skills deemed to be important.

7. Sessions on using hearing-aids, special languages and cards should be designed by a panel of experts on these. These could then be evaluated for hospital and district nurses who work in rather more isolated settings.

REFERENCES

Aronson A (1983) *Aphasic Therapy on Trial*. Proceedings of 1st European Conference on research in rehabilitation, Edinburgh.

Bridge W, Macleod Clark J (1981) *Communication in Nursing Care*. H M & M, London.

Burchett D (1967) *Factors Affecting Nurse–Patient Interactions in a Geriatric Setting*. ANA. Regional Clinical Conferences. Appleton-Century-Crofts, New York.

Carpenito LJ (1983) *Nursing Diagnosis: Application to Clinical Practice*. J B Lippincott Co, Philadelphia.

Chest, Heart and Stroke Association (1986) *Word and Picture Chart*. CHSA, London.

Clifford-Rose FR (1981) *Stroke: The Facts*. Oxford University Press, Oxford.

Cullinan T (1986) *Visual Disability in the Elderly*. Croom Helm, London.

Drane L (1986) Watch my lips. *Nursing Times* **82**(20), 52.

Eaton Griffith V, Miller CL (1980) Volunteer stroke scheme for dysphasic patients with stroke. *British Medical Journal* **281**, 1605–1607.

Fielding P (1981) Communicating with geriatric patients. In: Bridge W, Macleod Clark J (eds) *Communication in Nursing Care*. H M & M, London.

Isted CR (1979) *Learning to Speak Again After a Stroke*. King's Fund, London.

Lanceley A (1985) Use of controlling language in the rehabilitation of the elderly. *Journal of Advanced Nursing* **10**, 125–135.

Le May A, Redfern S (1987) A study of non-verbal communication between nurses and elderly patients. In: Fielding P (ed) *Research in the Nursing Care of Elderly People*. John Wiley & Sons Ltd, Chichester.

Leutenegger R (1975) *Patients' Care and Rehabilitation of Communication Impaired Adults*. Charles C Thomas, Springfield, Illinois.

Lincoln NB, Mulley GP, Jones AC, McGuirk E, Lendrem W, Mitchell JRA (1984) Effectiveness of speech therapy for aphasic stroke patients: A randomised controlled trial. *Lancet* **i**, 1197–1200.

Macleod Clark J (1982) *Nurse Patient Verbal Interaction: Analysis of Recorded Conversations in Selected Surgical Wards*. PhD Thesis, University of London, London.

Macleod Clark J (1985) Communicating with elderly people. In: Redfern S (ed) *Nursing Elderly People*. Churchill Livingstone, Edinburgh.

Macleod Clark J, Walton L (1986) Making contact—communication with stroke patients. *Nursing Times* **82**(33), 28–32.

Magilvy JK (1985) Quality of life of hearing-impaired women. *Nursing Research* **34**(3), 140–144.

Meikle M, Wechsler E, Tupper M, Benenson M, Butler J, Mulhall D, Stern G (1979) Comparative trial of volunteer and professional treatments of dysphasia after stroke. *British Medical Journal* **1**, 87–89.

Murphy K (1986) Noises off. *Nursing Times* **82**(17), 16–17.

Porch BE (1971) *Porch Index of Communicative Activity*. Consulting Psychologists Press, Palo Alto, California.

Royal College of Physicians (1986) Physical disability in 1986 and beyond: a report of the Royal College of Physicians. *Journal of the Royal College of Physicians of London* **20**(3), 160–194.

Sawyer J (1986) Speech impairment after a stroke. *Nursing Times* **82**(3), 39–41.

Sessler GJ (1981) *Stroke – How to Prevent it/How to Survive it*. Prentice Hall Inc, Hemel Hempstead, Herts.

Skelly M (1975) Aphasic patients talk back. *American Journal of Nursing* 77(7), 1140–1144.
Stockwell F (1971) *The Unpopular Patient*. Royal College of Nursing, London.
Wells TJ (1980) *Problems in Geriatric Nursing Care*. Churchill Livingstone, Edinburgh.

Chapter 6
Sexual Problems

INTRODUCTION

The subject of sexuality and sexual activities, like other human functions, is highly complex, involving a full range of biopsychosocial factors. Sexual functioning tends to be viewed as a higher function in the Maslow hierarchy, disturbance may be related to one's state of health, physical or psychological. Sexuality is seen to reflect aspects of the human character or individuality and gender (Lion, 1982), confidence and self-esteem influencing an individual's sexual behaviour. A healthy adult person is usually expected to have a sexual appetite although this may be reduced by lack of a partner or stimulus, by worries, fatigue or 'minor' physical illness (Webb, 1985).

Information on sexuality, sexual intercourse and sexual relationships has only relatively recently become widely available to members of the general public. Hence many people laboured under ignorance, misunderstanding and prejudice when reviewing their own or others' behaviour and attributes. Publications by Masters and Johnson (1966), Kinsey et al (1953) and Hite (1976) helped to dispel much ignorance and 'legitimise' such habits as masturbation. These works also demonstrated that the nature of sexual relationships was extremely varied, with a wide range of practice. Discontent among many respondents was also fairly evident, expectations were frequently unmet, and self-blame was a common reaction to unsatisfactory sexual intercourse and other activities.

Nurses and other health workers may be called upon to give advice if they express their readiness and knowledge. In primary care, general medical practitioners and those working in family planning may receive questions or comments which reflect relationship concerns. Severity of problems for clients who are generally quite healthy, should be assessed. If these problems are enduring concerns which are likely to damage an apparently successful life and partnership a nurse or doctor may need to explore them systematically with the individual. Referral to a 'sex' clinic may then be necessary, but many specialist nurses in primary care can act as valuable counsellors. Concerns may only be raised within the context of a consultation focused on another topic. A sensitive nurse therefore needs to be aware of 'veiled' comments, using open questions and follow-up probes to uncover these worries.

In other areas of practice, nurses may be more likely than their patients to raise the subject of sexual matters, as part of their counselling or rehabilitation role. For patients who have experienced long-term sickness or major surgery, advice on resuming sexual activities or on areas that have actually proved problematic, may be required. Evidence on the frequency of such problems for certain patients exists (reviewed below) and suggests that improved 'recovery care' may reduce this. Sensible and knowledgeable advice is, of course, required and reports from some research (Webb and Wilson-Barnett, 1983) reveal that alleviation of worries can do much to prevent and resolve sexual problems during convalescence.

Excellent reviews of sexual physiology are available for those wishing to revise this area (see Bancroft, 1983; Masters and Johnson, 1970).

DEFINITIONS

Unhappiness or a sense of frustration and inadequacy may accompany an individual's 'ability' to give and receive sexual pleasure. This is rarely due to a physical cause, more often being due to psychological and relationship factors. However, this only becomes a problem when it is defined as such by an individual or couple and the extent to which treatment or advice is sought depends on the motivation and priority given to this area of human functioning.

Carpenito's (1983) nursing diagnosis defines sexual dysfunction thus:

'The state in which an individual experiences or is at risk of experiencing a change in sexual health function that is viewed as unrewarding or inadequate.' (p. 407)

Causes listed include those which are pathophysiological such as endocrine, neuro-muscular and cardiovascular. Genito-urinary complications are sub-classified as chronic renal failure, premature or retarded ejaculation, priapism, chronic vaginal infection, decreased vaginal lubrication, vaginismus, altered structures and venereal disease. Psychological problems include fear of failure, fear of pregnancy, depression, anxiety, guilt, and vulnerability. Situational factors are sub-categorised under unwilling, uninformed or abusive partner or lack of partner, unfamiliar environment e.g. hospital, other stressors or events, and also, lack of knowledge, fatigue, obesity, pain, alcohol consumption, medications, radiation treatment and altered self-concept from change in appearance or trauma of surgery.

RANGE OF SEXUAL PROBLEMS

Primary sexual problems are sometimes due to pathological or structural problems, but these should always be initially assessed and eliminated by medical examination. Surgical treatment may be indicated, in which case nursing care will be directed towards helping the client to prepare for and recover from the operation(s). This chapter deals with problems which arise due to or subsequent to illness and may be called secondary sexual dysfunctions. In summary these problems may be classified as:

1. Primary impotence—a male never able to achieve and/or maintain an erection of the quality necessary for intercourse. This is a serious problem which is difficult to treat.
2. Secondary impotence—difficulty in getting or maintaining an erection sufficient for intercourse, but with a history of previous successful intromission. This is the most common problem occurring after illness often through anxiety or through physical

deterioration in old age. High levels of success have been achieved with relatively simple behavioural treatment.

3. Primary anorgasmia—a woman's inability to achieve orgasm. Often due to inappropriate sexual education or her partner's inadequate efforts to ensure arousal; this too may be successfully treated by educational techniques.

4. Situational anorgasmia—inability to achieve orgasm at times or with a particular partner. This may relate to interpersonal dynamics and be amenable to psychotherapeutic interventions.

5. Vaginismus—involuntary spastic contraction of the vaginal outlet stimulated by anticipated, real or imagined attempts at vaginal penetration. This may be primary or secondary arising after stressful experiences at any time in a woman's life but is usually treatable.

6. Premature ejaculation—inability to control ejaculation either until pleasure or orgasm has been achieved by the partner, or prior to intromission, or after minimal thrusting. This also has fairly good results with various measures if it is identified as a problem by both partners.

7. Dyspareunia—difficult or painful intercourse. This may occur after childbirth or gynaecological surgery, where insufficient dilatation or lubrication has occurred. This may however be as much due to anxiety on the part of the woman, causing frigidity (when the vagina remains tight), as to her ability to engage in sex without harm to herself or rather too rapid and vigorous attempts at penetration by the man. Advice, understanding and time usually resolves this.

8. Ejaculatory incompetence—a man's inability to ejaculate intravaginally is often a complex problem which requires correct analysis and sensitive psychotherapy.

PREVALENCE

Sexual functioning is affected by many aspects of life, and is rarely seen as a generally acceptable topic for detailed conversation as it is bound up with sensitivities and loyalties within partnerships. For these and other reasons accurate reports are rarely available and a figure for overall prevalence is therefore unobtainable. Different sexual problems also vary in their prevalence. Primary disorders (e.g. impotence, ejaculatory incompetence) in men tend to be quite rare yet some secondary disturbances (impotence) tend to affect most men at some time in their life. Many women are thought to suffer from anorgasmia, yet this may now be becoming less common as more educative literature and advice are available and greater expectations exist. Many problems occur with a particular relationship which have not been experienced with other partners. Nowadays sexual experience with different partners during a lifetime is providing individuals with their own estimates as to the nature and extent of their problems.

Estimates of sexual problems after serious illness and treatment demonstrate that quite a substantial proportion of patients are affected. This could be seen as an indicator of recovery: when problems resolve, patients' psychological, social and physical function has returned to normal. However proportions of patients with problems can reach between one-third and one-half for certain conditions and may persist for several months or even years.

ASSESSMENT

Interviewing and counselling skills are essential when exploring sexual problems. This should be done in a quiet, private situation. Same-sex counsellors are usually more acceptable to clients and co-counselling teams (nurses often acting as the female counsellor) are useful in order to facilitate simultaneous individual assessment of both members of the partnership. Sensitive yet direct interview approaches are necessary.

Comprehensive interviews, covering a wide area of questioning are necessary to explore the full range of biographical, health and relationship details. See Tables 1 and 2 for assessment and identification of sexual problems.

Table 1. Assessment of Sexual Problems

Criteria	Methods
Psycho-social	*Interviews*
Nature, permanence of relationship	Use systematic schedules e.g. Masters
Recent life events	and Johnson, 1970 or Kaplan, 1974
Perception of problem, gravity	
Level of knowledge	
Motivation to give time to resolving problem	
Self-concept and image	
Emotional predisposition and current mood state	
Physical	
Signs of ill health	General physical health assessment
Evidence of genito-urinary infection or discomfort	Direct examination of genitals
Males: erectile, ejaculatory capacity	If necessary: artificial stimulation to assess function
Females: vaginal muscularity, contraction reflex dilatory capacity	If necessary: use of dilators for assessment

PRIMARY ANORGASMIA (see Table 2, section 1)

Inability to achieve orgasm is often associated with inability to become sufficiently aroused. It is the most common female sexual problem, but woman often consider themselves unusual and imperfect as a result. Physical reasons for this include rare pelvic musculature or structural damage and drug effects. Most frequently the male is not aware of what is needed to stimulate his partner. Poor sexual education and an insufficiently affectionate relationship may lead to this problem.

Sexual education, in the past, may have concentrated on the mechanics of intercourse and contraception, and even this was often not provided in many schools. Recent controversies over whether or not sex education should be included in school curricula suggest that fewer young people will remain completely ignorant. However, instruction on the importance of attention and sincerity within a relationship is less easy. Loving attention and a real concern for the enjoyment of the partner is often surpassed for a young man by his bravado to 'score' and perform well.

Anxiety and a fear of not being attractive and sexually responsive is very common

Table 2. Identification of Sexual Problems

Criteria	Measures and findings	Diagnosis
Female	Use Masters and Johnson interview.	
Relationship	Permanent but 'unaffectionate'.	
	Woman feels it is insecure.	
	Male erection sustained, no premature ejaculation.	
Life events		
Perception of problem	Grave, affecting relationship.	Primary anorgasmia.
Level of knowledge	Poor.	
Motivation	Strong: feels man is losing sexual interest unless resolved.	
Self-image	Weak: 'not a proper woman'.	
Predisposition and moods	Nervous and slightly depressed.	
Physical examination	No abnormalities or discomfort and dilation and lubrication satisfactory.	
Both Partners	Use Masters and Johnson interview, and Derogatis sexual adjustment schedule.	
Relationship	Longstanding—supportive and sexually active.	
Life event	Surgery: hysterectomy for localised carcinoma, six months ago.	
Perception of problem	Serious inability, relevant to complete relationship.	
Level of knowledge	Previously good, but now confused and apprehensive.	
Motivation	Strong—important to rectify this.	Dyspareunia following woman's serious physical illness.
Self-image	Woman feels less feminine although outward appearance is relatively unchanged i.e. a small scar. Man is reassuring about this.	
Predisposition	Both partners stable and adjusted to diagnosis.	
Physical examination	No discharge, but vagina slightly tight and dry. No adhesions or infection.	
	Male partner normal.	
Male	Use Masters and Johnson interview.	
Relationship	Longstanding, supportive, sexually active.	
Life events	Myocardial infarction 4 months ago.	Secondary impotence after hospitalisation for myocardial infarction.
	Returned to work for 2.5 months.	
Perception of problem	Important—'part of being a strong man'.	
Level of knowledge	Generally good, but does not understand reason for this problem.	
Motivation	Strong—'willing to do anything'.	
Self-image	Affected—weakened by heart attack and impotence.	
Predisposition and mood	Unemotional but was slightly depressed for two months after heart attack.	
Physical examination	Generally fit—tolerating high levels of exercise.	
	Degree of erection achieved by artificial stimulation.	

for members of both sexes but females, being less dominant, are often blamed (by themselves also) if sexual intercourse is unsatisfactory. Orgasm watching and the anticipation of 'failure' increases anxiety, the root of this problem.

Goals

This is a resolvable problem but motivation in both partners is essential for a successful outcome. Resolution may be intentionally postponed until the couple understand the nature of the problem and can spend time relaxed and intimately affectionate without attempting intercourse. A few weeks are usually needed.

SEXUAL PROBLEMS AFTER SERIOUS ILLNESS (see Table 2, section 2)

Disturbance in self-concept is particularly relevant as a cause for problems in sexual relationships, defined by Carpenito (1983, p. 389) as the state in which the individual experiences or is at risk of experiencing a negative state of change about the way he feels, thinks, or views himself. It may include a change in body image, self-esteem, role performance, or personal identity. This commonly occurs during and after serious illness, or after a major life event or transition. Careful assessment and record of a patient's account of his feelings and reactions is necessary to help someone. Sexual identity and performance are closely linked to the concept; someone who feels changed or maimed is likely to lose confidence in his general appeal, as well as his sexual attractiveness. The concept of body image (Schilder, 1950) is centrally related to self-concept, our mental image or body perception is dependent on emotional feelings toward the body. As bodily perception changes so emotional attitude changes. Such changes may evoke a grief or mourning reaction, with the well-recognised associated emotional reactions. Constant attention to restoring a positive self-concept is necessary.

Cancer and gynaecological treatments

Sexual functioning and drive may well be unimpaired in many cancer patients. A few cancers affecting hormones or sex organs may interfere with functioning but otherwise staff, patients and their partners should never assume that sex is inappropriate or impossible. Certain treatments may also reduce libido but individual disorders and treatment factors should obviously be assessed for such effects before explanations and advice are given. Those who are suffering from pain or nausea are also unlikely to feel able to enjoy sex but this may vary throughout the course of treatment, rehabilitation or even terminal stages. Lamb (1985) discusses that this situation pertains even for patients with gynaecological cancers. As always the partner's reaction and understanding are essential to resumption of sexual relations after illness.

Hysterectomy should not really be seen as 'mutilation' although others have so labelled it in the past (e.g. Raphael, 1978; Dalton, 1957). Psychoanalytical interpretations of the supposed significance of removing the 'heart of womanhood' and retrospective uncontrolled research were responsible for many negative reports on the effects of hysterectomy. Many patients were reported to become depressed post-operatively but samples included those with malignant disorders and subjects who on further investigation may also have had 'neurotic' problems before surgery. Subsequent more recent research showed that depression and deterioration in sex life were not influenced by hysterectomy, in a controlled comparison by Gath (1980). However this does represent loss of child-bearing capacity and those who have no children or wish for more may suffer a real loss. Post-operative experiences however do tend to show that the quality of a woman's sex life after surgery tends, in general, to either continue in the same way or improve. A woman's 'self-identity' and satisfaction is not found to be threatened or reflected in a lack of interest in sex, as the psychoanalyst would suppose (Webb and Wilson-Barnett, 1983).

Cardiac problems (see Table 2, section 3)

Physiological responses to sexual arousal and intercourse include a rise in blood pressure, pulse rate, cardiac volume and respiration rate. Those with grave cardiovascular or respiratory incapacity may find sexual intercourse difficult or impossible. However sexual intercourse is rarely the cause of death through increased exertion, therefore those pleasures which are gained with a comfortable level of exertion should be encouraged for those who desire them (McCary, 1973).

Unfortunately it is sometimes the drug therapy itself which impairs sexual function in cardiovascular patients, hypertensive agents particularly affecting the mechanism necessary for erection. However, this should never be assumed until after particular effort has been made and failed. More generally however it tends to be emotional problems which are most pertinent for those with heart pathology. Fears associated with the heart failing may affect both individuals in a couple, the spouse is tense and takes longer to excite and the partner is aware of this and may also become afraid and impotent. Very careful counselling is indicated and clear information and guidance as part of the rehabilitation programme is required. For instance for post-coronary infarction patients, Hellerstein and Friedman (1970) have established clear safe physical limits for activities which are much higher than those involved in normal marital intercourse. They also found that even with reduced oxygen capacity, 80% of post-coronary subjects can meet the requirements for the physical activity of sexual intercourse. But they emphasise that patient and spouse should always be given the opportunity to discuss this with a doctor or prepared nurse.

Goals

The outcome for specific sex therapy interventions for those who have had serious illnesses will understandably be affected by the physical condition, treatments and general speed of rehabilitation. General counselling and support for couples usually has more long-term goals than are relevant to the more structural behavioural sex therapy approach. Despite this, satisfactory sexual activity and ultimately intercourse is usually achieved after 6–10 weeks.

RATIONALE FOR SEX THERAPY AND NURSING INTERVENTIONS

Formal treatments for sexual problems have been devised by psychologists and psychiatrists, but some techniques may be amenable for use by nurses and those in other health care professions. Masters and Johnson (1966) formulated their famous approach based on desensitisation and anxiety reduction which has been applied and adapted by many. However, psychiatrists warn that this approach is really only appropriate for a limited spectrum of patients within a broad class of sexual disorders, as it excludes issues of psychodynamics and transference. Meyer et al (1975) only had success on a small series of couples, and warn that this type of sex therapy could evoke grave psychological problems and damage relationships. Psychotherapy on the other hand would identify and try to deal with deep-seated problems which manifest themselves as sexual dysfunction. Masters and Johnson (1966) in contrast assume that the sexual problem is the 'disease' itself, of primary importance, usually based on fear of failure and maintained by habit, inadequate or misleading information, and problems of communication within a relationship. Sexual partners are treated together and given basic information on methods of giving pleasure to each other and being honest about what actually gives pleasure. (This approach is relevant to all three nursing diagnoses mentioned previously.) A discreet set of sessions is prescribed which aims to teach partners about each other and associate sex with fun and relaxation through a set of exercises. Typically intercourse is forbidden at first and couples engage in body massage, focusing on areas which range from particularly pleasant to erotic, other than the genital areas. This is called non-genital sensate focusing, which requires that couples give time to each other, being non-demanding and relaxed. Genital massage is then planned and in this exercise partners learn mutually to masturbate while communicating on what is particularly arousing. Where necessary women are taught to squeeze the man's erect penis either to postpone ejaculation, when this is usually premature, or when the husband is fearful of not retaining or regaining his erection. In later sessions intercourse may occur in a controlled and gentle manner with the 'woman in control' or on top. Such a course of sessions is particularly indicated where couples are ill-informed or nervous, where the woman tends to lack satisfaction or the man has erection problems.

Rates of success vary with the skill of the counsellor or therapist, simplicity of the problem, but above all commitment of the partners to adhere to advice. In Meyer et al's (1975) study of 52 couples presenting for sex therapy 16 were treated by Masters and Johnson's therapy over 10 weeks (not in the intense 2-week course that they have devised). There was 'improvement' or 'marked improvement' in half of them, equivocal results in one-third and deterioration in three couples after this 10-week period.

Despite Masters and Johnson's (1970) reports of very high success rates, outcome studies vary according to homogeneity of problems and interventions and measures used to follow up patients. One study dealing with anorgasmic women, for instance, combined other techniques with the behavioural desensitisation and found after 20 to 22 sessions, that 60% of women with secondary anorgasmia were achieving orgasm for over half the episodes of coitus after treatment (Munjack et al, 1976). Some recent reviews tend to show that the majority of problems without organic cause can be cured for good (see Bancroft, 1983).

Kaplan's (1974) most readable book on a slightly more eclectic mode of therapy is a great contribution to the literature. Her application of psychotherapy to help couples understand each other, in combination with desensitising routines, seems most convincing. She claims that 80% of patients with the complete range of sexual problems can be relieved of symptoms without 'concomitant changes in basic personality structure or of the fundamental dynamics of the marital relationship' (p. 190). Essentially Kaplan views her therapy as 'a type of crisis intervention which presents an opportunity for rapid conflict resolution' (p. 199). Evaluations show that premature ejaculation can be cured in an average time of 6.5 sessions, while vaginismus usually takes 10. Sensate focusing is seen as essential:

1. to alleviate the couple's anxiety about physical intimacy and closeness,
2. to counteract the defensive avoidance of sensuous and erotic feelings, and
3. to break the pattern of excessive preoccupation with orgasm and performance and lack of awareness of pleasure.

Positive sexual experience encouraged in these 'controlled' or prescribed sessions is said to dispel fears about and anticipation of injury, failure or rejection which might have hampered the relationship (Kaplan, 1974). Functioning well on even one occasion is used as a positive experience on which to build confidence and skills. Reassurance to talk about and enjoy sex, or to be told to forgo coitus for a time, or to use fantasy or a vibrator can be all that is necessary to help those who are having problems. For instance impotence, which is perhaps the most common problem, is often due to anxiety although the foci or reasons for this vary. Overriding aims of treatments are to alleviate anxiety and prevent its occurrence. Cooper (1971) has shown that brief symptom-focused treatment is superior to lengthy insight therapies for erection problems. As previously stated, for women, orgastic inhibition or insufficient arousal can be the most common problem for which relaxation, maximal clitoral stimulation and gradual build up exercises to non-demand coitus are indicated. Kaplan has rarely failed to alleviate this problem. Likewise with vaginismus Masters and Johnson and Kaplan report total success with gradual clitoral and sexual sensitivity exercises.

These therapists have not indicated group therapy, sexual matters being seen as private and intimate. However those without partners may also well have problems and wish to discuss them. Women in particular have recently become more open and willing to share problems. Webb (1985) describes group sessions for 'pre-orgasmic' women who are taught to become more aware of their own anatomy, sensations and reactions to stimulation. Apparently, this is found to be a successful and supportive medium for them, although it has not been formally evaluated in terms of orgasmic success.

Although nurses have not been particularly active in this area of research, their rationale for practice should explore all the principles on which sex therapy is based. Their contribution to the literature on sexual problems reflects a holistic view of health, frequently in the context of recovery from major illness. As this is the subject of Chapter 2, only a few specific points will be made here.

When discussing sexual problems among people who have had cancer, interventions are prescribed by Carpenito (1983) but little evaluative work has systematically assessed how these affect a patient. She suggests that sharing feelings of shock and anger should be encouraged and role play possibly used to anticipate how a patient may react to the partner at home or, particularly, in intimate situations. However, constructive suggestions for sexual activity with a changed body may need to be made by a nurse to help a patient realise that sex is still possible. All such interventions should be realistic and should explore the patient's strengths and resources. Possibilities for plastic surgery, prosthesis or acceptable coverage of certain drainage equipment should be investigated and effected early on. Professionals should never forget to mobilise other successfully rehabilitated patients to give helpful suggestions or share reactions and also aid the partner adjust to him or herself so they can achieve the confidence to provide reassurance and affection. Most authorities have agreed that a strong supportive partner and a previously fulfilling sex life will lead to a satisfactory recovery of self-concept and subsequent sexual relationship.

Open communication and feedback should be encouraged between the couple and reassurance given that as long as sex is comfortable and enjoyable for the patient it is a constructive way for them to confirm their love for each other. This in turn helps the patient to endure changes in self-concept or body image as discussed earlier. Fears of contamination or harming the patient should of course be allayed (Hogan, 1980, pp. 530–2). Any susceptibility to infection from the patient need not prevent active sex; the couple can engage in careful cleansing before or after and any danger of contamination should be prevented.

After surgery, even for benign conditions of the sexual organs, it has often seemed that many problems have been over-emphasised by some staff. For instance early rather misleading research on the effects of hysterectomy has led to nurses attempting to help women by providing controlled pre-hospital discharge advice to alleviate this supposed psychological morbidity (Webb and Wilson-Barnett, 1983). In patients treated for benign conditions it was found that of 76 women with a partner and sex life, 66 said that sex was the same or better after surgery. This was attributed to lack of either pain or concern for conception. For the few who reported that sex was worse, pain was said to be responsible in four cases and others cited a problem with their husband. In the study husbands were not included in any pre-hospital discharge talk and some were not found particularly supportive to women during the recovery period. Quite specific instructions to have sex after six weeks however were given to the women by surgeons. Similar findings were discussed by Krueger's team (1979), in which pre- and post-sexual adjustment were highly significantly correlated. Only 11% of this sample of 108 patients mentioned the nurse as supplying most useful information post-operatively although half these patients wrote comments urging nurses to adopt this role in discussing sexuality.

The intervention designed for the Webb and Wilson-Barnett study aimed to provide correct appraisals and understanding of anatomical changes and give women a clear picture of their ability to resume sex without being fertile, as soon as physical healing had occurred. Possible physical symptoms which could be expected were also explained to prevent unnecessary fearful reactions. Although women were very positive about this intervention and enjoyed asking questions there were no positive findings on their sexual readjustment or recovery four months later when compared to those who did not receive such information. This was partly accounted for by lack of morbidity and possible experimental design factors.

In research on patients with cardiac conditions nurses have been involved in providing interventions to prevent problems and encouraging active rehabilitation and sexual fulfilment. Such interventions tend to include a package of advice and supportive counselling, with information on how and when to resume sexual activity. Less vigorous intercourse, perhaps in a side-to-side position, may seem appropriate to begin with, usually after 6–8 weeks. But as long as this does not cause symptoms couples should feel secure enough to continue happily. However, sensible precautions of avoiding prior heavy meals, alcohol consumption or concurrent emotional excitement should be heeded. Uncomplicated myocardial infarction patients often tend to have nervous reactions when sex is recommended and may suffer impotence (Weiss and English, 1957) but now there is sufficient evidence to show that informative explanations can alleviate this problem (Thompson, 1980), although nurses are not generally providing this support in a systematic and planned way. Watts (1976) has devised clear guidelines for graduated sexual activity for post-coronary patients, which nurses can employ during teaching, incorporating many of Masters and Johnson's techniques and emphasising the warm up (foreplay) activities to help alleviate any possible circulatory problems which may impede erection.

PHYSICALLY HANDICAPPED PEOPLE

This group of people have been rather neglected despite their particular need for help in managing sexual relationships. In a survey for the association for Sexual Problems of the Disabled (SPOD) by Stewart (1975), it was found that 52% of such people experienced some sort of sexual problem. Such people suffer from strokes, cardiac problems, amputations and rheumatoid arthritis. Help in the form of a multi-disciplinary counselling team is available in some centres. For instance Stuckey and Dickerson (1979) report on a service which aims:

1. to provide awareness among hospital staff of possible sexual problems of such patients in their care,
2. to enable some staff to feel comfortable initiating discussion of sexual matters and where necessary make referrals to the counsellors,
3. to provide some staff with skills and knowledge to become counsellors dealing with the sexual problems of the disabled, and
4. to provide a resource centre for others.

Evaluation of the service, in which nurses also act as counsellors, has been informal. The educational methods, in particular a film and small group teaching process, have been found particularly helpful for patients.

In such programmes it is essential to assess levels of impairment by medical examination to provide realistic goals for treatment and activity. For spinal injury in particular, the level of lesion will determine sexual function, yet despite quadriplegia some people gain a great deal from bodily contact and sexual activity by using imagination and effort and with support from partners (Cole, 1975). Obviously the message for nurses is clear. Many patients seek to engage in sex, wish to talk about their problems and need encouragement and positive attitudes from professionals.

IMPLICATIONS FOR PRACTICE

Despite equivocal effects from counselling found in some studies, there is no doubt that many individuals and in particular patients and their partners need information and guidance on resuming sex post-illness or surgery. They appreciate this when it is provided and feel lost and rather helpless when it is not. As some are reticent about raising the subject themselves, nurses should do this and ensure discussion is carried out in a systematic and supportive way. The research evidence is clear that patients have this need.

NURSES AS SEX THERAPISTS

Recognising and being sensitive to people's needs for support, reassurance, guidance or advice on sexual matters is claimed to be an important role for the nurse (Webb, 1985; Eisenberg, 1980; Hogan, 1980). Some sexual problems or concerns can be resolved merely by providing the patient with accurate information couched in understandable language. Explanations on anatomy, methods of arousal and coital positions may be helpful to some (Eisenberg, 1980). Even though general sex education has improved in some schools one can never assume accurate understanding or utilisation of this. Eisenberg also advocates relaxation training as a useful technique which may be taught to patients or couples to help alleviate anxiety related to sexual intercourse.

However, there is grave concern that nurses are usually inadequately prepared to perform this role of sex counsellor or supporter, and particularly helpless when faced by those with physical handicap. In a review by Fisher (1985) several studies showed that specialist oncology nurses were lacking in relevant knowledge and skills to advise their patients. Nurses' attitudes and knowledge need to be explored and courses designed to make their attitudes more liberal and specific knowledge more relevant for this group of patients. Hogan (1980) reiterates these recommendations for all nurses. Even nursing instructors have been found to be aware of their own knowledge deficits and many schools in both the UK and USA are incorporating more sessions on sexuality into the basic curriculum. Other methods for effecting rapid education in this area have been advocated by Smith Santopietro (1980) who designed and evaluated a self-instructional module on human sexuality counselling for nurses with 161 students. Not only were impressive increases in knowledge achieved but also confidence in dealing with patient problems was significantly raised. Another competent guide, suitable for those applying principles in general practice, is provided by Hawton (1985).

FUTURE RESEARCH

Exploratory, descriptive and evaluative work is needed, such as:

1. Descriptive studies with different client and patient groups documenting sexual activity and problems.
2. Descriptive studies on patients' views about the nurse's role in sex counselling.
3. Comparative studies on ways of introducing sex counselling for hospitalised and follow-up patients with different health problems.

4. Evaluative studies on the effect of more systematic education for nurses on skills in discussing sexual matters with patients.
5. Evaluative research on nurse-run pre-discharge counselling for couples with a range of illness experiences.
6. Evaluative studies of nurse counsellors utilising behavioural sex therapy for clients in well-people clinics and for patients with declared sex problems in the general hospital setting.

REFERENCES

Bancroft J (1983) *Human Sexuality and its Problems*. Churchill Livingstone, Edinburgh.

Carpenito LJ (1983) *Nursing Diagnosis in Application to Clinical Practice*. JB Lippincott Co, Philadelphia.

Cole TM (1975) Sexuality and physical disabilities. *Archives of Sexual Behaviour* 4(4), 389–403.

Cooper AJ (1971) Treatment of male potency disorders: the present status. *Psychosomatics* 12(4), 235–244.

Dalton K (1957) Discussion on the aftermath of hysterectomy and oopherectomy. *Proceedings of the Royal Society of Medicine* 50, 415–422.

Derogatis LR (1980) Breast and gynaecologic cancers: their unique impact on body image and sexual identity in women. In (Ed) Vaeth JM, *Frontiers of Radiation Therapy and Oncology*. Karger, Basel.

Eisenberg MD (1980) Therapeutic approaches to counselling. In: Hogan RM (ed) *Human Sexuality: a Nursing Perspective* pp. 275–294. Appleton Century Crofts, New York.

Fisher SG (1985) The sexual knowledge and attitudes of oncology nurses: implications for nursing education. *Seminars in Oncology Nursing* 1(1), 63–68.

Gath D (1980) Psychiatric aspects of hysterectomy. In: Robins L, Clayton P, Wing J (eds) *The Social Consequences of Psychiatric Illness* pp. 33–45. Brunner/Mazel Inc., New York.

Hawton K (1985) *Sex Therapy: A Practical Guide*. Oxford University Press, London.

Hellerstein HK, Friedman EH (1970) Sexual activity and the post-coronary patient. *Archives of Internal Medicine* 125, 991.

Hite S (1976) *The Hite Report*. Macmillan, New York.

Hogan RM (1980) *Human Sexuality: A Nursing Perspective*. Appleton Century Crofts, New York.

Krueger JC, Hassell J, Coggins DB, Ishimatsu T, Pabulo MR, Tuttle EJ (1979) Relationship between nurse counselling and sexual adjustment after hysterectomy. *Nursing Research* 28(3), 145.

Kaplan HS (1974) *The New Sex Therapy*. Brunner/Mazel Publications and Quadrangle, New York.

Kinsey AC, Pomeroy WB, Martin CE, Gebhard PH (1953) *Sexual Behaviour in the Human Female*. WB Saunders, Philadelphia.

Lamb MA (1985) Sexual dysfunction and the gynaecological oncology patient. *Seminars in Oncology Nursing* 1(1), 9–17.

Lion EM (1982) (ed) *Human Sexuality in the Nursing Process*. John Wiley & Sons, New York.

Masters M, Johnson V (1966) *Human Sexual Response*. Little Brown, Boston.

Masters M, Johnson V (1970) *Human Sexual Inadequacy*. Little Brown, Boston.

McCary JL (1973). *Human Sexuality*. Van Nostrand, New York.

Meyer JK, Schmidt CW, Lucas MJ, Smith E (1975) Short-term treatment of sexual problems: interim report. *American Journal of Psychiatry* 132(2), 172–176.

Munjack D, Cristol A, Goldstein A, Philips D, Goldberg A, Whipple K, Staples F, Kanno P (1976) Behavioural treatment of organic dysfunction: a controlled study. *British Journal of Psychiatry* 129, 497–502.

Puhaty HD (1977) Confronting one's changed image, two rehabilitative approaches. *American Journal of Nursing* 77, 1437.

Raphael B (1978) Psychiatric aspects of hysterectomy. In: Howells JG (ed) *Modern Perspectives in the Psychiatric Aspects of Surgery*. Macmillan, London.

Schilder P (1950) *The Image and Appearance of the Human Body*. International Universities Press, New York.

Smith Santopietro M-C (1980) Effectiveness of a self-instructional module in human sexuality counselling. *Nursing Research* **29**(1), 14–19.

Stewart WFR (1975) *Sex and the Physically Handicapped*. National Fund for Research into Crippling Diseases, Horsham, Sussex.

Stuckey N, Dickerson M (1979) Sex counselling and the disabled. *British Journal of Sexual Medicine* **June**, 45–48.

Thompson DR (1980) Sexual activity following acute myocardial infarction in the male. *Nursing Times* **November 6**, 1965–1967.

Watts RJ (1976) Sexuality and the middle-aged cardiac patient. *Nursing Clinics of North America* **11**, 357.

Weisse E, English OS (1957) *Psychosomatic Medicine* p. 216, 3rd Edition, Saunders, Philadelphia.

Webb C, Wilson-Barnett J (1983) Self-concept, social support and hysterectomy. *International Journal of Nursing Studies* **20**(2), 97–107.

Webb C (1985) *Sexuality Nursing and Health*. John Wiley & Sons, Chichester.

Chapter 7
Urinary Incontinence

As an embarrassing, socially isolating and debilitating problem incontinence requires major careful study and intervention. Its widespread occurrence in those of most age groups, its personal and taboo nature and importance to patients and their families has led to much research by nurses and others. Although, as always, more needs to be done there are several clinical studies which give indications for methods of preventing and treating urinary incontinence.

NURSING DIAGNOSES

Voith and Smith (1985) attempted to gain agreement on a classification system for urinary incontinence by asking nurses about its aetiology, management and occurrence. They devised and validated four 'diagnoses'.

1. Stress incontinence. Urine is lost involuntarily when intra-abdominal pressure exceeds urethral pressure.
2. Urge incontinence. Involuntary urination occurs soon after a strong sense of urgency to void.
3. Reflex incontinence. This occurs as a spinal cord reflex in a predictable pattern.
4. Uncontrolled incontinence. Urine control is lost below the spinal reflex arc resulting in an unpredictable or continuous loss of urine.

Norton (1986a) explains that urgency, frequency, nocturia and nocturnai enuresis are usually symptoms of an unstable bladder (detrusor instability). Other (diagnoses) problems (excluding stress incontinence) suggest incompetence of the urethral sphincter.

CONTINENCE AND THE CAUSES OF URINARY INCONTINENCE

As the bladder fills, sensory messages are relayed to the cerebral cortex (part of the frontal lobe). Awareness and inhibition of micturition by motor impulses occurs until voiding is 'possible' in the conventional place. Micturition is made possible when the inhibitory mechanism is released, the bladder contracts and completely empties. Contraction of the bladder occurs simultaneously with sphincter relaxation. In the normal healthy state, adults usually void six or seven times a day. They also have the capacity to do this in the absence of any sensation of fullness (Norton, 1986a).

In discussing causes of incontinence Norton (1986a)* divides these into three categ-ories: physiological bladder dysfunction, factors directly influencing bladder functioning and factors affecting the individual's ability to cope with bladder function.

Physiological dysfunction

This includes:

1. Detrusor instability leading to frequency, urgency and urge incontinence due to involuntary contractions of the bladder during filling. Inhibitory impulses have been destroyed, although sensation is present. Instability may also occur due to neuro-logical deterioration in old age.
2. Genuine stress incontinence upon physical exertion, due to an incompetent urethral sphincter mechanism.
3. Outflow obstruction which leads to overflow or dribbling incontinence. Obstruction in the urethra from stricture, spasm, or external pressure (prostatic enlargement) is most usual. Persistence of this problem may result in an atonic bladder.
4. Atonic bladder or inadequate contraction of the muscle results in residual urine leading to infections, and sometimes overflow and frequency.

Factors influencing bladder function

1. Urinary tract infection may occur in someone with bladder dysfunction and by compounding this, cause incontinence. Frequency and dysuria accompany most urinary infections.
2. Faecal impaction, leading to voiding difficulty, may act as an obstruction to outflow. It may also weaken the pelvic floor, inhibiting contraction. This problem is often found among the elderly and immobile, on a poor diet.
3. Norton (1986a) also mentions other factors such as sedatory drugs which blunt bladder sensations, endocrine imbalance and other bladder pathologies.

Factors affecting ability to cope with bladder function

1. Immobility (for whatever cause) may lead to an inability to cope with a mild or potential bladder condition, resulting in urge incontinence. Hence many people rely on a commode nearby and become excessively anxious without this.
2. Environmental factors, linked to mobility problems, include poor eyesight and inad-equate toilet facilities.
3. Disturbed cognition or emotions may lead to unacceptable behaviour of many kinds as well as incontinence. Most sufferers can however be encouraged and motivated to be continent.
4. 'Carers' are given as Norton's last category of causal factors. Without due attention and care to promoting continence, many vulnerable people may no longer be able to cope with a potential problem.

For further information on the causes, assessment and treatment of incontinence,

* The author acknowledges Christine Norton's extensive work in this area, for this introductory section.

readers are strongly recommended to augment the information in this chapter by studying Christine Norton's (1986c) book *Nursing for Continence*.

PREVALENCE OF URINARY INCONTINENCE

Due to difficulties in defining incontinence and individuals' reluctance to mention the problem, true prevalence is difficult to ascertain. Different rates are therefore calculated. Research by Thomas et al (1980) with 22,430 people contacted by postal questionnaire, found that 6.9% of males over 65 years suffered from an involuntary loss of urine twice or more per month. For females percentages increased with age from 5.1% for those aged 5–14 years, 8.5% for those between 15 and 64 years and 11.6% for those over 65. These researchers also conducted interviews and showed that 22% of those regularly incontinent required pads and extra laundry and were very restricted in activities, frequently needing others to help in dealing with this problem. Lack of identification of many such cases of hardship by local services was also documented.

This study showed that incontinence is certainly not only a problem for the elderly, although its frequency increases with age. This was also highlighted by an in-patient hospital population census by Egan et al (1983) which found high rates of incontinence. Five to seven per cent of all hospital patients aged between 5 and 64 years and 18–21% of those over 65 are incontinent. For general wards the average prevalence was 9–10%.

For the general population many problems can be prevented for both young people (particularly women) and the elderly if due care and consideration is taken. Stress incontinence, suffered by 30% of young women at least occasionally and 50% of those over 50 years of age, is preventable or treatable by correct posture and pelvic floor exercise (Blannin, 1985). Yet thousands fail to report this and, when they do, receive unsympathetic responses from their doctors. So many mothers do not apparently realise the importance of postnatal exercises in preventing this problem.

ASSESSMENT

Careful assessment of the problem is required, as always, to arrive at an accurate diagnosis. One study evaluating methods for assessment by Robb (1985) found that most clients can record their 'amount' and 'frequency' of urination. An absorbent pad can be worn for 60 minutes as a screening test and if dry a three-day record chart can be employed to detect infrequent involuntary urine loss. This three-day record was found to be as reliable as charting for seven days.

Charting episodes of micturition and of incontinence is especially important for the diagnosis and management of incontinence as Robb (1985) and Norton (1986a) suggest. Hourly records should be completed, possibly with different coloured pens to indicate continence, incontinence or no voiding (see Table 1). A normal daily diary of micturition can then be devised indicating the frequency of incontinence and usual times for voiding.

Table 1. Criteria for Assessing Urinary Incontinence

Criteria	Methods
Severity—volume 'lost'	Patient or relative reports. Pads—supplied kept in plastic bag— weighed before and after set period of time.
—frequency and situation of occurrence	Diary or chart should be kept to monitor incontinence and normal voiding.
Physical status/problems	Physical examination e.g. for constipation, procidentia, mobility. Use Norton's assessment tool (see Appendix 1).
Environmental factors	Assess home or hospital for barriers to reaching the toilet.
Perception of problem	Interview patient about incontinence regarding understanding, distress, depression, practical and financial effects.

However, Norton (1986a) reinforces the need for urodynamic investigations (cystometry) to reach accurate diagnoses, as well as a full assessment of other related factors, as included in her assessment check-list (Appendix 1). Bowels, (possible impaction), mobility, eyesight, understanding and diet should all be assessed for possible causes of incontinence. Proximity of toilets should also be reviewed, and their signposting and availability should always be sufficient when assessing incontinence and preventing this for any patient group.

Although initial assessment may be done by nurses prior to referral to a more specialised team, it is possible to gain pertinent information and sometimes prevent further intractable problems by quite straightforward measures related to the criteria in Table 1. Obvious problems (like constipation or distance to the toilet) may be overcome.

For those being cared for in an institution, it may also be relevant to assess staff motivation and knowledge on this subject.

STRESS INCONTINENCE (see Table 2, section 1)

Weakening of the pelvic floor muscles through childbirth, injury or surgery may result in involuntary loss of urine at times of increased abdominal pressure, caused by such activities as coughing, running or laughing.

Goals

Alleviation of this bothersome problem is possible with strong motivation and participation by the afflicted individual. As treatment is directed towards muscle retraining, it may take several weeks to resolve, but improvement may be noted in 3–4 weeks.

Table 2. Identification of Different Types of Urinary Incontinence

Criteria	Measures and findings	Diagnosis
Severity	Small quantities. During running, coughing.	Stress incontinence.
Physical/environment	Poor muscle tone related to birth of second child—('too busy to do exercises').	
Perception	Understands aetiology. Distressed as it inhibits much social and sporting activity.	
Severity	Use Norton's interview schedule. Large amounts frequently lost. Pads worn, 5 daily Chart shows 5 days—clear pattern for micturition (see Appendix 2). Can hold for 2 minutes.	Urge incontinence (elderly resident in a rest home).
Physical	Slightly stiff and slow to move.	
Environmental	Toilet two rooms away—although clearly marked.	
Perception	Distressed and nervous. History shows long-term urgency, but worsened since admitted. Motivated and orientated, 'try anything'.	
Severity	Use Norton's interview schedule. Constant—catheter has been tried. Sometimes manages to express. No muscle tone, cystometric tests conclusive.	Uncontrolled incontinence (e.g. young, female multiple sclerosis victim).
Physical	Wheelchair bound, but good arm and hand co-ordination.	
Environmental	Extensive modifications already made. Clean environment and special bathroom.	
Perception	Well adjusted—eager to avoid pads and odours, has tried self-catheterisation once.	

Nursing interventions

Well-tried interventions of muscle tensing exercises (say four times each hour) may prevent this postnatally and resolve this in sufferers. In addition to this Montgomery (1986) advises that these muscles can be tensed in anticipation of activities which usually cause leakage. The writer advocates a set of progressive exercises involving the perineal and pelvic floor muscle group—contraction is practised for progressively longer periods. Correct posture with pelvis not tilted forward (as sometimes occurs in the obese) is also encouraged. Younger women may regain control in 2–3 weeks whereas older women may need to persist for months. Blannin (1985) also advises that all women should practise exercises when voiding by stopping midstream and intentionally moderating urine stream to strengthen future control.

Several successful evaluative studies of sessions for women taught by physiotherapists or nurses have been published (e.g. Kegal, 1951; Harrison, 1975) but it needs initial care to ensure that women really do these exercises correctly. Both individual and group instruction has been demonstrated with successful results for a majority of subjects.

URGE INCONTINENCE (see Table 2, section 2)

Usually occurring in the elderly, more often when cared for in institutions, this problem is heightened by anxiety that there is insufficient time to reach the lavatory. This is both preventable and treatable. Therefore, another professional indictment is earned when services and care of the institutionalised elderly are reviewed. Millard (1986), for instance, states that lack of facilities is the commonest cause for incontinence in the elderly in hospitals. Patients seem to be encouraged to become incontinent from insufficient help. Because patients are unable to find or reach the lavatory or do not receive assistance quickly enough incontinence develops. Sat on pads, without knickers or decent clothes, it would appear staff are expecting incontinence. Inadequate staff, improper dress necessiting draped blankets, and overcrowded facilities also encourage this problem. All this contrasts with the picture of most elderly people living at home having *not* lost control of their bladder.

Goals

Specific goals to ameliorate incontinence of this type are set in conjunction with retraining programmes. With well-orientated and motivated individuals the problem may be substantially reduced in the course of one week. It may take slightly longer to restore continence if there are other problems of immobility, poor facilities or disorientation and lack of understanding. Primary goals for enabling the person to recognise and respond appropriately to the need to void and reach the toilet promptly need to be understood by that individual and others who care for her.

Rationale for nursing interventions for urge incontinence

The incidence of incontinence in institutions is higher than for those at home (Millard, 1986). The unfamiliar, stressful and often thoughtless barriers to managing a visit to the lavatory must be removed to avoid the problem. Nurses are responsible for maintaining a safe comfortable environment and should use every method possible to stimulate and orientate the residents. This has been shown to reduce incontinence (Storss, 1982). Effective, dignified and scientific practice is possible with the growing body of research which should guide both prevention and treatment measures.

Specific interventions

Bladder training

Little research has evaluated the best methods of 'bladder training', but a majority of those with bladder instability are usually helped by this sort of approach. For instance Jarvis and Millar (1980) achieved an 80% success rate for their patients. They were given a careful explanation of their condition and by keeping a chart were encouraged to extend intervals gradually between visits to the lavatory. An alternative to this approach by a nurse, Clay (1978), was called habit retraining. In a small study with elderly patients she found greater success when nurses charted patients' own natural pattern of diuresis for a few days and then prevented incontinence by facilitating visits just before these times to regain 'habit'. She was successful as long as a pattern was observed and re-established.

As Norton (1986a) says, individualised patterns for guiding people to use the lavatory at appropriate times are much more likely to be successful than bladder drill or two hourly 'potting'.

Biofeedback

Autonomic functions can be brought under voluntary control by using techniques of biofeedback. This approach may be useful for urge or urgency incontinence which results in detrusor instability. Cardozo et al (1978) used auditory and visual feedback of bladder pressures to successfully treat female patients during 4–8 hour sessions. Changes in pressures indicated by monitors were associated with changes in bladder sensations, patients being taught to inhibit such sensations. However, this intervention is only possible when specialists and monitoring equipment are available. It is possibly only appropriate when other more routine 'training' approaches have been employed without success, and then only for particular patients.

UNCONTROLLED INCONTINENCE (see Table 2, section 3)

In those who have not learned to urinate in a lavatory, for instance the mentally handicapped or those who have local neurological cerebrospinal or muscular defects, uncontrolled incontinence results.

Approaches and goals for nursing interventions will vary according to the cause of the problem. For those who cannot be trained to void a few measures are usually available, but if these fail, appliances and sometimes catheterisation are advised.

Goals

For those with physiological deficits (neurogenic bladder) methods such as simple pressure on the lower abdomen or auditory cues (running water) may help but may also take weeks to perfect.

Lengthy training approaches are often required for this problem. With the mentally handicapped, programmes may take months, but they are usually completely successful as long as correct behaviour is constantly reinforced.

Rationale for nursing interventions

There is little research relating to nursing care of the physically handicapped, but experienced practice shows that when the bladder cannot be 'trained' as for some patients with cerebrospinal damage, patients may be helped to anticipate needs themselves and encourage voiding by certain trigger mechanisms such as stimulation or pressure. However, Norton (1986a) concludes that effecting methods of self-catheterisation for these problems is the most significant advance for such patients. (Catheterisation will be discussed at length below.) Careful advice and patient help for those learning these techniques is necessary.

Behaviour therapy

Tierney's (1973) study with mentally handicapped children demonstrated how these techniques could be used for groups of incontinent patients who were totally untrained. By careful reinforcement and encouragement of each step of the procedure of voiding in the toilet Tierney showed that an instructional group could become 'dry' as long as staff were co-operative and continuous therapy was applied. Such treatment can take several weeks but once successful can be the major factor in providing a more liberated, varied and stimulating life for individuals. It may even mean that more general education becomes possible. A typical model for this intervention is shown in Table 3.

Table 3. Model for Shaping Toilet Behaviour

Final target behaviour	Patient goes to the toilet independently	Patient removes his clothing independently	Patient sits down on the toilet independently	Patient eliminates only in the toilet and is otherwise continent
Intermediate target behaviour	Patient asks to go to the toilet	Patient removes or actively attempts to remove some of his clothing	Patient is helped to sit down on the toilet and sits unrestrained	Patient eliminates in the toilet regularly and has only infrequent episodes of incontinence
	Patient indicates his need to eliminate	Patient actively assists when clothing is removed by nurse	Patient is placed on the toilet and sits unrestrained	Patient has established some regularity and uses toilet more frequently than is incontinent
Base target	Patient is taken to toilet by nurse	Patient co-operates passively when clothing is removed by nurse	Patient is placed on toilet and is restrained to sit	Patient uses toilet when placed on it but is incontinent at all other times

From Christine Norton's chapter Training for urinary continence. In *Patient Teaching*. Edited by J Wilson-Barnett, Churchill Livingstone, Edinburgh, p. 166. Reproduced with kind permission of the author and publisher.

Various other studies have modified the approach, setting up rewards for such individuals, particularly for those with a mental handicap. Both nurses and psychologists have been active in designing programmes (see Norton, 1983). Such approaches of reward or punishment may also be applied to enuresis (Barker, 1979). Patients may be made to get out of bed and strip and remake their own bed when wet or alternatively incidents may be prevented by waking them prior to the usual time for such incidents. Apparently the first approach is most effective.

PRACTICAL IMPLICATIONS FOR THE MANAGEMENT OF INCONTINENCE

Even when these techniques are employed and every precaution is taken incontinence may persist. Norton's (1986c) text explains all the details of training and management for nurses who need to be aware of the most suitable aids and cleaning materials to use. Norton (1986a) suggests that these should be chosen for the individual: leakage often occurs and correct sizing and application are vital. Trial and (hopefully not) error is necessary. Unlimited use of disposable paper bed sheets should be avoided (wet and chaffing material soon lead to skin excoriation). Smith (1979) advises that Kylie sheets which are washable yet have a 'stay dry' surface are preferable. Trials of pads and pants are inconclusive, no one type being efficient for all patients (Shepherd and Blannin, 1980).

Any solution or material constantly applied to a skin surface may result in soreness or allergic reaction. Male appliances are perhaps more technically satisfactory and cheaper than pads. Yet dexterity and care is still needed to maintain this system. Condoms are said to be preferred to specially designed appliances (Norton, 1986a).

However, for the two-thirds of elderly incontinent patients who are female, constant washing and changing of pads may still be necessary. Trials of cleaning materials have been carried out in an effort to maintain a healthy skin condition. A trial by Willington et al (1981) for those who are faecally incontinent found a non-ionic detergent was preferable. Yet barrier creams may still be required to maintain skin integrity (Reid, 1974).

Ultimately, it may be necessary to catheterise patients if all other measures are unsuccessful and skin excoriation becomes severe. This is a major intervention which requires careful consideration.

CATHETERISATION OF THE BLADDER

Short-term

Inserting a sterile tube to drain urine from the bladder is a potentially dangerous procedure only indicated for those requiring particular types of surgery for accurate measurements of urine output, and for those with problems of acute retention or long-standing untreatable incontinence. It may be associated with infection, trauma and pain (Roe, 1985). This procedure is commonly undertaken by female nurses for female patients but male nurses or doctors are thought more suitable for undertaking catheterisation of males, although this arrangement may be questioned as unnecessary by some (Fader, 1986).

Infection and loss of bladder tone caused by inserting a catheter or retaining one is of grave concern to many, so research comparing the use and effects of different types of catheter for different periods, or the application of certain disinfectants prior to or during the procedure, is important. For instance, the effect of short-term catheterisation was investigated for patients scheduled for cardiac surgery by Jacques et al (1986). They found that there was no disadvantage to keeping a catheter in situ for 48 hours instead of 24 hours over the peri-operative period. Patients in different experimental groups voided similar amounts after removal of the catheter in the first or second post-operative day and they appeared to have generally less discomfort in re-establishing micturition on the second day. Neither group had any incidence of urinary infection. A similar lack of difference was found in regaining normal micturition after catheterisation in a small exploratory study by Williamson (1982). Catheters were removed without clamping for one group of surgical patients. Whereas clamping off the catheter for 3 hours and then releasing for 5 minutes (termed reconditioning treatment) was done for 9 hours for the other experimental group prior to removal of Foley's catheters. No significant differences in amounts of residual urine were found in the experimental group. The small number of patients (8) and the short period for total reconditioning may have influenced these results. This practice has therefore still not been indicated by research findings.

Long-term

Various parameters have been assessed as indicators for practice when dealing with catheters in the long-term, i.e. over several weeks. These usually concern infection rates but leakage, convenience and cost have also been considered as relevant to the evaluation of nursing care.

Nursing practice varies quite substantially between different hospitals and between hospital and community care. Kennedy and Brocklehurst (1982) surveyed 101 nurses in the hospital or home care setting to identify common problems with long-term indwelling catheters. Apart from very varied practice and advice given by this sample of senior nurses they found that infection and leakage were a great problem for a majority of patients. These nurses invariably expressed confusion and lack of knowledge on ways to cope with problems arising from catheterisation. In conclusion the researchers considered that some patients were catheterised needlessly and as a consequence suffered much indignity. Poor supply networks also resulted in inappropriate use of some catheters.

In a further detailed study of those requiring long-term catheters by Kennedy et al (1983) different problems were found for hospital and community. More hospital patients' problems were associated with larger catheters and being female, and the community sample factors were associated with frequent (daily) bag changing, immobility and use of very large (200 ml) drainage bags for bed attachment. Leakage, blockage, irrigation problems, irritation and offensive smell were frequently mentioned by patients. Researchers concluded from this study that:

> 'use of silicone catheters with small diameters left in situ for as long as possible, less frequent changing of drainage bags and mobilisation of patients whenever possible are suggested policies which may go a long way towards alleviating many of the problems discussed.' (p. 211)

However, careful experimental work does not uphold some of these recommendations for those patients in hospital.

INFECTION

It has been estimated that approximately 10% of patients admitted to hospital will have a urethral catheter inserted (Kunin, 1979) and research has indicated high infection rates as a consequence of this. The longer catheters remain in situ, the higher the risk of infection. Garibaldi et al (1980) found that each day the risk increased by 8.1% for their sample of 405 catheterised patients, and 50% were infected after the tenth day. This also increases the length of stay for post-operative subjects. Givens and Wenzel (1980) calculated a delay of 2–4 days.

Routes of infection are created during introduction of the catheter, through the peri-urethral space from the perineum, and via the drainage tube (Wilson and Roe, 1986). Each of these will now be considered with the implications and evidence for how infection can be avoided.

Garibaldi et al (1980) recorded 7.4% of infections were established within 24 hours of introducing the catheter, imperfect catheterisation techniques accounting for this. Ward catheterisations were found to be more likely to be associated with subsequent early infection (42.9%) when compared to the 10% rate for catheterisation in the operating room in a sample of 70 patients studied prospectively by Castle and Osterhout (1974). Introduction of a catheter into the bladder in an *aseptic* way is certainly not responsible for introducing infection. As Turck and Stamm (1981) explain, these are easily eliminated by antibacterial activity of the bladder wall or by voiding. Even infection rates of 6.9% after repeated aseptic instrumentation suggest that this alone cannot be accountable (Coyle and Macdonald, 1967).

Interventions to prevent infection

Attempts to reduce procedure-related infection have led to the application of antiseptic solutions/gels into the urethra prior to catheterisation. This has been found to be successful in a controlled study of 100 women, 50 of whom were treated with polymixin B as a urethral lubricant prior to catheterisation, while a matched control group of 50 were not. A significant reduction in the infection rate was established, seven experimental subjects contracting infections compared with 22 controls (Chavigny, 1975). Before this Gillespie et al (1962) also demonstrated, in a controlled study, advantages of using chlorhexidine to disinfect the urethra prior to catheterisation. Perineal disinfection has also been claimed as important (Wilson and Roe, 1986). However, the general consensus is that the benefit of prophylactic administration of antibiotics as a protective agent is transient and is accompanied by resistance (Kostiala et al, 1982).

The risk of infection on introduction of a catheter has to be weighed against the increasing risk with each additional day it remains in situ. Evidence is still incomplete although Lapides et al (1975) found that a particular group of patients with neurogenic bladder benefited from a repeated in-out procedure rather than an indwelling catheter.

On the basis of carefully reviewed research evidence, to prevent infection as a consequence of the catheterisation procedure, Wilson and Roe (1986, p. 90) advise that the environment should be clean and well lit, preferably a theatre or treatment room, handwashing and the performance of an aseptic procedure with minimal trauma is essential, and skin disinfectants, urethral lubricants and local anaesthetic should be used. The date, type and size of catheter and volume of water used to blow up the balloon should be documented.

Many studies evaluating catheter toilet and meatal cleansing have been carried out but findings are inconclusive. For instance Gibbs (1986) reported a small study comparing patients who received catheter care regularly with those who did not. This procedure was done twice daily aseptically using cetrimide solution to clean the meatus and adjacent area wearing sterile gloves. This did not provide any evidence that this prevented infections in either men or women. In contrast Seal et al (1982) found that combining daily cleansing of the meatal-catheter junction with chlorhexidine solution and applying chlorhexidine cream from a personal tube decreased the incidence of expected infections. Cleland (1977) compared four types of perineal cleansing in randomly divided groups of a sample of 184. In this highly controlled study no differences were found when compared to patients' own toilet. Wilson and Roe (1986) conclude that until further evidence exists meatal cleaning should occur once a day unless specially indicated when it should be more often. Special clean cloths are needed, hands should be washed rigorously or gloves should be worn, and thorough drying is indicated.

Drainage of urine

A closed system of drainage is obviously necessary but even this does not prevent infection, as rates of 23% were found by Newman and Price (1977) on a sample of patients for whom long-term closed drainage was used. Opening the system to drain or irrigate allows contamination. Gillespie et al (1967) showed that using bags which could be emptied rather than those which always required changing and replacing, halved the infection rate from the previous 53% to 23%. Sealed connections on drainage tubes which reduce the need to disconnect the system also halved the infection rate from 27% to 10% in a study by Platt et al (1982). Care with drainage equipment is necessary. Backflow and bubbles can transport bacteria up into the bladder (Roberts et al, 1965). Changing bags or emptying them can be associated with contamination of urine on to the hands. This procedure should be done wearing gloves. Scrupulous hand washing is also necessary.

Bags may also harbour and culture bacteria. In a controlled study to reduce this effect Islam and Chapman (1977) compared bags changed daily with those which were not changed but emptied and instilled with 10 ml of chlorhexidine. Once more no significant differences were noted. The 'daily change' routine was associated with infection of 30.4% and the chlorhexidine treatment with 33.3%.

Bladder irrigation as a prophylactic measure is also contraindicated from recent research (Dudley and Barriere, 1981). Breaking the closed system in order to administer washouts is also consistently disapproved of by microbiologists and other researchers (see Roe, 1985). If absolutely necessary to relieve blockage this should be done via a three-way tap to avoid breaking the seal.

Choice of size and type of catheter has also been found to affect both comfort and infection rates. Barnes and Malone Lee (1986) in a study devoted to this subject found that silicone-coated latex catheters remained patent with balloons inflated better than others, even the 100% silicone catheters which have been preferred by others. Catheters that are too large can lead to urethral damage and do not prevent (as some nurses think) but rather cause leakage. Choice should depend on length of time in situ and whether or not clots or debris will be passed (Jenner, 1983). Kennedy et al (1983) found great confusion among nurses on choice of catheters. They tended to precipitate problems by inserting catheters that were too large which caused leakage and blockage. Larger balloons may also cause bladder spasm which causes leakage. Small-sized catheters (12–18 Charrière) with balloon sizes of 5–10 ml are indicated to prevent these problems.

Implications for nursing practice

All these studies provide valuable evidence, although some need to be confirmed. Practice to prevent injury and infection can be based on findings now available and Gooch (1986) summarises in a clinical article, the risks of infection as open drainage systems, cross-infection through contact with careless handling of the bag and tubing, over-distension of bladder causing ischaemia of the bladder wall (therefore, avoid blockage or kinking of the tube), over-zealous cleansing of the meatal opening, holding the bag and tubing above the level of the bladder, bladder washouts, low urine output, and pH values below or above 6–7.

Positive recommendations for research-based practice would include:

1. Where possible catheterise in an operating room or separate 'treatment' room.
2. Apply a scrupulous aseptic technique with the use of an antiseptic gel or cream, i.e. polymixin B introduced into the urethra prior to catheterisation.
3. Do not clamp catheters (in short or long term).
4. Always have a good selection of different sized catheters between 12 and 18, never larger. Silicone-coated latex catheters are found to be best for indwelling long-term use.
5. For those with neurogenic bladders in-out (where possible self-catheterisation) rather than indwelling is safest.
6. Meatal cleansing once a day is indicated with clean materials, more is not needed unless particularly indicated.
7. Closed drainage systems are required. Do not break any seals and use bags which require emptying rather than changing.
8. Bladder irrigation is not indicated to prevent infection; if required as treatment, only do this using a three-way tap.

Discomfort and harm can be caused by catheterisation. It is often necessary but can be associated with great risk. Great attention to research is necessary to provide scientifically valid care. This should be combined with great sensitivity to the personal feelings of patients who have to tolerate bags and tubes. Methods for safe transport of these should be devised and disguised. Yet it seems from this review that more attention to instituting careful interventions to prevent both incontinence and the need for catheterisation is almost a greater challenge for the nursing profession than building on the substantial research evidence that exists. Changing routinised or ritualised care for the elderly by innovative schemes could be seen as a goal for clinicians, researchers and managers and therefore comes top of the list for future studies.

OVERALL NURSING POLICY FOR DEALING WITH THE PROBLEM OF URINARY INCONTINENCE

The enormous impact of urinary incontinence on individuals and the health services has led many to advocate a far more vigorous effort to educate both the lay public and doctors and nurses in preventing and coping with this problem. For instance, Isaacs (1979) proposes a specialist nurse as incontinence adviser, to act as a change agent. He or she could identify areas of need, liaise with the hospital and community services, provide updating courses and allay the general misconceived acceptance of incontinence as a long-term problem which cannot be prevented or improved. Likewise Friend, then Chief Nursing Officer (1977) for England, issued a letter urging nurse managers to appoint or designate nursing officers to become expert on incontinence aids and other resources to support patients and their families at home and in hospital. As a result there are presently over 40 nurse specialists in England (Norton, 1986a).

Research questions must be considered carefully, for despite a substantial literature there is still a great need for clear answers, as Norton (1986b) so rightly says:

'Research has suffered because too many studies have asked overly simplistic questions for an inherently complex and individualistic problem.' (p. 55)

FUTURE RESEARCH

In this vital area much more knowledge is needed, and studies may be rated thus:

1. Action research to evaluate change in routinised care to that which promotes continence in long-stay institutions for the elderly.
2. Evaluative and representative studies comparing the effectiveness of two-hourly bladder drill, with bladder retraining to an individual's normal pattern of micturition.
3. Evaluative and representative 'field' studies of behavioural techniques designed by ward staff for mentally handicapped incontinent individuals.
4. Evaluation of self-instruction booklets for women suffering from stress incontinence.
5. Evaluation of a nurse-run support group (a) for ambulant people suffering from incontinence, aimed to alleviate incontinence, and (b) for 'carers' or those with incontinent relatives to alleviate distress and provide more support and use of services.
6. Evaluate the effect of introducing regular audits to assess prevalence of preventable incontinence in hospital wards.

For assessing catheter care, studies should aim to:

7. Evaluate a ward- and a community-based teaching programme on correct catheterisation procedures and care, on nurse knowledge, behaviour and patients' urinary infection rates.
8. Replicate evaluations of a teaching programme for self-catheterisation for groups when this is indicated.
9. Survey wards where patients are catheterised and review to what extent alternative methods have been assessed for individual patients.

APPENDIX 1. INCONTINENCE ASSESSMENT CHECK-LIST

Name:	D.O.B.:
Address:	
General Practitioner:	
Assessed by:	
Date of assessment:	

1. Main complaint:

2. Urinary symptoms
Frequency
Nocturia   ? Woken.
Urgency   Average time of warning:
Urge incontinence
Stress incontinence
Passive incontinence
Nocturnal enuresis   Number of nights per week:

Symptoms of voiding difficulty:
Hesitancy
Poor stream
Straining
Manual expression
Post-micturition dribble
Dysuria
Haematuria

Incontinence:
Onset: When?   Circumstances:

Is incontinence improving/static/worsening?
How often does incontinence occur?
How much is lost?
Are aids or pads used?   Type:
   Number per day: Source of supply:
Are aids effective?   Problems:
Type and amount fluid intake.
Is fluid restriction used?

Other urinary symptoms:

3. Medical history
Previous illnesses/operations:
Parity.   Difficult deliveries?
Current medication.
Any previous treatment for incontinence?

4. Bowels
Usual bowel habit:
Constipation?
Laxatives or diet regulation used?
Faecal incontinence?

5. Mobility
Problems with mobility:
Aids used?:
Needs assistance: Who is available:

Difficulties in transfer to/onto lavatory.
Comments:
Foot problems.
Manual dexterity.
Clothing suitability.
Observe self-toiletting and comment on problems:
Eyesight.
Problems with personal hygiene.

6. Psychological state
Attitude to incontinence:
Anxiety?
Depression?
Impaired mental abilities?

7. Social network
Usual activities:
Are these restricted by incontinence?
Who does patient live with?
Who visits regularly?
Relationship problems because of incontinence?
Official services received:

8. Environment
Lavatory facilities:
Are urinals or commode used?
Obstacles to using lavatory.
Washing/laundry facilities.
Comments on general physical and social environment:

9. Results of physical examination
Skin problems:
Prolapse (women).
Atrophic changes (women).
Rectal examination.
Post-micturition residual urine volume:
MSSU/urine test result.
Other findings:

10. Results from Chart
Summary of Problems
1.
2.
3.
4.
5.

Aims/Goals
1.
2.
3.
4.
5.

Planned Action   Review date.
1.
2.
3.
4.

continued overleaf

5.
_____

Follow-up notes
_____

From Norton (1986a) with kind permission of author and publisher.

APPENDIX 2. HABIT RETRAINING CHART (a typical example)

Date	Day 8 9 10 11 12 1 2 3 4 5 6 7 8 9	Management	10 11 12 1 2
TUES	● + + ○ ★ x		
WED	● + ○ x ★ x		
THURS	x + + x + x		
FRI	x ○ ○ x ○ x		

8 9 10 11 12 1 2 3 4 5 6 7 8 9   10 11 12 1 2

KEY   State of Patient
Dry   = ○
Incontinent of urine   = ●
Result of toiletting
Urine passed in toilet   = x
Urine not passed in toilet   = +
Refused or absent   = ★

Based on method devised by nursing staff from West Birmingham Health Authority.

REFERENCES

Barker P (1979) Nocturnal enuresis: an experimental study involving two behavioural approaches. *International Journal of Nursing Studies* **16**, 319–327.
Blannin JP (1985) Promoting continence: What every woman should know. Patient Education. *The Professional Nurse* **Oct**, 10–11.

Cardozo L, Stanton SL, Hafner J, Allan V (1978) Biofeedback in the treatment of detrusor instability. *British Journal of Urology* 50, 250–254.

Castle M, Osterhout S (1974) Urinary tract catheterisation and associated infection. *Nursing Research* 23, 170–174.

Chavigny KH (1975) The use of polymixin B as a urethral lubricant to reduce the post-instrumental incidence of bacteriuria in females. An exploratory study. *International Journal of Nursing Studies* 12, 33–42.

Clay EC (1978) Incontinence of urine. *Nursing Mirror* 146, 23–34, 36–38.

Cleland VS (1977) Prevention of bacteriuria in female patients with indwelling catheters. In: Verhonick PJ (ed) *Nursing Research II*, pp. 53–75. Little Brown and Co, Boston.

Coyle JK, Macdonald DF (1967) The relationship between repeated instrumentation and urinary tract infection. *Journal of Urology* 98, 260–262.

Dudley MN, Barrière SL (1981) Antimicrobial irrigations in the prevention and treatment of catheter-related urinary tract infections. *American Journal of Hospital Pharmacy* 38, 59–65.

Egan M, Plymat K, Thomas T, Meade T (1983) Incontinence in patients in two district general hospitals. *Nursing Times* **Feb 2**, 22–23.

Fader M (1986) New thoughts on male catheterisation. *Nursing Times* 82(15), 64–66.

Friend PM (1977) *Standards of Nursing Care* CNO(SNO)(77)1. Department of Health and Social Security, London.

Garibaldi RA, Burke JP, Britt MR, Miller WA, Smith CB (1980) Meatal colonisation and catheter associated bacteriuria. *New England Journal of Medicine* 303, 316–318.

Gibbs H (1986) Catheter toilet and urinary tract infections. *Nursing Times* 82(23), 75–76.

Gillespie WA, Lennon GG, Linton KB, Slade N (1962) Prevention of catheter infection of urine in female patients. *British Medical Journal* 2, 13–16.

Gillespie WA, Lennon GG, Linton KB, Phippen GA (1967) Prevention of infection by means of closed drainage into a sterile plastic bag. *British Medical Journal* 3, 90–92.

Givens CD, Wenzel RP (1980) Catheter associated urinary tract infections in surgical patients: a controlled study on the excess morbidity and costs. *Journal of Urology* 124, 646–648.

Gooch J (1986) Catheter care. *The Professional Nurse* **May**, 207–208.

Harrison S (1975) Physiotherapy in the treatment of stress incontinence. *Nursing Mirror* 141(2), 52–53.

Hart JA (1985) The urethral catheter—a review of its implication in urinary tract infection. *International Journal of Nursing Studies* 22(1), 57–70.

Isaacs B (1979) Water, water everywhere . . . it's time we stopped to think. *Royal Society of Health* 4, 155–165.

Islam AKMS, Chapman J (1977) Closed catheter drainage and urinary infection. A comparison of two methods of catheter drainage. *British Journal of Urology* 49, 215–220.

Jacques L, McKie S, Harries C (1986) Effects of short-term catheterisation. *Nursing Times* 82(25), 59–62.

Jarvis GJ, Millar DR (1980) Controlled trial of bladder drill for detrusor instability. *British Medical Journal* 281, 1322–1323.

Jenner EA (1983) Prevention of catheter associated UTI. *Nursing Supplement* 2nd series **May 13**, 1–3.

Kegal AH (1951) Physiologic therapy for urinary stress incontinence. *Journal of the American Medical Association* 146, 915–917.

Kennedy AP, Brocklehurst JC (1982) The nursing management of patients with long-term indwelling catheters. *Journal of Advanced Nursing* 7, 411–417.

Kennedy AP, Brocklehurst JC, Lye MDW (1983) Factors related to the problems of long-term catheterisation. *Journal of Advanced Nursing* 8, 207–212.

Kostiala AAI, Nyren P, Runeberg L (1982) Effect of nitrofurantoin and methenamine hippurate prophylaxis on bacteria and yeasts in the urine of patients and an in-dwelling catheter. *Journal of Hospital Infection* 3, 357–364.

Kunin CM (1979) *Detection, Prevention and Management of Urinary Tract Infections*. 3rd Edition. Lea and Febiger, Philadelphia.

Lapides J, Dioko AC, Gould FR, Lowe BS (1975) Further observations on self catheterisation. *Transactions of the American Association of Genito Urinary Surgeons* 67, 16–17.

Millard P (1986) A programme for continence. *Nursing Times* **82**(15), 57–58.

Montgomery E (1986) Steps to regaining pelvic control. *Nursing Times* **82**, 58–60.

Newman E, Price M (1977) Bacteriuria in patients with spinal cord lesions: its relationship to urinary drainage appliances. *Archives of Physical Medicine and Rehabilitation* **58**, 427–430.

Norton C (1983) Training for urinary continence. In: Wilson-Barnett J (ed) *Patient Teaching*, pp. 153–175. Churchill Livingstone, Edinburgh.

Norton C (1986a) Nursing the incontinent patient. In: Tierney AJ (ed) *Clinical Nursing Practice* Recent advances in Nursing Vol **14**, 48–75. Churchill Livingstone, Edinburgh.

Norton C (1986b) Promoting research. *Nursing Times* **82**(15), 55.

Norton C (1986c) *Nursing for Continence*. Macmillan, London.

Platt R, Polk FB, Murdock B, Rosner B (1982) Mortality associated with nosocomial urinary tract infection. *New England Journal of Medicine* **307**, 637–642.

Reid EA (1974) *Incontinence and Nursing Practice*. M.Phil Thesis. University of Edinburgh, Edinburgh.

Robb SS (1985) Urinary incontinence verification in elderly men. *Nursing Research* **34**, 278–282.

Roberts JBM, Linton KB, Pollard BP, Mitchell JP, Gillespie WA (1965) Long-term catheter drainage in the male. *British Journal of Urology* **37**, 63–72.

Roe B (1985) Catheter care: an overview. *International Journal of Nursing Studies* **22**(1), 45–56.

Seal DV, Wood S, Barret S (1982) Evaluation of aseptic techniques and chlorhexidine on the rate of catheter associated urinary tract infection. *Lancet* **i**, 89–91.

Shepherd AM, Blannin JP (1980) A clinical trial of pads and pants used for urinary incontinence. *Nursing Times* **76**(23), 1015–1016.

Smith B (1979) A dry bed and save on costs. *Nursing Mirror* **148**(22), 26–29.

Storss AMF (1982) What is care? *British Journal of Geriatric Nursing* **Apr**, 12–14.

Thomas TM, Plymat KR, Blannin J, Meade TW (1980) Prevalence of urinary incontinence. *British Medical Journal* **281**, 1243–1245.

Tierney AJ (1973) Toilet training. *Nursing Times* **69**(51/52), 1740–1745.

Turck M, Stamm W (1981) Nosocomial infection of the urinary tract. *American Journal of Medicine* **70**, 651–654.

Voith AM, Smith DA (1985) Validation of the nursing diagnosis of urinary retention. *Nursing Research* **31**(1), 28–30.

Willington FC, Yarnell JWG, Sweetman DM (1981) Cleansing incontinent patients: an evaluation of the use of non-ionic detergents compared with soap. *Journal of Advanced Nursing* **6**, 107–109.

Wilson J, Roe B (1986) Nursing management of patients with an in-dwelling urethral catheter. In: Tierney AJ (ed) *Clinical Nursing Practice* Recent Advances in Nursing Vol **14**, pp. 76–104. Churchill Livingstone, Edinburgh.

Chapter 8
Pain

Pain is a symptom which humanity has tried to understand in terms of religion, philosophy and medicine from time immemorial. Sometimes the term pain is used to refer to suffering and distress of all kinds, including existential pain and aesthetic pain. Although this chapter focuses upon pain related to physical pathology, it is obvious that any attempt to compartmentalise human experience for the convenience of discussion is artificial. People can and do turn to medicine for help in existential anguish and also turn to priest, rabbi or other religious leader for help with pathophysiological pain. The divide is not so much in the personal experience of pain as in the specialisation of skills and knowledge of the healer. The current concern in medicine and nursing with holistic care is an acknowledgement of the total context in which human suffering is felt (Scott, 1982).

The normal state or the state to which we aspire for ourselves and our patients is to be pain free. However, the normal state includes the ability to feel pain. The rare state in which an infant is born, unable to perceive pain, is not compatible with long life as accidental injury goes unattended.

When then is pain a problem? When it interferes with physical and mental activities, slows the healing process, or is felt as unbearable in intensity or duration by the sufferer. In most circumstances, relief of pain is desirable and desired and in certain circumstances is absolutely vital. There are however some situations in which freedom from pain is not desired or not desirable.

PREVALENCE

Pain is a major reason for entry into the health care system (Kohn and Kerr, 1976) and for economic loss. Bonica (1982) states that pain is

'the most common cause of physiologic and psychologic stress and the most frequent reason patients seek medical counsel.' (p. 5)

He speculates that nearly one-third of people in industrialised countries have chronic pain and, of these, one-half to two-thirds are either partially or totally disabled for periods of days, weeks, months and sometimes permanently. Bonica (1982) further asserts that

'there is impressive evidence that a large percentage of patients with post-operative pain, post-traumatic pain, severe pain associated with visceral disease and most patients with post-burn pain are inadequately relieved.'

In addition,

'many patients with non-malignant chronic pain do not respond to the usual medical therapy and an impressive number are exposed to high risk iatrogenic complications, including drug toxicity, drug dependence, and multiple often useless and at times mutilating operations.' (p. 5)

The reasons suggested for the above by Bonica are:

1. great voids in knowledge about pain,
2. inadequate or improper application of knowledge and therapies available, and
3. communication problems.

Voids in knowledge about pain are being filled. In 1968 an Intractible Pain Society of Great Britain and Ireland was started. In 1974 the International Association for the Study of Pain was set up and a journal exclusively devoted to pain was launched. Pain clinics and hospices dedicated to the relief of chronic and terminal pain respectively have blossomed in the past decades. Although as recently as 1983, Twycross and Lack estimated that 25% of cancer patients in the UK died without pain relief.

It is possible that many people could be freed of their pain if the knowledge we now have was disseminated and utilised. However, we will not succeed in helping unless and until we accept a positive role. Sofaer (1983) begins her article *Pain relief—the core of nursing practice* with a quote from a patient who had emergency abdominal surgery:

'I don't think that nurses think it is their job to bother about pain relief.'

Sofaer (1985) suggests that

'the theoretical and practical implications of this new knowledge (about pain) have not affected practice to the extent where pain management is a specific part of nursing care.'

This view is borne out by studies such as Seers (1987).

The Delphi report on priorities in clinical nursing research identified pain as one of the priorities of nursing research (Lindeman, 1975). Open communication is needed between researchers and practitioners and all concerned with relief of pain including nurses and doctors, patients, priests and paramedics, patients' families, friends and employers.

Prevalence of children's pain

Estimation of the prevalence of pain in children is not available, though current statistics of child abuse suggest that at the least adult dealings with vulnerable children are inept. Children suffer pain inflicted by adults, by other children and by accidental injuries. Due to the advancement of medical science, survival of serious congenital abnormalities and heroic treatment of childhood malignancies may have shifted the causes of pain in industrialised societies from suffering resulting from child labour to medically inflicted and iatrogenic pains. Eland (1985) makes a plea for humane treatment for children, the use of appropriate anaesthesia and analgesia during painful procedures such as setting up intravenous infusions and inserting drains, helping children to keep still using minimal constraint, and teaching and encouraging the use of techniques such as imagery and relaxation. She states:

'After 10 years of research interviewing over 2000 children, one thing is clear—health professionals need to do a better job of working with children who hurt.' (pp. 29–30)

Eland found that for these 2000 hospitalised children aged between four and 10 years in the USA, 66% received no analgesics for the relief of pain. Eland and Anderson (1977) compared analgesia doses received by 18 adults with 18 children who had identical diagnoses and surgical procedures. The adults received 372 doses of narcotics and 299 non-narcotics, whereas the children received 11 doses of narcotics and 13 of non-narcotic analgesics.

Research findings and observations of children's responses to pain leave us with no excuse whatsoever for minimising or ignoring their suffering. The myth that children do not experience pain as do adults because of nervous system immaturity is not tenable. It has been known at least since 1968 that children are not neurologically defective as far as pain is concerned (Swafford and Allen, 1968).

DEFINITIONS OF PAIN

There are as many definitions of pain as there are theories about pain and it is important to recognise the relationship between definition and research, and definition and practice.

Purpose and nature of pain

One major difference exists between definitions (and theories) about the purpose of pain and the nature of pain. Purpose explanations may view pain as punishment for sin, or more pragmatically, as the consequence of certain behaviour and events. Indeed, the word pain is derived from the Greek *poine* which means punishment or penalty. Pain was viewed as punishment from the gods for wrong-doing. The Hebrew view of the pain incurred by men's work and women's birth-giving was explained as punishment for the sin of eating of the tree of knowledge (Genesis, 3). The purpose of pain in biological terms is as a useful warning of tissue damage. Part of Sternbach's (1968) definition of pain illustrates the most common 'purpose type' scientific view:

'. . . a harmful stimulus which signals current or impending tissue damage; a pattern of impulses which operate to protect the organism from harm.'

Explanations of the nature of pain define it in terms of the experience of the sufferer, including the sensory/perceptual, emotional/motivational and the cognitive/evaluative aspects (Reading, 1984; Fordham, 1986). Descarte's (1644) sensory model of pain influenced Western biomedical thinking to the point that the affective or emotional component was relegated to a reaction to pain rather than an integral part of pain. Aristotle regarded pain as a quality of experience, an affective state, the opposite of pleasure. Hardy et al (1952) viewed pain as a feeling state to be either avoided or terminated.

The definition of pain produced by the International Association for the Study of Pain Sub-committee on Taxonomy (1979) combines a nature and purpose view as follows:

> 'an unpleasant sensory and emotional experience associated with actual or potential tissue damage or described in terms of such damage.'

Wall (1984a) suggested that, instead of viewing pain as either a sensation or an emotional response, it may usefully be classified as a need state, analogous with thirst (for water) or hunger (for food). Thus pain would be 'one of many modes exhibited by a single sensory-emotional-behavioural system'—the need for stillness and recuperative rest. Sternbach (1984) points out however that acute pain may be logically regarded as both 'a sensation of actual or impending injury signals and as a need-state for rest', but chronic pain serves neither function.

Acute and chronic pain

A second and important difference exists between definitions of acute and chronic pain. Bonica (1982) describes acute pain as

> 'a constellation of unpleasant, perceptual and emotional experiences and associated auto-nomic (sympathetic) reflex responses and psychologic and behavioural reactions provoked by tissue damage inherent in injury or disease.' (p. 6)

Acute pain has an important biological warning function that something is wrong, in some instances it results in enforced stillness which promotes healing, and the anxiety reaction initially helps prepare for emergency response. Melzack (1981) states that acute pain is associated with a well-defined cause, has a characteristic time course and vanishes after healing. The rapid onset is called the phasic component and the continued variable time of pain the tonic component.

The American classification of nursing diagnoses (Carpenito, 1983) places pain under the heading of alterations in comfort, and defines acute pain as:

> 'A state in which the individual experiences an uncomfortable sensation in response to a noxious stimulus and as pain which can last from one second to six months, but subsides with healing or when the stimulus is removed.'

Chronic pain, according to Melzack (1981), begins as acute, but the tonic component persists long after the injury has healed and may spread to adjacent and distant parts of the body. Characteristic body movements and physiological responses are absent as they cannot be maintained indefinitely and chronic pain is associated with high levels of anxiety and depression. The diagnoses of chronic pain sufferers include cancer, herpes, arthritis, phantom limb, low back pain and chronic pain syndromes including causalgia, reflex sympathetic dystrophy, peripheral neuropathies and functional changes in the central nervous system following chronic deafferentation (Bonica, 1982). Chronic pain is defined in *Nursing Diagnoses* (Carpenito, 1983) as persistent or intermittent pain that lasts for more than six months. The tying of the difference between acute and chronic pain solely to a specific time period could be misleading; the cause and bodily reaction to pain may also be useful as criteria for distinguishing between the two types.

Tractable and intractable pain

It is sometimes more useful to distinguish between tractable and intractable pain than between acute and chonic. Intractable pain is defined by Wall (1986) as pain for which no therapy is effective and by Glyn (1987) as 'pain of at least one month's duration that has not been relieved by conventional techniques'. It is not pain without organic cause, indeed the cause may be obvious, including

> 'deep tissue damage as in arthritis, low back pain and cystitis, peripheral nerve damage as in causalgia and amputation pains, and dorsal root damage as in arachnoiditis and brachial plexus avulsion.' (Wall, 1986)

Wall further states that where clear organic diagnosis cannot be made, that does not constitute a reason for labelling the sufferer with a psychiatric diagnosis—rather the 'psychiatric problem' lies as much with the doctor (or nurse) obsessed with simple truths about complex problems. If there is one clear message coming from the research on pain it is that pain mechanisms and human experience are not simple.

Useful, useless and harmful pain

A further important distinction is made by Bonica (1982) between useful, useless and harmful pain. Generally acute pain is useful and chronic pain is useless in terms of biological warning. Harmful or potentially harmful pain is related to the cause and intensity of the pain and when it exists this means that pain per se is an emergency and must be relieved if the person is to avoid serious physiological complications and even death. Bonica (1982) describes harmful pain thus:

> 'Acute pain and reflex responses which develop in the post-operative period or after massive injury or burns have no useful function and if not promptly and effectively relieved produce progressively serious pathophysiological responses . . . excessive adrenergic activity, vagal inhibition and skeletal muscle spasm.' Central sympathetic stimulation induced by anxiety causes pulmonary complications, marked inhibition of gastro-intestinal and genito-urinary activity with consequent ileus and oliguria; marked increase in the workload of the heart and excessive increase in the metabolism and oxygen consumption.

plus

> Severe trauma can result in excessive splanchnic vasoconstriction and thus initiate and sustain shock.' (Bonica, 1980a)

Other examples of harmful pain include post-myocardial infarction pain in which sympathetic overactivity can increase the discrepancy between myocardial oxygen supply and the demand for oxygen and consequently increase the size of the infarct and the risk of death (Bonica, 1980a). The pain of severe acute pancreatitis, biliary and renal colic results in reflex spasm of abdominal and chest wall and hence provokes hypoventil-ation 'which unless promptly corrected may progress to death' (Bonica, 1982).

Other categories of pain include referred pain and phantom pain. *Referred* pain, or *transferred* pain as Procacci and Zoppi (1984) call it, classically arises when intense pain in viscera is prolonged. The pain is gradually felt in structures sometimes far away from the site of origin. The distribution of superficial referred pain to the skin is to the cutaneous distribution of spinal nerves (dermatomes) and of deep referred pain to the muscle distribution of spinal nerves (myotomes) or bone (sclerotomes). Examples include myocardial pain referred to chest wall and arm and sub-diaphragmatic pathology to the shoulder.

Phantom pain

'Deafferentation of part of the body due to loss of part of the body is almost invariably followed by an awareness of the deafferented parts.' (Jensen and Rasmussen, 1984)

The person can give a detailed description of limb image. Phantom limb is a normal phenomenon though the mechanisms are still hypothetical. Approximately 90% of amputees report phantom sensation during the first month post-amputation, although due to the lack of clarity in definition, the incidence ranges from 2 to 100% (Jensen and Rasmussen, 1984). Loss of other parts of the body including tongue, teeth, breast and penis also result in phantom sensations and pain.

The distinctions between acute and chronic, useful and useless serve, as do all classification systems, to help us make sense of the complexity of reality (see Figure 1). However, many pains do not fit neatly into categories. Long-lasting or intermittent pain, such as that of arthritis or deafferentation pain, may result from continued tissue damage or abnormal neural structure or function, so being chronic in terms of time, but acute in terms of warning. Acute pain felt by empathetic carers in the same site as their patients' pain or that of 'fathers to be' with their wives may be acute in terms of duration, but arise without pathological cause.

Acute–Chronic

Useful–Useless–Harmful

Tractable–Intractable

Referred–transferred

Phantom

Figure 1. Classifications of pain

Injury without pain is a paradoxical state, but one which occurs not only 'in the heat of battle' when conscious attention is focused on staying alive or winning the match, but is also experienced by between 28 and 53% of injured casualty patients (Melzack et al, 1982). The body is capable of producing a state of instantaneous analgesia at specific injured sites, allowing the injured person to carry on their current activity or seek help and evaluate the consequences of injury in a detached manner.

However, whilst acknowledging the need to use categorical labelling with due caution, the importance of the acute-chronic pain differentiation is crucial for both research and practice. By far the majority of research has been on acute pain, whilst the greatest challenges to pain relief are of chronic pain. Most laboratory studies of both human and animal pain have been of transient acute pain. Recently animal models of chronic pain have been devised (Hallin and Torebjörk, 1980; Vyklicky, 1984), and research on patients in pain clinics and hospices has been on chronic pain sufferers. As Cervero (1987) points out,

'Although visceral pain is the most common form of pain produced by disease and [accounts for] a substantial proportion of recurrent and persistent pain syndromes, yet little of the underlying neurophysiological mechanisms are understood as traditional pain studies examine immediate reaction of the central nervous system to acute skin injury.'

When considering the implications of research on pain for nursing practice, we need to bear in mind a number of caveats. Firstly, although we owe an enormous debt to the animals who have endured pain to enhance our understanding, for example of the neurophysiology of pain (Lindblom, 1982), the conceptual leap from another species to humans is likely to be a minefield of misinterpretation. We have also to be aware of the fact that, much as we might wish otherwise, we are not entirely rational or logically consistent. On the one hand, we justify ethically the use of animals rather than humans for some pain researches and extrapolate rodent responses to humans, on the other hand we doubt that animals experience pain to the same extent as ourselves. Children and mentally handicapped people also tend to be assumed to feel less pain than the average adult, because their behavioural expression and logic differs (Eland, 1985).

Secondly, laboratory research on human pain may give misleading results compared with 'real life' pain because of differences in the cognitive meaning to the sufferer and in his control over his pain. In addition, many subjects of laboratory research are healthy and young whereas many patients in pain are sick and elderly. However, as Reading (1984) states,

'Laboratory pain-induction methods have become important tools in furthering our knowl-edge and understanding of pain mechanisms . . .' and 'are useful for human analgesic assays with drugs and other pain relieving treatment modalities, such as acupuncture, transcutaneous electrical nerve stimulation, hypnosis, relaxation and cognitive strategies.'

Thirdly, when caring for an individual in pain who can communicate with us, our safest way to proceed may be on the basis of McCaffery's (1972) definition of pain that it 'is whatever the experiencing person says it is, and exists whenever he says it does', and in addition heed Sofaer's (1985) suggestions that we:

'1. Do not judge the appropriateness of a patient's behaviour in relation to his pain, and
2. Have no expectations in relation to a patient's response to a particular pain therapy.'

These may seem very difficult views to accept when we want to use research findings to understand, predict and control pain, but if we assess, intervene and evaluate our care with blinkers on, we will be unlikely to see the reality. The experience of pain is dependent upon the integrated functioning of pain receptors, afferent peripheral nerves, and the dorsal horn of the spinal cord including the substantia gelatinosa; the ascending neural pathways, particularly spino-thalamic, spino-reticular, spino-mesencephalic, spino-cervical and dorsal tracts; the thalamic nuclei, the somatosensory and frontal cortex, the hypothalamus and the whole limbic system, the descending pathways, including the dorsolateral fasciculus and efferent motor and autonomic nerves (Willis, 1984). The interplay of inhibition and excitation throughout the nervous system is such that neither sensory, nor emotional, nor cognitive aspects of pain are predictable from the apparent cause(s) of pain or even from the apparent lack of causation of pain. However, alteration in any or all levels of the nervous system has the potential to reduce or eliminate pain.

Neurophysiological (and psychological) pain theories which have arisen from research

'describe and explain the mechanisms of pain and to some extent increase the likelihood of correct prediction of the effectiveness of pain reducing strategies. However, recognition of the complexity of pain mechanisms, including the ability of the nervous system to modulate pain and to change and adapt following injury should increase our willingness to accept the patient's perception of his pain and reduce the inclination to approach patients with our own preconceived dogma about the patient's pain. Accurate prediction of pain requires knowledge of *all* the facts about the state of a person's nervous system. We will *never* be able to know fully the state of a person's nervous system however much our knowledge expands, because the state is transient, changing and complex. With increased knowledge we may be able to make a more educated prediction, but we will always need to listen to and accept the patient's perception of his pain.' (Fordham, 1986)

PAIN ASSESSMENT

Assessment of other people's pain is fraught with difficulties because 'pain is a personal, private sensation of hurt' (Sternbach, 1968). In other words it is a subjective experience which we attempt to understand and measure on the basis of indirect evidence. There will never be an instrument like a thermometer for temperature, which will perfectly transduce subjective pain into an objective form, although some researchers, for example Chen and Chapman (1980), have found that the amplitude of electrical potentials recorded externally on the scalp seems to reflect the subjective intensity of pain rather than the physical stimulus strength.

Pain threshold or the minimal stimulus felt as pain and pain tolerance or the duration or intensity of pain which a person is willing to endure can be objective about the stimulus applied, but this does not make pain into an objective phenomenon (Houde, 1982). Pain research is revealing many specific anatomical and physiological changes which arise from damage to tissues such as the release of bradykinin, histamine and prostaglandins and the release of chemicals from nerves such as substance P, neurokinins, noradrenaline, acetylcholine and other peptides (Wall, 1986). Complex interplay of excitation and inhibition in the peripheral and central nervous system and nervous system's networks, such as the endorphin-mediated analgesic system (EMAS) (Fields and Basbaum, 1984), is known to exist. However, although invasive medical investigations of neuro-anatomy and neurophysiology, plus estimations of blood or cerebrospinal fluid levels of chemicals such as endorphins are sometimes an essential part of the assessment of intractable and chronic pain, nursing assessment is generally confined to overt manifestations of these covert changes using non-invasive methods.

Pain, like any other human experience, is capable of expression in three major ways, that is by physiological response, by behavioural response and by verbal description. Therefore the criteria used to estimate pain are based on these responses.

Physiological responses

The most obvious physiological changes arise from the autonomic nervous system response. In acute pain this is sympathetic adrenergic dominance plus vagal inhibition resulting in increased heart rate and stroke volume, plus peripheral vasoconstriction, palmar and plantar sweating, glycogen release from the liver to the blood and inhibition of gastro-intestinal motility. However, in some visceral pains blood pressure and pulse fall rather than rise and in chronic pain autonomic responses may be absent.

Gross physiological changes alone are not adequate criteria for the diagnosis of pain, for a number of reasons. Firstly, the human body has a limited repertoire of responses, such that the autonomic response to many stressors, including blood loss, fear, pain and the anticipation of pain may be indistinguishable. Heart rate, for instance, is the final common effector of responses to multiple influences i.e. muscular exercise, digestion, posture, altitude, climate, noise, psychosensory activity, drugs and emotion. Vogt et al (1973) state that heart rate

'should be used as an index of a particular physiological or psychological stress factor only if the simultaneous influence of all other factors is properly taken into account.'

Secondly, 'initial values' affect the possibility for change; for example, a person with pre-existing hypertension or tachycardia has little leeway for increase in these parameters due to pain.

Behavioural responses

By behavioural is meant any non-verbal reaction to pain, for example facial expression, vocalisation, bodily posture, movement or abnormal stillness. Typical responses to acute or recurrent intermittent pain include gross hypermotility, rocking, rubbing, moaning, screaming, screwed up closed eyes, frowning, or total immobility, freezing of all movement, and muscle spasm of local skeletal muscles. Responses to chronic pain are generally more subtle including decreased mobility, cautious or restricted movement and more or less constant tension in facial muscles.

Behavioural responses may give direct clues to the site as well as the felt intensity of pain, for example abdominal wall guarding of peritoneal pain. The sufferer may look directly at the site or hold it, or he/she may rub an adjacent skin area.

It would be wonderful if differences in autonomic or behavioural responses accurately reflected different types and intensities of pain, particularly when we aim to assess pain in those who are totally or partially inarticulate, such as the unconscious, the mentally handicapped, the newborn or those whose language we do not share, but as Houde (1982) stated both behavioural and autonomic signs are unreliable indices of pain severity and may be absent in patients with chronic pain. It is therefore obvious that we have to be particularly vigilant about potential causes of pain in the above groups of patients and sensitive to their non-verbal responses.

Researches into the facial expressions accompanying pain have and are being undertaken. Darwin noted the facial expression of pain in 1872 (Darwin, 1965). Le Resche (1982) found from analysis of photographs of adults in acute, intense pain that the typical expression was of

'brow lowering with skin drawn in tightly around closed eyes, accompanied by a horizontally stretched open mouth, sometimes with deepening of the nasolabial furrow.'

Izard et al (1980) described the facial expression of infants during medical procedures such as inoculation as

'brows down and together, nasal root broadened and bulged, eyes tightly closed, and the mouth angular and squarish.'

These expressions of pain were followed by anger expressions in which the eyes are open and staring.

If physiological response such as increase in heart rate and respiratory rate is taken as a criterion of pain, then Williamson and Williamson (1983) suggest that circumcision pain response in unanaesthetised babies (i.e. without a penile block) is similar to that of adults who are in extreme pain. Haslam (1969) and Jay et al (1983) concluded from observations of overt distress caused by laboratory induced pain and painful medical procedures, that the younger the child, the more pain they seem to experience.

In all age groups the experience of pain disrupts ongoing behaviour, habitual responses and life-style, such that the aftermath of severe acute pain is a recovery phase when the person becomes quiet, solitary and antisocial with prolonged sleep and minimal movement. When assessing the efficacy of pain-relieving strategies and particularly narcotics, it is crucial to remember that hypersomnolence is not necessarily a sign of overdose, but of the need to make up for lost sleep. Many a patient has had their analgesic dosage reduced and suffered the return of pain because of misunderstanding of the cause of their sleep.

The adult with chronic pain may become dysphagic or hyperphagic and suffer sleep disturbance, may seek seclusion or abdicate social responsibilities and interact solely in the 'sick role'. Children's response to chronic pain parallels their response to other stressful events. Stoddard (1982) summarises these as follows:

'Infants withdraw and develop eating and sleeping difficulties. Pre-school children lose motor and toilet training milestones. School-age children become increasingly aggressive or withdrawn or out of control. Adolescents become depressed, withdraw socially or develop oppositional behaviour.'

Verbal description

Verbal responses to pain may be spontaneous or solicited and they may refer to the sensory, emotional or cognitive aspect of the person's experience. A huge area of pain research has been devoted to the development of assessment tools which aim to enhance the person's verbal expression of their suffering so that they can convey in a pseudo-objective way their subjective experience. Crawford-Clark (1984) says that reports of pain are a 'noisy' source of information since they represent a complex sensory and emotional experience.

A now classic tool for pain assessment is the McGill–Melzack Pain Questionnaire (Melzack, 1975). It has been widely used in research and clinical practice. Information sought includes the site(s) and extent of the pain, the subjective feeling of the pain, the way in which the pain changes over time, the intensity of the pain and accompanying symptoms and activities. Background information enables the findings to be related to age, diagnosis, and analgesia. The number of components into which the clusters of words have been analysed depends on the subjects, their pain type and the research protocol. Melzack (1981) suggests that there are four major classes: sensory, affective, evaluative and miscellaneous. Dubuisson and Melzack (1976) found that the pain descriptions derived from use of this questionnaire differentiated in a statistically significant way between eight pain syndromes: metastatic carcinoma, post-herpetic neuralgia, phantom limb pain, toothache, degenerative disc disease, rheumatoid or osteoarthritis, labour pain, and menstrual pain. Reading (1982) in comparing the words chosen by women who had undergone episiotomy with women who had pelvic inflammatory disease or dysmenorrhoea, suggested that

'it is possible that acute pain leads to less differentiation of sensory, affective and evaluative reaction components than chronic pain.' (p. 190)

In a clinical setting we do rely to some extent on the choice of descriptor word to diagnose the likely cause of pain, including the fact that people with severe visceral discomfort and pathology often decline to use the word pain, preferring pressure, tightness or squeezing instead. Much research has investigated the meaning of different words to describe pain and not surprisingly the findings depend upon the population studied, their educational level and their experience of pain (Gaston-Johansson, 1984).

Body outlines

The use of front and back outlines (as in the McGill–Melzack Pain Questionnaire, Melzack, 1975) by patients and nurses has revealed that the extent and location of pain is often underestimated by nurses. For example, post-operative pain is generally assumed to be at the site of the incision, but may be widespread and include throat, neck and back. The London Hospital Pain Observation Chart (Raiman, 1986) includes a body outline and a rating scale and a diary of measures to relieve pain. Developed initially for cancer patients, it has been successfully used on in-patients of all sorts and the 'Home Diary' also containing body outlines has facilitated assessment of patients in pain in the community. The importance of enabling patients to draw and describe their own pain is obvious when we consider the nature and localisation of visceral pain. Cervero (1987) describes typical visceral pain as

'dull, aching, badly localised and often referred to a part of the body away from the diseased organ, varying in intensity with time, but seldom disappearing completely within a short period of time and often accompanied by general increased excitability of the central nervous system as shown by tenderness of skin, general discomfort, muscle spasms and increased autonomic reflexes.'

Body outlines are also helpful in assessing children's pain. Eland's Colour Tool uses body outlines and eight coloured crayons. The child is asked to select the colours which are like

1. the event which the child said hurt most, so representing severe pain,
2. not quite as much as the event which the child said hurt most, so representing middle pain,
3. the colour which is like 'hurts a little', representing little hurt, and
4. the colour which is like 'no hurt at all'.

This assessment tool has been used by many researchers and is said to be a reliable and valid instrument (Eland, 1985, p. 33).

Scaling techniques

The McGill and the London Hospital pain questionnaires contain categorical scales of pain intensity. Scales used in experimental pain studies and in clinical research and practice have been developed from psychophysical research (Stevens, 1975). Psychophysical scales are used to ask people to estimate other subjective experiences such as fatigue or exertion (Borg, 1970). Mathematical assumptions are sometimes made about the equidistance of intervals and ratios of the scale. The ability being tested is a complex one. Hallsten (1980) in his discussion of the puzzle of ratio scaling describes the task which the subject or patient is asked to perform, i.e. to compare some internal state with an external numbered and symbolically worded scale. He states that

> 'not only do we not know what the person is doing when making the comparison, but neither do we know what he is measuring (in his internal milieu) . . . yet it is a task which subjects are willing to undertake, do not regard as an unreasonable request, and furthermore provides data which are reasonably consistent with the experimenter's expectations.'

In some pain studies, people are asked to match clinical pain with induced pain (Sternbach, 1974) or with light or sound intensity. Most often in clinical settings patients are asked to compare their pain with so-called visual analogue scales (VAS) such as line length with anchor words at each end (see Figure 2) or verbal pain scales which may attach behavioural consequences to each rating number (Linton and Gotestam, 1983, p. 60), or patients may be asked to use pain intensity descriptors, such as no pain, just noticeable, weak, mild, moderate, strong, severe and excruciating (Tursky, 1976), or none, slight, moderate or severe (Houde, 1982). Bourbonnais (1981) developed a pain assessment ruler for use by nurses. Research findings suggest that verbal scaling can distort by forcing patients to choose a category and that visual analogue scales are more sensitive indicators of patients' pain experiences (Ohnhaus and Adler, 1975). By no means all people understand what is being required of them when asked to compare an internal state with a visual analogue or verbal pain scale. Urban et al (1984) found that around 85% of 20 patients with chronic pain could reliably scale intensity words, but only 50% could do so for unpleasantness descriptors. Urban et al drew two conclusions which are potentially relevant for clinical application of analogue scaling. Firstly, patients with chronic pain were generally less able to make required proportional judgements than healthy people, and secondly training did not eradicate the relatively poor performance. Carlsson (1983) found that patients differed considerably in their ability to use a VAS reliably. Research into the application of psychophysical scaling to the accuracy of pain assessment has attempted to answer such questions as 'Are VAS's valid and reliable measures of pain intensity?' (Scott and Huskission, 1976), and 'do they validly and reliably measure both experimental and chronic pain?' (Price et al, 1983). The answers are a qualified yes, depending upon the exact protocol of experimentation or assessment and the extent to which subjects/patients understand what they are being asked to do.

---

1. A visual analogue scale

    o _____ o

    No pain   100 mm line   Unbearable
                                                                   pain

2. A verbal pain rating scale (Linton and Gotestam, 1983)

Rating	Definition
0	No pain.
1	Pain present, but can easily be ignored.
2	Pain present, cannot be ignored but does not interfere with everyday activities.
3	Pain present, cannot be ignored, interferes with concentration.
4	Pain present, cannot be ignored, interferes with all tasks except taking care of basic needs (eating, toilet visits).
5	Pain present, cannot be ignored, rest or bedrest required.

Figure 2. Pain scales

Raiman (1986) describes a Pain Symbol Chart which is being developed for use with patients who have language or comprehension difficulties in place of the verbal pain severity scale in the London Hospital Observation Chart.

In discussing the inappropriateness of using adult assessment tools for children, apart from finding that over half of children between 5 and 8 years did not know what the word pain meant, 'hurt' or 'owie' were young American children's words for pain (Eland and Anderson, 1977), Eland (1985) suggests that numerical rating scales are useful. The person rating, whether he/she is a child or an adult must understand the concepts of lesser and greater, or if numbers are used, that two is less than eight. Eland supports the use of a five-point scale for older children with words attached so that one is 'no hurt' and five 'the worst you have ever hurt in your life'. A pain thermometer has been used successfully with children who understand numbers (Molesberry, 1979).

In conclusion, as Price et al (1983) point out, although there is agreement that the principal criteria for pain assessment should be validity, that is unequivocal measurement of pain, and reliability or consistency over time, 'there is controversy regarding which pain assessment procedures satisfy these criteria' (p. 46). Research findings suggest that accuracy of assessment requires the use of more than one index of pain (Carlsson, 1983) and that there is a lack of correspondence between non-verbal behaviour and patients' self-report of pain. Furthermore, the discrepancies between observers and patients' ratings of pain are greater for chronic than acute pain sufferers (Teske et al, 1983).

Timing of pain assessment

This depends upon the reason for assessment, and most often in clinical settings this is to evaluate the change in the nature and intensity of pain as a result of some form of pain intervention. In these circumstances, at least two assessments are needed— before and after. The choice of time will depend upon the expected efficacy of the intervention. In the case of analgesia, for example, the time when it is expected to have maximum effect and/or the time when a repeat dose can be taken, may be appropriate. An alternative to selecting a set time interval for evaluation is to select an intensity level such that the patient agrees to report pain if it reaches a predetermined level. The logic for this is that less analgesia is needed to obliterate low level pain.

Sometimes assessment of pain is undertaken to gain information about its periodicity or relationship to other events or activities. It is important to note that 'many painful diseases have definite patterns of circadian variation in the intensity of pain' (Domzal et al, 1983, p. 67). Typically intractable pain increases throughout the day, reaching a peak in late evening (Glyn et al, 1976). Also, the highest sensitivity to experimentally induced pain has been found to occur in the evening (Procacci et al, 1974). In such circumstances it may be desirable to ask patients to record the pain at hourly intervals prior to planning logical interventions.

We need also to be aware of the effect of the task of assessment per se on the patient. Self-assessment of pain is incompatible with some techniques of pain management, such as distraction or hypnosis. In other words, it is not possible to both ignore and introspect pain at the same time. Finally, the person in severe pain is likely to have difficulty concentrating so that a long questionnaire assessment may not be acceptable or appropriate until some measure of relief has been obtained.

Problems inherent in pain assessment

The main problems are those of communication—difficulty in expressing pain, limitations of observation, failure to listen and hear, and difficulty in interpretation. Patients' attempts to please medics and nurses can lead some to suppress their non-verbal responses and tone down their verbal expressions of pain, being afraid of disappointing the staff in their attempts to relieve their pain. Communicating in public may deter truthful expression. As Proshansky et al (1970) remark, privacy removes social constraints and permits behaviours such as vocalisations, body movements and vomiting, which the sufferer would not wish to perform in public. The rationale patients and staff use for limiting expression of pain was graphically described by Fagerhaugh and Strauss (1977) when discussing open burns units:

'It becomes essential that pain expression be kept within reasonable limits. A patient who, without inhibition, cries, screams, moans, groans and constantly complains of pain is intolerable and devastating both for the staff and for other patients.'

Stoicism is seen as a positive virtue in many cultures. Zborowski (1969), in his discussion of culture and pain responses, includes this category of response as 'absence of manifest behaviour', hiding of pain or suppressing extreme signs of pain. Sargent (1984) describes the centrality of non-expression of pain to the Bariba culture of northern Benin and Nigeria. For them the ideal behaviour is endurance without expression of pain during childbirth, accidental wounds and initiation ordeals. The admission of pain is shameful. Craig (1978) discusses cross-cultural studies of patients in pain. There is a certain consistency within subcultures, but also considerable individual differences within particular groups. Lipton and Marbach (1984) also found inter-ethnic differences in patients' stoicism and expressiveness in response to pain. In our multi-ethnic societies we need to be mindful of the personal consequence of eliciting admissions of pain and remember that for some (maybe rare) individuals the consequence of admitting behaviourally or verbally that they are in pain may 'unman' them far more than the pain itself. Jacox (1979) studied 102 patients and found that 70% did not like discussing their pain with others. They felt other people would not like a complainer or hypochondriac and denied the existence of pain at the start of the interview.

Children may have particular difficulty in expressing pain. Eland (1985) has found that children can tell the truth about their pain if they are given appropriate ways to express their hurt. However, they may not admit to pain if they associate the admission of pain with the infliction of more pain (by intramuscular injection) and Eland found that intramuscular injection is classed by most children as the worst hurt they experienced in hospital. Also it is possible that some children may not recognise their discomforting symptoms as pain or hurt if the onset is insidious—accepting the status quo as normal or inevitable. Eland (1985) describes one such child, a 13-year-old with advanced sarcoma who, when given regular analgesia, stated

'I really did not think I hurt until you took it (the pain) away. Now I really feel great and I sleep a lot better. I had kind of forgotten what it was like not to hurt.'

Eland makes further important points about children in pain. Parents tend to think that nurses automatically know when their child is in pain and the parents' personal distress can result in failure to recognise their own child's hurt. Many children are actively discouraged from discussing pain by their parents. Ross and Ross (1984) found this to be true of the 66 parents they interviewed.

The socialisation and experiences of different professions result in differences in the attribution of pain. When descriptive vignettes of patients' suffering were compared, Lenburg et al (1970) found that nuns and teachers inferred most pain and nurses and doctors least. The balance and credence which observers put on non-verbal and verbal expressions of pain is complex. Past research found that nurses believed that physiological and non-verbal behaviours are better indices of pain than verbal reports (Johnson, 1977) possibly because they are less easily subject to what is termed 'motivated dissimulation' (Kraut, 1978). This attitude leads to a failure to recognise the extent of chronic pain (Teske et al, 1983) and to the current plea to first and foremost believe the patient's verbal description of his/her pain.

It is obvious that there is enormous room for improvement in our assessment of patients' pain. One way of improving communication would be to use deliberative nursing interventions for pain, as described by Horsley et al (1982). The underlying proposition comes from Orlando (1961) and is that, in order to do what the client needs, the nurse must first know what is needed. This requires the nurse to explore and test (validate) their thoughts, feelings and perceptions *with* the patient before coming to a conclusion about the patient's pain. The use of a pain assessment chart reportedly improved communication between nurses and patients with chronic cancer pain (Raiman, 1986).

The purpose of clinical pain assessment is problem identification, such that logical interventions may be taken. The existence and nature of the patient's pain are not however sufficient information to form the basis of decision taking (Houde, 1982). The major factors which need to be assessed are listed in Table 1.

Table 1. Pain Assessment

Physiological responses Sympathetic-adrenergic dominance in acute pain resulting in change in heart rate, respiratory rate, blood pressure, sweating, pupil size.
Behavioural responses Facial expression, vocalisations, posture, movement or stillness, life-style changes such as eating habit, sleep disruption, social withdrawal, fatigue, irritability, aggression, anxiety, depression.
Verbal responses Spontaneous or elicited views enhanced by use of questionnaires, interview schedules, body outlines, analogue and categorical scales.
Major areas to be assessed Nature, intensity and site of pain(s). Precipitating factors and circumstances e.g. movement, posture, time of day, month of year. Likely cause including medical diagnosis. Associated symptoms e.g. nausea, anxiety, insomnia, breathlessness. Meaning or significance to the patient i.e. purpose of pain, usefulness, uselessness. Patient's desired goal.
Resources. Patient's coping methods. Nurses' knowledge and skills in using/teaching non-pharmacological methods of pain relief. Medical and paramedical knowledge and skills in use and provision of pharmacological and non-pharmacological methods of pain relief. Availability of time, special equipment, drugs, privacy, etc.

GOAL SETTING

Whenever possible, goal setting should be agreed with the pain sufferer, not imposed. The goal or expected outcome should also be realistic. Hanks (1983) suggests that the goal of pain relief should not be confined simply to the effectiveness, but also related to the time of day and activity of the patient. He suggests as progressive goals for cancer pain, firstly, to be free of pain at night, secondly, to be free of pain when at rest and thirdly, to be pain free on movement. The first two goals are almost always achievable, the third more difficult.

Goal setting could logically be related to the category of pain. The obliteration of useful pain before arriving at a conclusion about its cause may be counter-productive. Sometimes for short periods the continued evaluation of the site of the pain, its intensity, spread, precipitating factors, etc, may be crucial to accurate diagnosis and decisions about appropriate medical, surgical or nursing intervention.

Useless pain, including most post-operative pain and chronic pain, where the causes are iatrogenic and/or known, should logically be completely relieved. Research leaves us in no doubt that patients regard unrelieved post-operative pain as highly stressful (Volicier and Bohannon, 1975) and a serious complication (McConnell, 1983). The goals of both patients and nurses range from complete relief to just enough for the patient to tolerate it. Both Cohen (1980) and Sofaer (1984) found a higher percentage of patients wanted complete relief than did the nurses, though more nurses aimed to relieve pain as much as possible than did patients. It may be that nurses do not believe total pain relief is possible and therefore do not aim high enough. Sometimes patients use their pain to self-monitor progress post-operatively (Fordham, 1985) and although the eventual expected outcome is 'no pain', they do not wish to be pain-free immediately.

The goal for harmful or potentially harmful pain should be immediate reduction or elimination if the dangerous sequelae are to be avoided (Bonica, 1982).

Realistic goal setting for chronic pain is far from straightforward. Multi-disciplinary assessment and discussion of available interventions and likely outcomes are essential to realistic goal setting for these patients (Glyn, 1987).

PAIN INTERVENTIONS

It is not proposed in this chapter to reproduce the existing comprehensive reviews of particular interventions, but rather to attempt to put nursing interventions into some context.

As pain is one of the most common reasons for individuals to seek medical aid, the overwhelming majority of surgical and medical interventions aim to remove or alleviate the cause(s) of pain. Most surgery, be it to remove diseased viscera such as inflamed appendices or tumours, or replace clogged blood vessels, is highly successful in eliminating pain, as is much radiotherapy of primary and secondary tumours. New non-invasive treatments, such as lithotripsy, can even remove the cause of pain without incurring post-operative wound pain. Doctors, nurses, physiotherapists and others expend much of their time and energy in 'putting the patient in the best condition for nature to heal itself'—in the mostly realised expectation that, when healing occurs, pain will disappear. Suturing, splinting, positioning, providing appropriate nutrition, judicious exercise, adequate rest and many other caring activities are all grist to the mill in aiding rapid healing and so reducing the initial cause(s) of pain and avoiding the iatrogenesis of further pain(s).

However, as discussed at the beginning of this chapter, there are many pains which are endured unnecessarily, including those caused by acute injury, serious pathology and operation. There are chronic pains arising from pathological processes which medical science does not yet know how to reverse, and most problematic of all there are intractable pains arising from central and peripheral nerve damage.

In almost all situations, we are part of a team of carers with different skills and opportunities to help. Anaesthetists have developed special skill in, for example, local and regional block analgesia (Bonica, 1984) and epidural anaesthesia (Bromage, 1984). Neurosurgeons can treat central nervous system lesions with percutaneous cordotomy

(Lipton, 1984), brain stem surgery (Sweet and Poletti, 1984) and psychosurgery (Bouckoms, 1984) with variable success in eliminating or reducing intractable pain. Radiotherapy, chemotherapy and hormone therapy may be used to reduce pain (Hoy, 1984). Orthopaedic surgeons and other medics use their skills in an attempt to reduce or obliterate pain. Many physiotherapy techniques such as ultrasound, shortwave, microwave, heat and cold treatments, massage and manipulation are all pain treatments (Lehmann and de Lateur, 1984). Psychotherapy (Pinsky and Crue, 1984) and complementary therapies, such as music therapy and relaxation techniques (Benson et al, 1984) also aim to reduce the causes or the adverse consequences of the experience of pain.

Where then does the nurse's role in intervention lie? What skills do they have or should they have? Do they behave as Sofaer (1983) suggests they should, accepting that 'pain relief (is) the core of nursing practice'? Most nursing interventions are non-invasive, therefore apart from the medically delegated task of drug administration, nurses mainly use psychosocial interventions and physical or environmental manipulations (see Table 2).

Table 2. Nursing interventions

---

1. Assessment and advocacy.
2. Analgesic and other drug administration.
3. Support of patients' own methods of pain control.
   Externally focused such as rocking, rubbing 'flight into activity', seeking companions.
   Internally focused such as vigilant focusing, mind-body separation, fantasy.
   Avoidance strategies such as posture, stillness, sleep.
4. Teaching of, and assisting with, cognitive and behavioural coping strategies.
   Distraction techniques such as guided imagery, mental focusing.
   Relaxation techniques.
5. Non-invasive physical therapies.
   Cutaneous stimulation such as pressure, massage, vibration, heat, cold, external analgesia, transcutaneous nerve stimulation.

Assessment and advocacy

Assessment has been discussed at length. Osler in 1947 said,

> 'I envy for our medical students the advantages enjoyed by the nurses who live in daily contact with the sick.'

The shorter working hours of nurses and the rapid discharge rate of patients from hospital have eroded this advantage, but still we accompany our patients as they attempt to carry out their normal activities—we still have rich opportunities to assess in detail the incidence of pain and the effect of pain on a person's life. If we develop our skills in assessment and help the patient to communicate, we can fulfil our role as advocate to other team members, be they nursing colleagues or members of other professions. Three conditions are necessary for advocacy to be realised—firstly, a belief in the patient's communication of his/her pain experience, secondly, the sensitivity to recognise pain provoking situations, especially for those who cannot communicate verbally, and thirdly, the fostering of a multi-disciplinary approach which includes the patient.

Bagley et al (1982) remarked that pain in a hospice is not only more likely to be considered a multi-dimensional concept, but also to be managed in a multi-disciplinary way. Foley (1985) discusses the importance of a multi-disciplinary approach for cancer pain. Sofaer (1985) in her discussion of the issue of nurse education about pain, points out the truism that

> 'one of the major barriers to caring for patients in pain is poor communication between patients, nurses and doctors.' (p.71)

Policy interventions are also needed at management level to facilitate good practice, including participation in pain control teams (White, 1985) and multi-disciplinary teaching forums. One finding which is evident from the research literature is the paucity of multi-disciplinary research. Following the suggestion made in the childish hymn that everyone should shine 'you in your small corner and I in mine' just will not do for the relief of pain. The conventional way of describing the behaviour of the patient with chronic and intractable pain who goes from one medical specialist to another, then to alternative or complementary practitioners, is of someone who fails to understand the nature and purpose of their pain (Pilowsky and Spence, 1976). At the least, such a person is likely to be called irrational, and at worst to acquire a more pejorative psychiatric label. An holistic approach and interdisciplinary co-operation could undoubtedly reduce the need for such patient behaviour and would also help the helpers to cope with the despair of failure to remove everyone's pain.

Analgesic and other drug administration

Research on analgesic and other drug therapy has been sufficient to lead to a number of recommendations for practice. Marks and Sachter (1973) surveyed medical patients and found that three-quarters of those with severe pain continued to experience moderate to severe distress, despite narcotic use. They suggest that doctors prescribed narcotics at half to two-thirds the required dose for pain relief and nurses under-administered the drugs by another half to one-third. Underestimation of the effective dose range, overestimation of the duration of action and exaggeration of the dangers of addiction and respiratory depression were cited as causes for this failure. There is little excuse for these misconceptions and myths, but they persist (Weis et al, 1983). Hoskins et al (1985) found a lack of knowledge in a substantial proportion of nurses.

Severe pain is a powerful respiratory stimulant, so it is usually possible to achieve pain relief without dangerous compromise of respiration (Twycross, 1984). Also, narcotics reduce voluntary muscle immobility and so many increase chest movements. In the case of agonist narcotics, an antidote, nalorphine, exists. Appropriate medical selection of patients (Hanks et al, 1981) and vigilant post-analgesic monitoring of patients at particular risk of respiratory failure is obviously prudent. Walsh et al (1981) found that clinically important respiratory depression rarely occurred in patients with severe pain due to malignant disease, even when they received large doses of morphine. Chapman (1984) says that recent clinical trials have shown that narcotic analgesics carefully titrated to the needs of the patient provide good pain relief 'without producing respiratory depression and indeed a narcotic-induced analgesia results in improvement of ventilation' (p. 1268).

As long ago as 1943, Himmelsbach reported that (a) physical dependence requires regular routine administration of the optimum therapeutic dose of narcotics four–six times per day for six weeks, and (b) the incidence of addiction was 1 in 4,000 of hospitalised patients who received narcotics. Porter and Jick (1980) in a survey of 12,000 adults and children found that addiction was similarly rare in patients treated with narcotics. Some patients are labelled as addicted when they demand injections and clockwatch anxiously. Such patients typically have gained inadequate analgesia from their current regime and/or have experienced long delays in the administration of drugs. They are not demanding narcotics to gain psychological effects, but to be relieved of pain (Twycross, 1984). Reassessment and replanning of drug therapy and other care is indicated.

The avoidance of breakthrough pain is an important aim in pain control (Coyle et al, 1985). Lower doses of drugs will control lower levels of pain, and, for this reason regular, not as necessary (p.r.n.), prescription and administration of analgesia is more successful in controlling severe continuous pain. In any case p.r.n. analgesia does not have fewer side-effects than routine administration (*British Medical Journal*, 1978). Effective relief of pain may be achieved by the use of both centrally acting narcotics and peripherally acting non-narcotics or non-steroidal anti-inflammatory drugs (Tammisto and Tigerstedt, 1982). Adjuvant analgesic drugs including tricyclic antidepressants, anticonvulsants and diuretics have been found to be effective in controlling certain chronic pains and their accompanying symptoms. There are many excellent reviews of current knowledge of drug actions on pain, for example Goodinson (1986), Huskinson (1984), Twycross (1984), and Monks and Merskey (1984). Foley (1985), Coyle et al (1985) and Melzack (1981) discuss the logic of analgesia for cancer pain and Latham (1983a,b,c and d; 1985a and b; 1986a and b) in her series of articles discusses the work of pain clinics and the control of pain. Research findings on the actions and efficacy of newly developed analgesia appear in the *Drug and Therapeutics Bulletin* (see, for example, June 17, 1985 on buprenorphine). Pharmacological developments aim to produce drugs which have less side-effects, especially on the nervous and gastrointestinal systems, and can be absorbed from external sites such as skin and mucous membranes. Two points are noteworthy regarding the use of analgesia. Firstly, it is not reasonable to expect any drug or any dose level to be equally effective in all patients. Drugs are manufactured and marketed on the basis that they are effective in 50% of cases. Secondly, the patient's need for analgesia cannot be inferred from his/her diagnosis.

Support of patients' own methods of pain control

Pain is a stress and there are three main ways in which a person may respond to or cope with stress — active cognitive coping, active behavioural coping and avoidance (Billings and Moos, 1981). Nurses could view their role as helping the pain sufferer to choose the most appropriate ways of coping, and aiding and abetting their responses (Broome, 1986). Patients with acute and chronic pain develop ways to tolerate, minimise or reduce their pain (Tan, 1982). Copp (1974) interviewed over 100 acute and chronic pain patients and reported that most of them used both cognitive and behavioural coping strategies. Children used similar coping strategies to adults.

Research findings suggest that coping strategies effective in experimentally induced pain are not effective in chronic pain (Rosensteil and Keefe, 1983), and that it does not always follow that, because a person uses a particular strategy, it is necessarily the most effective response (Chapman, 1984).

The literature on cognitive and behavioural coping strategies is bedevilled with inconsistency in classification and use of terminology. Copp (1985) categorises pain coping strategies used by patients as either externally or internally focused. Externally orientated strategies include the use of the muscles of the body to inflict counter pain on themselves, to rock, rub, or take 'flight into activity'; to seek the presence of other persons with whom to talk, use as a witness, or strength lender or validator of their suffering; and to use, wear or touch specific objects associated with pain relief in a sort of superstitious way. Internally orientated strategies require concentrated thinking. Copp describes five categories: vigilant focusing, mind-body separation, spatial relationships, tropistic yearning (e.g. for the feel of the sun, or sound of running water), and dreams. Fernandez (1986) classifies pain management in a trimodal system according to the source of control: cognitive strategies (self-controlled), behavioural manipulations (externally controlled initially), and physical interventions (completely externally controlled). Cognitive strategies in this classification include imagery and fantasy (Horan et al, 1975), self-statements (Worthington, 1978), and attention diversion (Kanfer and Goldfoot, 1966).

Avoidance strategies are used in both acute and chronic pain and may be achieved by, for example, the use of drugs and by keeping still. Broome (1986) found that patients with chronic orthopaedic pain did use avoidance strategies, finding a comfortable position, resting, taking analgesics. However, excessive reliance on avoidance strategies in chronic or intractable pain may in the long run be counter-productive. Avoiding activities, exercise and work may lead to an unnecessarily curtailed life-style without achieving pain relief. Some people may have to unlearn maladaptive and learn adaptive behaviour (Lethem et al, 1983).

A number of explanations are put forward for why particular strategies work. As the pain experience includes sensory, emotional and cognitive aspects, alteration in any or all of these aspects can be beneficial. Reducing anxiety and tension levels can break the pain-tension-anxiety cycle and potentially reduce pain. The self-appraisal of power has been found to be a major determinant of emotional state (Russell, 1978) so maintaining or regaining control is considered an important determinant of pain, especially chronic pain which otherwise can result in helplessness, despair and pessimism. Fernandez (1986) suggests that as psychological variables influence pain, including anxiety, predictability, perceived controllability, attention, personality attributes and sociocultural factors, cognitive strategies which influence these variables constitute a major approach to the management of pain. Many of the active cognitive and active behavioural strategies capture the focus of attention and so displace pain from the centre of consciousness, at least for a while.

Teaching of and assisting with cognitive and behavioural coping strategies

There are many circumstances in which nurses can assist the patient in using mental focusing and other distraction strategies, for example when coping with brief painful procedures, by talking or doing mental arithmetic, etc. We can help patients to use guided imagery (Gollop, 1983) and teach breathing and relaxation techniques. Midwives have been doing so for generations. Eland (1985) supports the usefulness of teaching such techniques to children whose rich imagination can be harnessed positively. Aiding and abetting the use of coping strategies includes providing the right environment. This may be quietness, privacy or group activities. It may mean giving permission and acceptance to patients to do whatever they find helpful. Helping may require us to contact the person whom the patient most wants by his side. The one thing children wanted most when they were in pain was their parents (Ross and Ross, 1984) even though Eland (1983) suggests that parents did not always understand their child's pain and mostly had great faith that the nurse did and would know what to do about it. Interestingly, many researchers including Vorchol (1983) have found that children do not necessarily know that they may hurt less if they keep still. Eland (1985) suggests that children's early post-operative mobility may be an attempt to escape from the place, the people and the procedures which add to their hurt. The action of intramuscular analgesia is not instantaneous, so if they do not understand the reason for an injection and expect causal connections to be close in timing, it may be logical to try to avoid nurses. The importance of teaching and assisting patients to use coping strategies is that it returns some control of the situation to the sufferer and raises their self-esteem.

Non-invasive physical therapies

The most common non-invasive physical therapy is massage (Tappan, 1984), an ancient art practised by specialists, physiotherapists and increasingly by nurses. McCaffery (1983) describes the use of numerous methods of cutaneous stimulation for pain relief, including pressure, massage, vibration, heat, cold, external analgesia and transcutaneous nerve stimulation (TENS). Some of these interventions are merely extensions of the behavioural strategies used by people in pain. These touch therapies may be effective in relieving pain when used either at its site, in adjacent and/or in contralateral areas, or far distant parts of the body, and their effectiveness is not only dependent upon what is done, but also by whom (Beard and Wood, 1974). It is important that the recipient wishes and consents to try these therapies as imposing them may be perceived as assault.

In addition to the interventions so far mentioned in this chapter, there are others which nurses may learn to use or assist other professions in using, such as hypnosis (Hildegard, 1975), biofeedback (Flor et al, 1983), acupuncture (Price et al, 1984), and operant conditioning (Fordyce, 1976). Behaviour therapy is sometimes used as a method of unlearning maladaptive and learning adaptive behavioural responses to chronic pain (Turk and Flor, 1984).

CONCLUSION

There are many hypotheses about the physiological mechanisms of pain relief. The most clearly supported by evidence are the actions of analgesics and physical therapies. However, there is also dispute and contradictory evidence in the literature about the ways in which interventions work and the most commonsensical explanations are not always supported by findings (Flor et al, 1983). Current understanding of the multiple influences on the pain experience and the complexity of the nervous system interactions should lead us to abandon 'one-cause-one-effect' explanations of pain and therapeutic interventions. Gate control theory can be invoked to explain any successful strategy post hoc — but prediction is still a lottery. Willingness to be open-minded, accepting and adventurous in the use of pain-relieving strategies is likely to be more useful to the pain sufferer than premature ossification of explanations of why or how they work.

Sometimes just having an hypothesis about how pain relief may work is sufficient to give respectability and acceptance to an intervention. It is therefore not always the case that proof of how or why a method works is considered necessary prior to using it. This is true of pharmacological as well as other methods. Knowledge of the many physiological actions of aspirin has taken time to emerge and has followed rather than preceded the use of the drug. The understanding of the actions of morphia and the relationship with morphine receptor sites and the naturally occurring endorphins is very recent, but the use of morphia goes back to earliest history.

It seems however that there is a breakthrough or threshold level of understanding required before a method of relieving pain acquires respectability. The acceptance of acupuncture by Western cultures illustrates this point—first of all being dismissed or doubted by most Western medicine, then grudgingly thought to have something to do with gate control theory or endorphin levels (Clement Jones et al, 1980), so let us use it and see if and when it works and try to tease out the mechanisms. The overwhelming need of people for pain relief is such that it is just as unethical to withhold a method of treatment because we are unsure of how it works as it is to use a method which has iatrogenic side-effects which outweigh the benefits.

What is regarded as acceptable also seems to depend on the circumstances. In hospital, pharmacological relief seems to have greater credence and efficacy than non-pharmacological methods. In a large study of 454 medical/surgical patients in the USA, analgesia was reported by the patients as the most effective intervention, followed by sleep, immobilisation and distraction (Donovan et al, 1987).

Pain is both a formidable foe and an essential ally. Pain perception is vital for survival and the nervous system responds in such a way as to maintain this ability despite our best efforts to obliterate the experience. As Wall (1984b) concludes:

'The brain specialises in dynamic homeostatic controls. Unfortunately those controls may change to a pain producing pathological setting . . . Combination, alternation and circulation of therapies may well be the best tactic to defeat the homeostatic abilities of nervous mechanisms to restore pathological states.' (p. 840)

Nurses have an important part to play in helping patients to use and lose their pain.

FUTURE RESEARCH

There is a need for further fundamental research, particularly into the phenomena and alleviation of chronic and visceral pain. As in sleep and other areas of research, there is a relative lack of longitudinal studies and of multi-disciplinary research compared with cross-sectional studies and single discipline research. Possible areas of future nursing research include:

1. Longitudinal studies of individual patient's pain careers both in hospital and the community.

2. Descriptive studies for example of patients' understanding of the meaning and significance of their pain experience.
3. Evaluation studies, particularly of nursing interventions for people with chronic pain, and research into the effectiveness of supporting patients' own choice of methods of pain relief, of teaching cognitive and behavioural methods of pain alleviation, and the use of non-invasive physical therapies.
4. Comparative studies, for example to elucidate the similarities and differences between patients' desired outcomes and nurses' expected outcomes and between patients' views of nurses' behaviour and interventions and nurses' expectations of their own interventions to relieve pain.
5. Cross-cultural studies, for example to compare the expectations and interpretations of pain by successive generations of different ethnic groups in the same society.

REFERENCES

Bagley CS, Falinski E, Garnizo N, Hooker L (1982) Pain management: a pilot project. *Cancer Nursing* **June**, 191–199.

Beard G, Wood EC (1974) *Massage: Principles and Techniques*. WB Saunders, Philadelphia.

Benson H, Pomeranz B, Kutz I (1984) The relaxation response and pain. In: Wall PD, Melzack R (eds) *Textbook of Pain*. Churchill Livingstone, Edinburgh.

Billings G, Moos RH (1981) The role of coping responses and social resources in attenuating the stress of life events. *Journal of Behavioural Medicine* **4**(2), 139–157.

Bonica JJ (1980a) Introduction to pain. *Pain* **58**, 1–17.

Bonica JJ (1980b) Pain research therapy: past and current states and future needs. In: Bonica JJ, Ng Lorenz KY (eds) *Pain Discomfort and Humanitarian Care*, 1–136. Proceedings of the National Institute of Health, Bethesda, Maryland, USA. Feb 15–17, 1979. Elsevier North Holland, Amsterdam.

Bonica J (1982) Introduction. Narcotic analgesics in the treatment of cancer and post-operative pain. Proceedings from symposium. Stockholm. Nov 12–14, 1980 *Acta Anaesthesiologica Scandinavia* Supplement 74. **26**, 5–10.

Bonica JJ (1984) Local anaesthesia and regional blocks. Chapter 1, Section 3B. In: Wall PD, Melzack R (eds) *Textbook of Pain*. Churchill Livingstone, Edinburgh.

Borg G (1970) Perceived exertion as an indicator of somatic stress. *Scandinavian Journal of Rehabilitative Medicine* **2–3**, 92–98.

Bouckoms AJ (1984) Psycho-surgery. In: Wall PD, Melzack R (eds) *Textbook of Pain*. Churchill Livingstone, Edinburgh.

Bourbonnais F (1981) Pain assessment: development of a tool for the nurse and the patient. *Journal of Advanced Nursing* **6**, 277–282.

British Medical Journal (1978) Editorial, post-operative pain. *British Medical Journal* **8**(6136), 517–518.

Bromage PR (1984) Epidural anaesthetics and narcotics. In: Wall PD, Melzack R (eds) *Textbook of Pain*. Churchill Livingstone, Edinburgh.

Broome A (1986) Coping with pain. Strategies for relief. *Nursing Times* **Apr 16**, 43–44.

Carlsson AM (1983) Assessment of chronic pain 1. Aspects of the reliability and validity of the visual analogue scale. *Pain* **16**, 87–101.

Carpenito LJ (1983) *Nursing Diagnoses; Application to Clinical Practice*. JB Lippincott Co, Philadelphia.

Cervero F (1987) Visceral pain. Fifth world congress on pain of the International Association for the Study of Pain. *Pain* Supplement **4**, 51–54.

Chapman R (1984) New directions in the understanding and management of pain. *Social Science and Medicine* **19**(12), 1261–1277.

Chen ACN, Chapman CR (1980) Aspirin analgesia evaluated by event-related potential in man: possible central action in brain. *Experimental Brain Research* **39**, 359–364.

Clement-Jones V, McLoughlin L, Tomlin S, Besser GM, Rees LH, Wen HL (1980) Increased beta-endorphin but not met-enkephalin levels in human cerebrospinal fluid after acupuncture for recurrent pain. *Lancet* **ii**, 946–949.

Cohen FL (1980) Postsurgical pain relief: patients' status and nurses medication choices. *Pain* **9**(2), 265–274.

Copp LA (1974) The spectrum of suffering. *American Journal of Nursing* **74**(3), 491–495.

Copp LA (1985) Pain coping. In: Copp LA (ed) *Perspectives on Pain. Recent Advances in Nursing* 11, pp. 3–16. Churchill Livingstone, Edinburgh.

Coyle N, Monzill E, Loscalzo M, Farka C, Massie MJ, Foley KM (1985) A model of continuity of care for cancer patients with pain and neuro-oncologic complications. *Cancer Nursing* **8**, 111–119.

Craig KD (1978) Social modelling influences on pain. In: Sternbach RA (ed) *The Psychology of Pain*. Academic Press, New York.

Crawford-Clark W (1984) Applications of multidimensional scaling to problems in experimental and clinical pain. In: Bromm B (ed) *Pain Measurement in Man: Neurophysiological Correlates of Pain*, pp. 349–369. Elsevier, Amsterdam.

Darwin C (1965) *The Expression of the Emotions in Man and Animals*. University of Chicago Press, Chicago. (Originally published 1872)

Descartes R (1644) L'homme, In: *Lectures on the History of Physiology during the 16th, 17th and 18th Centuries*. (translated by Foster M), Cambridge University Press, Cambridge.

Domzal T, Szczudlik A, Kwasucki J, Zaleska B, Lypka A (1983) Plasma cortisol concentrations in patients with different circadian pain rhythms. *Pain* **17**, 67–70.

Donovan M, Dillon P, McGuire L (1987) Incidence and characteristics of pain in a sample of medical-surgical in-patients. *Pain* **30**, 69–78.

Drug and Therapeutics Bulletin (1985) *Stronger Analgesics with Low Risk of Dependence—Buprenorphine, Meptazinol and Nalbuphine*. Consumers Association 23(12), 45–46.

Dubuisson D, Melzack R (1976) Classification of clinical pain descriptions by multiple group discriminant analysis. *Experimental Neurology* **51**, 480.

Eland JM, Anderson JE (1977) The experience of pain in children. In: Jacox A (ed) *Pain: a Source Book for Nurses and other Health Professionals*. Little Brown, Boston.

Eland JM (1983) Children's pain: developmentally appropriate efforts to improve identification of source, intensity and relevant intervening variables. In: Felton G, Albert M (eds) *Nursing Research: A Monograph for Non-nurse Researchers*.

Eland JM (1985) The role of the nurse in children's pain. In: Copp LA (ed) *Perspectives on Pain. Recent Advances in Nursing* 11. Churchill Livingstone, Edinburgh and London.

Fagerhaugh SY, Strauss A (1977) *Politics of Pain Management: Staff Patient Interaction*. Addison-Wesley, California.

Fernandez E (1986) A classification system of cognitive coping strategies for pain. *Pain* **26**, 141–151.

Fields HL, Basbaum AI (1984) Endogenous pain control mechanism. In: Wall PD, Melzack R (eds) *Textbook of Pain*. Churchill Livingstone, Edinburgh.

Flor H, Haag G, Turk DC, Koehler H (1983) Efficacy of EMG biofeedback, pseudotherapy and conventional medical treatment for chronic rheumatic back pain. *Pain* **17**, 21–31.

Foley KM (1985) The treatment of cancer pain. *New England Journal of Medicine*, **313**(2), 84–95.

Fordham M (1985) Deconditioning and reconditioning following elective surgery. Thesis (unpublished), University of London.

Fordham M (1986) Psychophysiological pain theories. *Nursing* **3**(10), 360–364.

Fordyce WE (1976) *Behavioural Methods for Chronic Pain and Illness*. Mosby, St. Louis.

Gartside G (1985) Alternative methods of pain relief. *Nursing* **3**(11), 405–407.

Gaston-Johansson F (1984) Pain assessment: differences in quality and intensity of the words pain, ache and hurt. *Pain* **20**, 69–76.

Glyn CL, Lloyd JW, Folkard S (1976) The diurnal variation in perception of pain. *Proceedings of the Royal Society of Medicine* **69**, 369–372.

Glyn C (1987) Intractable pain: a problem identification and solving exercise. *Hospital Update* **13**(1), 44–54.

Gollop SM (1983) Pain and pain control. In: Wilson-Barnett J (ed) *Patient Teaching*. Churchill Livingstone, Edinburgh.

Goodinson SM (1986) Pain relief: pharmacological intervention. *Nursing* **3**(11), 395–403.

Hallin RG, Torebjörk EH (1980) Activity in unmyelinated nerve fibres in man. In: Bonica J (ed) *Advances in Neurology 4*, pp. 19–27. International Symposium on Pain, Raven Press, New York.

Hallsten L (1980) The puzzle of 0.7. and some other issues of ratio scaling. *Report 80*. Institute of Applied Psychology, University of Stockholm.

Hanks GW (1983) Management of symptoms in advanced cancer. *Update* **26**(10), 1691–1702.

Hanks GW, Twycross RG, Lloyd JW (1981) Unexpected complications of successful nerve block: morphine induced respiratory depression following removal of severe pain. *Anaesthesia* **36**(1), 37–39.

Hardy J, Wolff H, Goodell H (1952) *Pain Sensations and Reactions*. Williams and Wilkins, Baltimore.

Haslam DR (1969) Age and the perception of pain. *Psychosomatic Science* **15**, 86.

Hildegard ER (1975) The alleviation of pain by hypnosis. *Pain* **1**, 213–231.

Himmelsbach CK (1943) Further studies of the addiction liability of demorol. *Journal of Pharmacology and Experimental Therapy* **79**, 5.

Horan JJ, Laying FC, Pursell CH (1976) Preliminary study of effect of 'in vivo' emotive imagery on dental discomfort. *Perceptual and Motor Skills* **42**, 105–106.

Horsley JA, Crane J, Reynolds MA (1982) *Pain: Deliberative Nursing Interventions*, CURN Project, Grune and Stratton, New York.

Hoskins JM, McFarlane EA, Rubenfeld MG, Walsh MB, Schreier AM (1985) Nursing diagnosis in the chronically ill: methodology for clinical validation. *Advances in Nursing Science* **8**(3), 80–89.

Houde RW (1982) Methods for measuring clinical pain in humans. *Acta Anaesthesioligica Scandinavica Supplement* **74**, 25–29.

Hoy AM (1984) Radiotherapy, chemotherapy and hormone therapy; treatment for pain. In: Wall PD, Melzack R (eds) *Textbook of Pain*, Churchill Livingstone, Edinburgh.

Huskinson EC (1984) Non-narcotic analgesica. In: Wall PD, Melzack R (eds) *Textbook of Pain*. Churchill Livingstone, Edinburgh.

International Association for the Study of Pain Sub-Committee on Taxonomy (1979) Pain terms: a list with definitions and notes on usage. *Pain* **6**, 249–252.

Izard CE, Huebner RR, Risser D, McGinnes CG, Dougherty LM (1980) The young infant's ability to produce discrete emotion expressions. *Developmental Psychology* **16**, 132.

Jacox A (1979) Assessing pain. *American Journal of Nursing* **79**(5), 895–900.

Jay SM, Ozolins M, Eliot CH et al (1983) Assessment of children's distress during painful medical procedures. *Health Psychology* **2**, 133–147.

Jensen TS, Rasmussen P (1984) Amputation. In: Wall PD, Melzack R (eds) *Textbook of Pain*, Churchill Livingstone, Edinburgh.

Johnson M (1977) Assessment of clinical pain. In: Jacox AK (ed) *Pain: a Sourcebook for Nurses and Other Health Professionals*, pp. 139–166. Little Brown, Boston.

Kanfer FH, Goldfoot DA (1966) Self-control and tolerance of noxious stimulation. *Journal of Personality and Social Psychology* **25**, 381–389.

Kohn R, Kerr LW (eds) (1976) *Health Care: an International Study*. Oxford University Press, London.

Kraut RE (1978) Verbal and non-verbal cues in the perception of lying. *Journal of Personal and Social Psychology* **36**, 380–391.

Latham J (1983a) The pain relief team. *Nursing Times* **Apr 27**, 54–57.

Latham J (1983b) The nervous system. *Nursing Times* **May 4**, 57–60.

Latham J (1983c) Complications. *Nursing Times* **May 11**, 36–38.

Latham J (1983d) The nurses' role. *Nursing Times* **May 18**, 33–35.

Latham J (1985a) Pain control: an introduction. *Professional Nurse* **Oct**, 17.

Latham J (1985b) Functional anatomy and physiology of pain. *Professional Nurse* **Nov**, 42–44.

Latham J (1986a) Assessment, observation and measurement of pain. *Professional Nurse* **Jan**, 107–110.

Latham J (1986b) Pain relief unit techniques: neural blockage. *Professional Nurse* **Mar**, 151–154.

Lehmann JF, de Lateur BJ (1984) Ultrasound, shortwave, microwave, superficial heat and cold in the treatment of pain. In: Wall PD, Melzack R (eds) *Textbook of Pain*. Churchill Livingstone, Edinburgh.

Lenburg CB, Glass HP, Davitz LJ (1970) Pain in relation to the stage of the patient's illness and occupation of the perceiver. *Nursing Research* **19**, 392–398.

Le Resche L (1982) Facial behaviour in pain: a study of candid photographs. *Journal of Non-verbal Behaviour* **7**, 46.

Lethem J, Slade PD, Troup JDG, Bentley G (1983) Outline of a fear-avoidance model of exaggerated pain perception, 1. *Behaviour Research Therapy* **21**(4), 401–408.

Lindblom U (1982) Neurophysiological measurement of pain. *Acta Anaesthesiologica Scandinavica Supplement* **74**, 30–32.

Lindeman CA (1975) Delphi survey of priorities in clinical nursing research. *Nursing Research* **24**(6), 434–441.

Linton SJ, Gotestam KG (1983) A clinical comparison of two pain scales: correlation, remembering chronic pain and a measure of compliance. *Pain* **17**, 57–65.

Lipton JA, Marbach JJ (1984) Ethnicity and the pain experience. *Social Science and Medicine* **19**(12), 1279–1298.

Lipton S (1984) Percutaneous cordotomy. In: Wall PD, Melzack R (eds) *Textbook of Pain*. Churchill Livingstone, Edinburgh.

Loan WB, Morrison JD (1976) The incidence and severity of post-operative pain. *British Journal of Anaesthesia* **39**, 695–698.

McCaffery M (1972) *Nursing Management of the Patient in Pain*. JB Lippincott, Philadelphia.

McCaffery M (1983) *Nursing the Patient in Pain*. Adapted for the UK by Beatrice Sofaer. Lippincott Nursing Series, Harper & Row, London.

McConnell EA (1983) After surgery: how you can avoid the obvious . . . and the not so obvious hazards. *Nursing* (US) **13**(875), 8–15.

Marks RM, Sachter EJ (1973) Undertreatment of medical in-patients with narcotic analgesia. *Annals of International Medicine* **78**, 173.

Melzack R (1975) The McGill pain questionnaire: major properties and scoring methods. *Pain* **1**, 277–299.

Melzack R (1981) Current concepts of pain. In: Saunders Dame C, Summers DH, Teller A (eds) *Hospice: the Living Idea*, Edward Arnold, London.

Melzack R, Wall PD, Ty TC (1982) Acute pain in an emergency clinic: latency of onset and descriptor patterns related to different injuries. *Pain* **14**, 33–43.

Molesberry D (1979) *Young Children's Subjective Quantification of Pain Following Surgery*, unpublished Thesis, University of Iowa.

Monks R, Merskey H (1984) Psychotropic drugs. In: Wall PD, Melzack R (eds) *Textbook of Pain*. Churchill Livingstone, Edinburgh.

Ohnhaus EE, Adler L (1975) Methodological problems in the measurement of pain. A comparison between the verbal rating scale and the visual analogue scale. *Pain* **1**, 379.

Orlando IJ (1961) *The Dynamic Nurse–patient Relationship*. Putnam's & Sons, New York.

Osler W (1947) *The Hospital as a College*. Aequanimatas, The Blackstone Co, Philadelphia.

Pilowsky I, Spence ND (1976) Illness behaviour syndromes associated with intractable pain. *Pain* **2**, 61–71.

Pinsky JJ, Crue BL (1984) Intensive group psychotherapy. In: Wall PD, Melzack R (eds) *Textbook of Pain*. Churchill Livingstone, Edinburgh.

Porter J, Jick H (1980) Addiction rare in patients treated with narcotics. *New England Journal of Medicine* **302**, 123.

Price DD, McGrath PA, Rafii A, Buckingham B (1983) The validation of visual analogue scales as ratio scale measures for chronic and experimental pain. *Pain* **17**, 45–56.

Price DD, Rafii A, Watkins LR, Buckingham B (1984) A psychophysical analysis of acupuncture analgesia. *Pain* **19**, 27–42.

Procacci P, Corte MD, Zoppi M, Maresca M (1974) Rhythmic changes of the cutaneous pain threshold in man. A general view. *Chronobiologia* 1, 77–96.

Procacci P, Zoppi M (1984) Heart pain. In: Wall PD, Melzack R (eds) *Textbook of Pain*. Churchill Livingstone, Edinburgh.

Proshansky HM, Ittelson WH, Rivlin LG (1970) *Experimental Psychology*. Holt, Rinehart and Winston, New York.

Raiman J (1986) Towards understanding pain and planning for relief. *Nursing* 11, 411–423.

Reading AE (1982) A comparison of the McGill Pain Questionnaire in chronic and acute pain. *Pain* 13, 185–192.

Reading AE (1984) Testing pain mechanisms in persons in pain. In: Wall PD, Melzack R (eds) *Textbook of Pain*, Churchill Livingstone, Edinburgh.

Rosenstiel AK, Keefe FJ (1983) The use of coping strategies in chronic low back pain patients: relationship to patient characteristics and current adjustment. *Pain* 17, 33–44.

Ross DM, Ross SA (1984) Childhood pain: the school-aged child's viewpoint. *Pain* 20, 179–191.

Russell JA (1978) Evidence of convergent validity on the dimensions of affect. *Journal of Personality and Social Psychology* 30, 1152–1168.

Sargent C (1984) Between death and shame: dimensions of pain in Bariba culture. *Social Science and Medicine* 19(12), 1299–1304.

Scott J, Huskisson EC (1976) Graphic representation of pain. *Pain* 2, 175–184.

Scott WE (1982) The continuing problem of pain: a discussion paper. *Journal of the Royal Society of Medicine* 75, 117–120.

Seers C (1987) *Pain, Anxiety and Recovery in Patients undergoing Surgery*. PhD thesis (unpublished), University of London, London.

Smith G (1983) Advances in morphine therapy. International Congress and Symposium Series 6A. Royal Society of Medicine, pp. 11–17.

Sofaer G (1983) Pain relief—the core of nursing practice. *Nursing Times* Nov 23–29, 79(47), 38–42.

Sofaer B (1984) *The Effect of Focused Education for Nursing Teams on Post-operative Pain of Patients*, PhD thesis (unpublished), University of Edinburgh, Edinburgh.

Sofaer B (1985) Pain management through nurse education. In: Copp LA (ed) *Perspectives on Pain*, Recent Advances in Nursing 11, Churchill Livingstone, Edinburgh and London.

Sternbach RA (1968) *Pain: a Psychophysiological Analysis*. Academic Press, New York.

Sternbach RA (1974) *Pain Patients—Tracts and Treatment*. Academic Press, New York.

Sternbach RA (1984) Acute versus chronic pain. In: Wall PD, Melzack R (eds) *Textbook of Pain*. Churchill Livingstone, Edinburgh.

Stevens SS (1975) *Psychophysics*. Introduction to its perceptual, neural and social prospects. Wiley, New York.

Stoddard FJ (1982) Coping with pain: a developmental approach to the treatment of burned children. *American Journal of Psychiatry* 139, 736–740.

Swafford LI, Allen D (1968) Pain relief in the paediatric patient. *Medical Clinics of North America* 48, 131–133.

Sweet WH, Poletti CE (1984) Operations of the brain stem and spinal canal, with an appendix on open cordotomy. In: Wall PD, Melzack R (eds) *Textbook of Pain*. Churchill Livingstone, Edinburgh.

Tammisto T, Tigerstedt I, Korttila K (1980) Comparison of lysine acetyl salicylate and oxycodone in postoperative pain following upper abdominal surgery. *Annales Chirurgiae et Gynaecologiae* 69(6), 287–292.

Tammisto T, Tigerstedt I (1982) Narcotic analgesics in postoperative pain relief in adults. *Acta Anaesthesiologica Scandinavica Supplement* 74, 161–164.

Tan SY (1982) Cognitive and cognitive-behavioural methods for pain control: a selective review. *Pain* 12, 201–228.

Tappan F (1984) Massage. In: Wall PD, Melzack R (eds) *Textbook of Pain*, Churchill Livingstone, Edinburgh.

Teske K, Daut RL, Cleeland CS (1983) Relationships between nurses' observations and patients' self reports of pain. *Pain* 16, 289–296.

Turk DC, Flor H (1984) Etiological theories and treatments for chronic back pain. 11. Psychological models and interaction. *Pain* **19**, 209–233.

Tursky B (1976) The development of a pain perception profile: a psychological approach. In: Weisenberg M, Tursky B (eds), *New Perspectives in Therapy and Research*. Plenum Press, New York.

Twycross RG, Lack SA (1983) *Symptom Control in Far Advanced Cancer*. Pitman, London.

Twycross RG (1984) Narcotics. In: Wall PD, Melzack R (eds) *Textbook of Pain*. Churchill Livingstone, Edinburgh.

Urban BJ, Keefe FJ, France RD (1984) A study of psychophysical scaling in chronic pain patients. *Pain* **20**, 157–168.

Vogt JJ, Meyer-Schwertz MT, Foehr R (1973) Motor, thermal and sensory factors in heart rate variation. A methodology for indirect estimation of intermittent muscular work and environmental heat loads. *Ergonomics* **16**, 45–60.

Volicier BJ, Bohannon MW (1975) A hospital stress rating scale. *Nursing Research* **24**(5), 352–359.

Vorchol DA (1983) The relationship between nurses' and children's perceptions of pain in the acute and chronic pain experiences of children. PhD Thesis (unpublished), University of Cincinnati, Cincinnati.

Vyklicky L (1984) Methods of testing pain mechanisms in animals. In: Wall PD, Melzack R (eds) *Textbook of Pain*. Churchill Livingstone, Edinburgh.

Wall PD (1984a) Introduction. In: Wall PD, Melzack R (eds) *Textbook of Pain*. Churchill Livingstone, Edinburgh.

Wall PD (1984b) Summary and conclusion. In: Wall PD, Melzack R (eds) *Textbook of Pain*, p. 840. Churchill Livingstone, Edinburgh.

Wall PD (1986) Causes of intractable pain. *Hospital Update* **12**(12), 969–974.

Walsh TD, Baster R, Bowman K, Leber R (1981) High-dose morphine and respiratory function in chronic cancer pain. *Pain Supplement* **1**, 39.

Weis OF, Sriwatanakul K, Alloza JL, Weintraub M, Lasagna L (1983) Attitudes of patients, house staff and nurses towards postoperative analgesic care. *Anaesthesia and Analgesia* **62**(1), 70–74.

White R (1985) Policy implications and constraints in the role of the nurse in the management of pain. In Copp LA (ed) *Perspectives on Pain*. Recent Advances in Nursing 11, Churchill Livingstone, Edinburgh.

Williamson PS, Williamson ML (1983) Physiologic stress reduction by a local anaesthetic during newborn circumcision. *Paediatrics* **71**, 36–40.

Willis WD (1984) The origin and destination of pathways involved in pain transmission. In: Wall PD, Melzack R (eds) *Textbook of Pain*. Churchill Livingstone, Edinburgh.

Worthington Jr EL (1978) The effects of imagery content, choice of imagery content and self-verbalization on the self-control of pain. *Cognitive Therapeutic Research* **2**, 225–240.

Zborowski M (1969) *People in Pain*. Jossey-Bass, San Francisco.

Chapter 9

Sleep Disturbance

Sleep is regarded as such an idyllic state that, like love, it has been the topic of much romantic poetry:

'I fellowed sleep who kissed me in the brain, let fall the tear of time.' (Dylan Thomas)

'Balm that tames all anguish, saint that evil thoughts and aims takest away.' (William Wordsworth)

Unusual states of sleep have been observed and carefully described in fairy tales, notably the excessive sleep of Rip van Winkle and the Sleeping Princess. From classical literature the Pickwickian syndrome, a form of sleep apnoea described by Charles Dickens, and the sleepwalking of Shakespeare's Lady Macbeth are well known. Aristotle also wrote about sleep.

Despite this long history of observation and the fact that most of us spend about a third of our lives asleep, there is little consensus about why we sleep. There are however theories, both philosophical and scientific, and the vast majority of people are convinced that sleep is necessary to rest their weary bodies and unravel their addled brains.

This chapter is primarily concerned with the relationship between sleep and illness and the sleep problems of the sick; however the implications of some of the research are as great for the carers as for the sick. Oswald (1986) suggested that, if we want to sleep well, we should lead a regular life and forgive our enemies, amongst other things. The former is well nigh impossible for those who care for the sick, the latter the achievement of saints.

THE NORMAL STATE

Sleep is a normal state for humans, provided it alternates with periods of wakefulness. People differ considerably in the length and timing of sleep. There are fairly stable interindividual differences in length of sleep such that some adults consistently sleep less and others more than the average of 6–9 hours in 24 hours. The distinction between morningness and eveningness (Horne and Ostberg, 1976) types or 'larks' and 'owls' is another normal variation. Sociocultural 'norms' such as taking a siesta (Smirne et al, 1983) or going to sleep at sundown contribute to our view of what is normal. The age of an individual also leads to expectations of normality; for instance neonates sleep for 14–18 hours in every 24 hours and gradually acquire their mono- or biphasic adult pattern during childhood and adolescence. The sleep of many elderly is polyphasic in

148

that night-time sleep is broken and daytime naps occur (Webb, 1982). What is considered normal is related both to the usual sleep of that individual when in health and to the length and timing of sleep which results in feeling refreshed and efficient during waking hours. Although humans usually take the majority of their sleep at night, it is also normal to be able to alter times of sleeping to suit work and leisure activities. Regular night-time sleep is synchronised with other circadian rhythms such as hormone levels, temperature and metabolic rate but major determinants of human sleeping are external time cues (Zeitgebers) light-dark and particularly social events (Weitzman et al, 1983).

WHEN IS SLEEP A PROBLEM?

Sleep problems exist either if a person is unable to sleep when they wish to be asleep or if they are unable to stay awake when they wish or need to be awake. Very often people present with both problems. Most people complain about their sleep if they have difficulty in falling asleep or staying asleep, have reduced or excessive overall length of sleep and/or do not feel alert and refreshed when they awaken. According to Dement et al (1982) and in agreement with common belief,

> 'it is axiomatic that there is a relationship between sleep at night and the way we feel during the day'. (p. 30)

Although sleep problems have been recognised from time immemorial, the centrality and seriousness of sleep abnormalities have been only slowly recognised by medical practitioners and they remain relatively overlooked patient problems by nurses. Roffwarg (1979) in his introduction to a system of diagnostic categories states:

> 'Disturbed sleep and inadequate wakefulness are inestimable sources of human misery . . . the general physician is not alone, however, in turning aside or misunderstanding patients' complaints about sleep . . . because of his customary uncertainty about the significance of sleep symptoms (he) has a tendency to treat sleep complaints as trifling or annoying. Characteristically he both underestimates the etiology of sleep disorders and overtreats the symptoms with drugs.' (p. 5)

Acknowledgement and increasing understanding of sleep disorders and sleep problems have occurred in the past few decades. Sleep has become a medical sub-specialty in some countries with the development of sleep laboratories and sleep clinics. An Association for the Psychophysiological Study of Sleep was set up in 1962 and an Association of Sleep Disorders Centres in 1975 in the USA. A specialist journal *Sleep* was launched in 1978. Much of this activity and progress in understanding sleep problems has arisen from the merger of two major strands of research — circadian physiology and sleep disorder medicine (Czeisler et al, 1983).

Although the nurse's responsibility for promoting sleep has long been recognised (Nightingale, 1969) and problem-orientated nursing models include sleep as an activity of living (Henderson and Nite, 1978, Roper et al, 1985) there is anecdotal and research evidence that sleep problems remain marginal in the planning of patient care by nurses (Dodds, 1980). Indeed, there is a tendency in hospital for staff to collude with patients' views that poor sleep is to be expected and so regarded as normal in that setting (Hopkins, 1980).

In American nursing diagnoses (Carpenito, 1983) sleep problems are defined as sleep pattern disturbances or

'the state in which the individual experiences or is at risk of experiencing a change in the quantity or quality of his rest pattern as related to his biological and emotional needs'. (p. 440)

The terminology of sleep problems is defined in Table 1.

Table 1. Terminology

The terminology used in discussion of sleep problems includes:
Insomnia—difficulty in sleeping. Disorders of initiating and maintaining sleep or DIMS. Initial insomnia—difficulty in falling asleep. Intermittent insomnia—difficulty in staying asleep, frequent awakening. Terminal insomnia—awakening too early. Subjective insomnia—appearing to sleep well but reporting poor sleep. Somnolence—sleepiness, tendency to sleep. Hypersomnolence—excessive sleep, maybe 16–18 hours per day. Disorders of excessive somnolence or DOES. Sleep latency—time taken to fall asleep. Narcolepsy—uncontrollable REM sleep attacks during waking activities. Cataplexy—attacks of abrupt weakness or paralysis of voluntary muscles. Hypnogogic hallucinations—disturbing or frightening dreams on falling asleep. Sleep paralysis—inability to move or speak on awakening. Parasomnias—waking behaviour during sleep such as sleep walking, talking, bruxism (teeth grinding), enuresis. Sleep apnoea—cessation of breathing during sleep; more than 5 episodes per hour and more than 30 episodes per night each lasting 10 seconds or more is considered abnormal (Parkes, 1985). Night terrors—intense short horror dreams, sometimes followed by shrieks, crying and sleep walking, occurring in non-REM sleep. Nightmare—a dream in which some powerful force threatens to harm or destroy the sleeper, occurring in REM sleep. Periodic movements in sleep (PMS)—stereotyped repetitive movements of legs and feet that are triggered by sleep. Restless leg syndrome—extremely disagreeable deep sensation of creeping inside the calves whenever sitting or lying, resulting in irresistible urge to move the legs.

DEFINITIONS OF SLEEP

Sleep per se is not a problem, but in order to understand sleep disturbance and abnormalities it is necessary to discuss first of all definitions and theories about the nature and possible functions of normal sleep.

The problem of definition of sleep was stated thus by Webb (1973):

'As with any complex but familiar biological process such as digestion, sexual behaviour or vision, a superficial definition is easy, but an ultimate definition may be impossible . . . Sleep, which involves changes ranging from degrees of consciousness through skeletal and physiological responses to biochemical and cellular changes, presents such a problem.' (p. 6)

It is important to note that there are two possible ways of defining sleep. Firstly as a discrete state, and secondly as part of continuous cyclical changes in level of consciousness. The significance of these two aspects of sleep lies in the fact that sometimes patients have problems with the state of sleep, sometimes with the scheduling of sleep, and sometimes with both.

The first type of definition describes sleep as a state of reduced responsiveness to external stimuli, an altered state of consciousness from which a person can be aroused if the stimulus is of sufficient magnitude. Usdin (1973) stated:

'The salient feature of wakefulness is the environmental engagement of the organism: he interacts with the world around him. The onset of slow wave sleep entails the cessation of such interaction. . . . The moment of sleep is best defined as the point of perceptual disengagement.' (p. 7)

A particular problem for nurses arises because sleep can be difficult to distinguish from abnormal states of hypoarousal such as coma and can be simulated deliberately.

The second type of definition describes sleep as the physically inactive part of the circadian (around a day) sleep-wake-activity cycle and is characterised by cyclical changes in electroencephalographic (EEG) and other physiological parameters (Webb, 1971).

Much research undertaken by psychologists and psychiatrists has sought to gain a greater understanding of the physiological correlates of sleep and the emotional and behavioural concomitants and consequences of normal and abnormal sleep patterns (Horne, 1983b; Oswald, 1980b). This research has attempted to describe the nature of sleep and indirectly to understand the purpose of sleep.

The way sleep is described has been determined by the technology of investigation. Although sleep is a relatively inactive physical state, it is not neurologically or physiologically passive. Recordings of the electrical discharges picked up from scalp and face electrodes have led to the distinguishing of sleep from wakefulness and to the definition of stages of sleep in terms of electroencephalograph (EEG) and electroocculograph (EOG) (Dement and Kleitman, 1957). The sleep stages thus defined include 0—eyes shut resting with alpha rhythms (8–12 Hertz and synchronised), a preparatory sleep stage; stages 1–4 termed non-REM (rapid eye movement) or orthodox sleep in which EEG waves become slower and more irregular until large slow delta waves ($\frac{1}{2}$–3 Hertz and five to 10 times the amplitude of wakefulness) occur, and periodically (4–6 times per night), REM or paradoxical sleep occurs in which the EEG is desynchronised and similar to wakefulness or stage 1 (Koreorgos, 1980).

Many other physiological and behavioural parameters have been investigated during sleep by using transducers to measure and record changes in cardiorespiratory responses, temperature, oxygen uptake, muscle tone (electromyography) and penile tumescence. By analysing blood and urine samples the levels of chemicals such as cortisol, growth hormone and catecholamines have been measured. The overall findings can be summarised as follows:

In non-REM sleep the metabolic rate slows, core temperature falls, heartrate, respiratory rate and blood pressure are low and steady, and muscle tone is reduced. In other words these orthodox stages of sleep accord with the general view of sleep as an hypoactive time. It becomes increasingly difficult to awaken someone as they pass into deeper stages of non-REM sleep and if they are awakened they may report that they recall thinking, but rarely report vivid dreaming. Peaks of growth hormone occur in slow wave sleep (stages 3 and 4).

During REM sleep heart and respiratory rate and blood pressure increase relative to non-REM, may be irregular and even exceed daytime levels. Oxygen uptake increases. Although rapid eye movements occur under closed eyelids and the EEG looks akin to waking patterns, skeletal muscle tone is almost abolished, resulting in physiological paralysis and the sleeper is variably responsive to external stimuli, he may awaken spontaneously, or may be very difficult to awaken. When awakened from REM sleep people frequently report dreaming. REM sleep is further subdivided into tonic and phasic components.

The passage through all the stages of non-REM and REM sleep is called a sleep cycle (Helton et al, 1980) and a complete cycle takes approximately 90 minutes. Indeed a 90–100 minute cycle of alertness seems to exist throughout the 24 hours, most clearly evident in the newborn.

CONTROL OF SLEEP

There has been a scientific search for a sleep centre in the brain and for a naturally occurring substance which produces sleep (Chen et al, 1974). Tryptophan and cholecystokinin have been contenders for the natural hypnotic role. Simple explanations or single controls of sleep do not however fit with the evidence. Current research findings suggest that the control of sleep is not confined to one localised part of the brain. Parkes (1985) concludes:

'The integrity of much of the brain stem, as well as the cerebral cortex, is necessary for normal sleep patterns.' (p. 105)

and

'The separation of separate systems for wakefulness (a reticular activating system), NREM sleep (forebrain and pontine areas), REM sleep (more specific pontine nuclei) and circadian sleep control (suprachiasmatic nucleus) is somewhat artificial, for all these states are interdependent.' (p. 106)

THEORIES ABOUT SLEEP

Theories about the purpose of sleep are concerned with explanations of why we sleep, and despite both lay and scientific assertions to the contrary Parkes (1985) suggests that no one is certain what sleep is for. Hartmann (1973) points out:

'In sleep research, as in other areas of scientific enquiry, "why" is often the first question asked and the last question answered or left unanswered.' (p. 3)

The reason for concern with theories of the function of sleep is that if sleep is essential for survival or health or recovery we need to take sleep problems very seriously. If sleep is just an unnecessary 'time filling behaviour' or luxury we could be justified in considering many sleep problems as trivial. As Webb (1983) put it:

'A theory or conceptualization is a belief and for all men, laymen and scientists alike, beliefs direct behaviour.' (p. 8)

There are two major sets of theories about the function of sleep:

1. Non-restorative, occupying unproductive hours, providing safety and conserving energy.
2. Restorative, body and/or brain restitution.

Horne (1983b) in his discussion of the functions of mammalian sleep proposes that these sleep theories should not be regarded as mutually exclusive, but that human sleep serves both functions. He uses the terms *obligatory sleep* for sleep which performs an essential restitutive function and *facultative sleep* for non-restorative sleep (p. 262).

Following prolonged sleep deprivation it has been found consistently that there is a failure to make up *all* lost sleep when given the opportunity to do so. Most of the lost stage 4 is recouped, only around one-third of REM, some of stage 3 and almost none of stages 1 and 2 (Bennot et al, 1980). This is one of the pieces of evidence which is used to argue for the view that some sleep is obligatory and some not.

Arguments for and against the restorative theory of sleep rest on interpretation of findings of a peak in human growth hormone in slow wave sleep (Takahashi, 1979), but no sleep-related insulin release (Jefferson, 1980); of cellular energy charge levels (Adam, 1980b); of mitosis peaks during the usual sleep period, but which are found even in the absence of sleep (Scheving, 1959; Parker et al, 1980), and of the effects of sleep deprivation (Horne, 1978; Martin, 1981). These arguments are well discussed by Horne (1983a and b), Adam and Oswald (1977), and Adam (1980b). On balance, the case for sleep as essential for body restoration is not proven. Food intake and bodily relaxation seem more important (Clugston and Garlick, 1982). However, the effects of sleep deprivation on mental functioning, particularly psychological performance decrements, behavioural irritability, tiredness, slurred speech, suspiciousness, mild paranoia and disorientation (Berger and Oswald, 1962) provide part of the arguments in favour of sleep as essential for brain restitution.

Whatever the outcome of this debate there are reasons other than or in addition to physical and mental restoration which lead to concern of the sick and their carers with sleep. Some sleep abnormalities such as sleep apnoea are life-threatening, indeed the commonest time of death is between 0400 and 0700 hours and may be sleep related. Some disease symptoms including cardiorespiratory symptoms may be exacerbated during sleep, and, subjectively, disturbance of sleep feels stressful.

CLASSIFICATION OF SLEEP DISORDERS

As in any branch of scientific knowledge, an agreed classification is fundamental to interpretation of observations. A number of different classification schemes are possible.

Primary and secondary sleep disorders (Williams and Karacan, 1973) distinguish between sleep entities such as narcolepsy and sleep disorders arising from pathological states or iatrogenesis. Classification based on polysomnography (EEG, EOG and EMG) has the merit of objectivity but such recordings are not made on the majority of people with sleep complaints. The Sleep Disorders Classification Committee (Roffwarg, 1979) produced a classification scheme based upon the sleep behaviour of the individual. It has four major groupings:

1. Disorders of initiating and maintaining sleep—DIMS or insomnias.
2. Disorders of excessive somnolence—DOES.
3. Disorders of the sleep–wake schedule.
4. Dysfunctions associated with sleep, sleep stages or partial arousals—parasomnias.

 No one classification scheme is entirely successful in producing mutually exclusive categories. As already noted night-time insomnia (DIMS) is frequently associated with daytime somnolence (DOES).

PREVALENCE OF SLEEP PROBLEMS

The exact prevalence of sleep problems is not easily determined. Webb (1983) states:

> 'Chronic and acute sleep disturbances are pervasive . . . Any one night millions and millions will struggle with their sleep. The Edison world of 24 hours of potential light has ripped away sleep's cocoon of darkness and cut sleep loose to float in a world of shiftwork and continuous entertainment. Airplanes toss sleep across time zones. Sleep stubbornly, defending its existence, needs all the help it can get.' (pp. 4–5)

Perhaps the rate of social evolution in industrial societies has far outstripped the rate of biological evolutionary adaptation. Lugaresi et al (1983) speculate as to whether insomnia is an effect of modern society or an inherent clash between instinctual behaviour and reason.

 General population studies have found between 14 and 35% of people complain of difficulty with sleep (Karacan et al, 1976a; Welstein et al, 1983). The overall prevalence of sleep problems is generally stated to increase with age (McGhie and Russell, 1962) although babies and young children (Guilleminault, 1983; Smirne et al, 1983), teenagers and young adults may have significant sleep problems (Price et al, 1978; White et al, 1980). Indeed Smirne et al (1983) did not find an increase in sleep problems with age.

 The prevalence of reported insomnia differs between men and women. Lugaresi et al (1983) from a sample of 5,713 found 14.7% of males and 23.1% of females over 20 years reported poor sleep. However, the difference in frequency did not appear until middle age, when female insomniacs increased from 20 to 40%. Over 60 years of age, male insomniacs increased from 20 to 30%. Insomnia was the third most frequent subjective complaint made to general practitioners, exceeded only by headaches and gastrointestinal disturbances. In young females pregnancy can be a temporary cause of sleep disturbance. Karacan et al (1968) found an increase in sleep problems from the first to the third trimester.

 The prevalence of sleep problems in the elderly may be high but as with other age groups findings will depend on the population studied (healthy or sick) and on what is considered normal for this group. There is a reported reduction in sleep efficiency (time in bed/time asleep) with increase in the number of nocturnal awakenings (Coleman et al, 1981). Loss of neurones and progressive failure of cyclical circadian organisation are possible explanations (Samis and Capobianco, 1978). The disturbance of sleep by physical symptoms increases with age (Carskadon et al, 1980).

Coleman (1983) investigated the diagnosis, treatment and follow-up of around 8,000 patients from sleep clinics in the USA, Canada and Italy. In contrast with general population studies in which insomnias (DIMS) of 14–35% greatly exceed complaints of daytime somnolence (DOES) of 0.3–4% as the primary problem; 25% of sleep clinic patients were diagnosed as having DIMS and 39% DOES. The majority of DIMS in sleep clinics were associated with psychiatric disorders, drug dependency, periodic movement and restless leg syndrome, sleep apnoea, psychophysiological conditions and circadian rhythm disorders. DOES were found to be twice as frequently related to sleep apnoea as to narcolepsy.

Smirne et al (1983) chose to study a population of particular relevance to hospital nurses — the in-patients in general medical, surgical and orthopaedic wards in Milan, *not* patients admitted with psychiatric or sleep disorders. Their questionnaire referred to sleep in the past three months — not on admission, in the hope of avoiding answers which related solely to the transient effect of current illness or surgery. The sample of 2,518 with an age range of 6–92 years was comprised of 1,347 females and 1,171 males. Smirne et al found that 25% of this population reportedly suffered from some persistent sleep disorder. The majority (around 13%) complained of insomnia, around 9% of parasomnias—mostly sleeptalking and bruxism, and 3.4% of hypersomnia.

Prevalence of sleep problems in children

Dramatic changes in sleep patterns occur in early childhood, with or without the prompting of parents. The length of sleep drops from an average of 16 hours (range 10–22 hours) in the first days after birth, to around 13.5 hours at 26 weeks to 12 hours by the age of two years. The percentage of REM sleep declines from 50% to 30% by the second year (Webb, 1975). Apart from the problem of clashes between adults and children about appropriate sleeping times, a number of sleep-related problems occur in childhood, the most serious of which is sleep apnoea, reportedly the cause of some sudden infant deaths (SIDS) (Guilleminault, 1983). Enuresis and other parasomnias such as night terrors and sleep-walking also occur in childhood, and may disappear in adulthood only to recur at times of great stress (Oswald and Adam, 1983).

Up until 1976 insomnia was considered rare in children, but since then studies have reported frequent sleep-related complaints in young people, although according to White et al (1980) teenagers are not always highly concerned by these problems. In a study by Price et al in 1978 of 627 American teenagers (aged 15–18 years) they found a prevalence of 12.6% of chronic poor sleepers and 37.6% occasional poor sleepers, whereas in an Italian interview survey Lugaresi et al (1983) only found 1.6% of the population complained of insomnia before the age of 20 years. The latter also found that post-prandial sleepiness was rare before 20 and almost the rule after 25–30 years. In contrast, a telephone survey in the USA by Welstein et al (1983) found that the highest reported sleep problems were in the age groups 6–14 and 15–19 years. The most common problems reported by children were taking a long time to fall asleep, early morning awakening and feeling tired by day.

Cross-sectional studies have found a dramatic decrease in sleep length from an average of 10 hours in 10-year-olds (Carskadon, 1982) to 7–8 hours in late teenagers (Webb and Agnew, 1973). However, Carskadon et al (1983) suggest that the reduction in sleep is related to social factors rather than changes in biological need, and results in increased daytime sleepiness. In a longitudinal study they report that, given the opportunity to sleep 10 hours a night, this level would be maintained throughout adolescence. This finding could be viewed as an example of obligatory and facultative sleep.

In conclusion, it would seem from these prevalence studies that as many as one-quarter of our patients may have chronic sleep problems, and as acute episodes of illness, surgery and hospitalisation provoke transient, sometimes severe sleep disruption, that sleep is likely to be a very frequent patient problem. However, useful though the prevalence literature is in alerting us to sleep problems, it is crucial to remember that in all groups there are considerable individual differences. Research findings may reveal statistically significant differences between the sleep of the young and old, and male and female, but we can never assume that the individual in our care conforms to a trend.

SLEEP AND ILLNESS

In this section the research findings on sleep will be discussed under four headings which arise from the sub-categories of the diagnostic classification of sleep and arousal disorders (Roffwarg, 1979), see Table 2.

Table 2. Sleep Problems

1. Associated with psychological and psychiatric states
2. Associated with physical illness
3. Associated with drugs
4. Associated with environmental factors

Sleep problems associated with psychological and psychiatric states

Any situation which causes emotional arousal, be it anxiety, fear, anger or exhilaration and joy, is likely to result in transient change in sleeping. Stonehill et al's findings (1976) suggest that sadness results in early falling asleep and early awakening; anxiety in difficulty falling asleep and later awakening, and anger in difficulty both in falling asleep and remaining asleep, resulting in repeated awakenings. Most insomnias arising from emotional shock or threat to one's security are transient, but sometimes chronic tension-anxiety states develop and sometimes failure to sleep becomes associated with, or conditioned to, aspects of the environment. Roffwarg (1979) states:

'The mental state that appears to be the most powerful disruptor of the sleep onset process is the internal arousal related to conscious and excessive "trying" to fall asleep.' (p. 21)

Such people fall asleep when not trying such as when reading or watching television but cannot sleep when they go to bed.

Excessive daytime somnolence may be the consequence of poor night-time sleep. However, in high states of arousal individuals may not fall asleep by day, but feel achy, washed out and unable to nap. A minority of people respond to threat by excessive sleep rather than insomnia, anger and fear resulting in central nervous system depression rather than arousal. Either reaction can be adaptive—insomnia maintaining vigilance of the situation and somnolence conserving energy. However, when unremitting or recurrent tension anxiety results in persistent tiredness, some fatigue-prone patients learn to 'take to their bed'. Such prolonged bedrest and napping becomes complicated by disorders of circadian rhythmicity.

Psychiatric disorders associated with insomnia include neurotic anxiety, panic attacks, phobia, obsessive-compulsive neuroses, depressions and schizophrenia. The severity of sleep problems is related to the severity of the psychiatric disorder. Acute psychiatric states can result in almost total insomnia and partial or complete inversion of the day-night cycle (Feinberg and Hiatt, 1978). Mania results in short sleep, as does anorexia nervosa, but the manic person typically feels refreshed on awakening and the anorexic may welcome awakening and exercise rather than attempt to sleep.

Excessive daytime sleepiness as well as prolonged night-time sleep may occur in mild depression and in bipolar depression. The most dramatic type of hypersomnolence is narcolepsy. This may be accompanied by cataplexy, sleep paralysis and hypnogogic imagery. Typically REM sleep occurs at sleep onset. The attacks of sleep occur in the middle of activities and may be triggered by certain emotions or behaviour such as laughter. Narcolepsy is a rare (4 per 10,000) but socially crippling and potentially dangerous condition (Roth, 1978). Approximately 1 in 8 patients who attend sleep clinics complaining of excessive daytime sleepiness are diagnosed as having idiopathic central nervous system (CNS) hypersomnolence. They constantly feel sleepy, sleep for long periods at night and fall asleep easily by day (Guilleminault and Dement, 1974).

Sleep problems associated with physical illness

Some sleep problems, such as sleep apnoea, do not fit entirely happily into this classification, and will be discussed under physical illness.

Sleep apnoea has been recognised as a significant and serious cause for concern, not only in early childhood, but also in adults. It may contribute to sudden unexplained death during sleep in adults and to chronic daytime sleepiness affecting work and recreation (Guilleminault, 1983). Daytime respiratory function is typically normal, but a significant proportion of such people develop pulmonary hypertension and cor pulmonale secondary to repeated hypoxia, and sleep apnoea is sometimes associated with systemic hypertension (Guilleminault et al, 1980). Bradycardia occurs during apnoeic attacks followed by tachycardia related to arousal of the patient. The occurrence of severe ventricular arrhythmias is one probable mechanism for death (Guilleminault, 1983). Three types of sleep apnoea have been classified—central apnoea in which respiratory effort stops; obstructive or upper airway apnoea in which airflow is blocked despite persistent respiratory effort, and mixed central and obstructive apnoea. The ratio of men to women is 30:1. In most cases no anatomical defect is apparent, though a high proportion of primary sleep apnoeic patients are overweight. Pathologies associated with non-obese obstructive apnoea include acromegaly, thyroid enlargement, neck irradiation, micrognathia, severe kyphoscoliosis, myotonic dystrophy, Shy-Drager syndrome, nasal polyps and enlarged tonsils. Snoring is common in obstructive apnoea.

Many sleep abnormalities are caused by or secondary to physical pathology. Conditions which increase intracranial pressure or alter CNS physiology are particularly liable to affect sleep adversely. Pathologies of the brainstem and hypothalamus, and cerebral atrophy may disrupt sleep onset and maintenance, whether they are due to neoplasms, vascular disorders, CNS infections, trauma, toxicity or degenerative changes. Excessive daytime sleeping or hypersomnolence typically occurs with increasing intracranial pressure from whatever cause, especially from tumours of the pineal and posterior hypothalamus and any which impinge on the third ventricle, and from subdural and subarachnoid haemorrhage. Incapacitating daytime somnolence sometimes develops gradually 66 to 18 months after head injury. Many toxic and infectious conditions result in excessive sleepiness whether caused by fungae, viruses or bacteria, and including neurosyphilis, encephalitis lethargica and trypanosomiasis. An unwanted side-effect of brain surgery performed to alleviate intractable pain, severe psychiatric disorders or parkinsonism is sometimes abnormal sleep patterns and somnolence. Major endocrine and metabolic diseases result in sleep abnormalities, including diabetes mellitus, Addison's disease and Cushing's syndrome. Hyper- and hypothyroidism result in reduced or excessive sleep respectively. Uraemia results in hypersomnolence, and hepatic failure is often accompanied by nocturnal delirium.

Many common symptoms are worse at night. Chronic pain may have a circadian rhythm of increasing intensity at night (Glyn et al, 1976). The incidence of asthma attacks is highest during the second half of the night. Sleep-related dyspepsia and gastric ulcer pain disrupt sleep. Patients whose cardiac or respiratory function is compromised by day are liable to a further deterioration during sleep, resulting in angina, palpitations, cardiac arrhythmias, myocardial incompetence, coronary artery insufficiency, nocturnal dyspnoea and hyperpnoea and worsening of Cheyne-Stokes respirations.

Sleep problems associated with drugs

All CNS stimulants and depressants alter sleep patterns, their effects being more dramatic on the functioning and the sleep of the elderly than on younger age groups. The effects of CNS drugs are well documented in pharmacology books so will only be summarised here.

Central nervous system depressants

These include sedatives, hypnotics, tranquillisers, anticonvulsants, antihypertensives, antidepressants, antihistamines, beta adrenergic blockers and alcohol, and all produce hypersomnolence. With sustained use CNS depressants generally become less effective in inducing sleep, thereby leading to physical and psychological dependence, increasing dosage plus intermittent attempts to reduce or withdraw the drugs. The person who has become tolerant to sedatives—including barbiturates and non-barbiturates, such as glutethamide, chloral hydrate, methaqualone, antihistamines, bromides, benzodiazepines and alcohol—develop long (more than five minutes) and frequent periods of awakening from sleep, especially during the second half of the night. The time to fall asleep also gets longer as the person gets used to the drug. If the drug is omitted, sleep latency may be several hours. Residual (hangover) effects during the day include sluggishness, poor co-ordination, ataxia, slurred speech, visual problems and, in the late afternoon, restlessness and nervousness. Gradual withdrawal from sedatives results in an improvement in sleep in many people, though after long habituation the individual may not return to an absolutely normal sleep pattern. Rapid reduction or abrupt withdrawal of CNS depressants almost completely disrupts sleep.

REM sleep is suppressed by these drugs and REM rebound can precipitate terrifying nightmare attacks. Withdrawal symptoms of nausea, muscle tension, aches, restlessness and nervousness are likely to occur in the succeeding days and sleep-related myoclonus may appear. It is interesting to note that the poor sleepers in Lugaresi et al's (1983) study typically used sleeping pills and felt that they could not do without them. Welstein et al (1983) found that of those who sought medical help for sleep problems, more females received prescriptions for tranquillisers and hypnotics than men.

Central nervous system stimulants

Amphetamines, methylphenidate, sympathomimetic drugs, analeptics and caffeine all cause delayed sleep onset and reduction in total sleep time. To overcome the resultant daytime sleepiness more stimulants may be taken. Sudden episodes of sleepiness by day—the 'crash' of the stimulant-dependent individual—occur from time to time. The person may also be anxious and irritable, have difficulty in concentrating and even become severely depressed and suicidal. A paradoxical finding in the prevalence study of Lugaresi et al (1983) was that there was no significant difference in smoking and alcohol intake between the good and bad sleepers, but the insomniacs aged 20–60 years drank significantly less coffee than the good sleepers, possibly in the hope of avoiding further sleep disruption.

Other drugs affecting sleep

In the 1979 classification of sleep disorders two other lists of drugs are mentioned, some of which are recognised for their psychotropic actions, others not.

Group 1

These cause delay in sleep onset, interrupted sleep and early awakening; the severity of the effect depending on the drug dosage.

Antimetabolites and other cancer chemotherapeutic agents, thyroid preparations, anticonvulsants such as phenytoin, monoamine oxidase inhibitors (MAOI), adrenocorticotrophic hormone (ACTH), alpha methyldopa, propranolol and many other drugs are in this group.

Group 2

These drugs improve sleep, but sleep disturbance occurs during withdrawal in the same way as withdrawal from other CNS depressants.

Major tranquillisers, sedating tricyclics, sometimes MAOIs, diazepam, marijuana, cocaine, phencyclidine, opiates and aspirin-containing drugs are included in this group.

Many, if not the majority of the sick, are prescribed drugs at some stage of illness and may suffer consequent sleep-related problems.

Sleep problems associated with environmental factors

On the face of it, environmental research evidence seems scarcely necessary other than to add scientific respectability to the obvious—that we seek somewhere which is quiet, warm, comfortable and dark when we wish to sleep for extended periods; and that if we are even slightly sleepy a modicum of comfort, a monotonous or boring environment (a train or a lecture) and a high probability that no one and nothing is going to demand a response from us is sufficient to encourage a nap. That hospitals in general provide both a poor environment for night-time sleep (Hopkins, 1980) and recurrent opportunities for daytime napping is almost beyond dispute. The most extreme sleep disruption is likely to occur in intensive care units, including deprivation of total sleep length, sleep fragmentation and desynchronisation of circadian rhythms. As Sanford (1982) remarked:

> 'The critical care patient is fortunate if the length of just one cycle (90 minutes) passes without interruption.' (p. 74)

The so-called 'intensive care syndrome' shows a remarkable similarity with the experimentally sleep-deprived subject and the sleep-disturbed seriously ill patient (Helton et al, 1980). The extent to which pathology, liable in itself to alter sleep and mental status, is controlled for in these studies probably accounts for differences in the percentage of patients found to develop intensive care syndrome.

Studies of environmental causes of sleep disruption in the sick sometimes recognise and admit the difficulty or inadmissibility of attributing findings to one cause. For instance, Pacini and Fitzpatrick (1982), in an investigation of the sleep of 38 elderly people, half at home and half during the first seven days of admission to medical/ surgical wards, found that hospital sleep was shorter, the time of going to bed and of being awakened was earlier, and daytime sleep occurred more often. However, the relatively poor sleep of the people in hospital was related both to environmental causes—being woken for recording of vital signs, medication and venesection—and to personal psychological status, notably anxiety. Institutional care per se may not constitute an environmental cause of sleep disruption. Indeed Wessler et al (1976) suggested that a strict institutional regime may be beneficial for those in long-term care.

Noise

Lugaresi et al (1983) found that 'good sleepers' regarded environmental noise as an important cause of sleep difficulty. Ogilvie (1980) compared noise levels in nightingale and cubicle race-track wards. Nightingale were noisier than cubicle wards but noise levels were above the recommended level of 35 decibels (dB(A)) for a bedroom at night—often by as much as 15 dB in both types of ward with noise comparable to 'a living room by day'. People—staff and patients—were the most frequent source of noise, but loudest noises came from equipment, e.g. telephones, trolleys and doors.

A fact known to almost everyone, especially parents of young babies, that humans are more likely to awaken in response to personally meaningful stimuli such as their name (Oswald et al, 1960), or an infant's cry (Poitras et al, 1973) has been confirmed by research. Auditory threshold depends to some extent on the sleep stage (Bonnet, 1986a). Rechtschaffen et al (1966) found that the level of disturbing noise tends to be lowest late in the night or rather early in the morning — at a time in hospital when potentially noisy preparations for the morning 'rush' are under way. They found that awakening threshold was lowest in stage 1, greatest in delta sleep (stage 3 and 4) and variable in REM sleep. However, arousal threshold is also dependent on the amount of prior sleep and is higher following sleep deprivation (Downey and Bonnet, 1987). There are obvious individual differences in noise threshold and some group differences are reported in the literature; for example, Dobbs (1972), in a study of the effect of aircraft noise, found that women were awakened more easily by sudden noise than men. Paradoxically, considering the hearing decline of age, the sleep of the elderly is more disturbed by noise than the young (Roth et al, 1972).

Nutrition

The relationship between sleep and nutrition has been extensively studied, particularly in relation to psychiatric diagnoses (Crisp and Stonehill, 1976). There are three main aspects of the relationship between nutrition and sleep which are of practical relevance. The first is the relationship between alertness and hunger, especially evident in the 90-minute cycle in infants (Kleitman, 1972) and conversely between satiation and sleepiness, or post-prandial sleepiness most evident in adults after lunch (Stahl et al, 1983). The second is the association between weight change and sleep. Many studies including those on treated anorexics support the conclusions of Crisp and Stonehill (1973) that weight loss is associated with reduction in total sleep compounded by more broken sleep and earlier waking; weight gain is associated with an increase in total sleep compounded by less broken sleep and later waking. It is important to note that the association is not between sleep and obesity or any particular weight. However, massive obesity, somnolence and respiratory insufficiency are characteristic of the so-called pickwickian syndrome, and the Klein-Levin syndrome is described as a profound disorder of weight with episodes of almost total somnolence and awakening solely to enable 'binging'. The findings of a study of people suffering prolonged post-war under-nutrition was that around 50% complained of fatigue, weakness, restlessness and irritability plus insomnia, particularly in the middle and second half of the night (Russell Davis, 1951). Depression, according to Crisp and Stonehill (1973), is sometimes associated with increased food intake, weight gain, and increased sleep, but typically with reduced food intake, weight loss and increased restlessness, especially sleep loss in the second half of the night in severe depression.

The third relationship between nutrition and sleep concerns the person's habitual eating habits. Although early studies suggested that specific food such as milky drinks (Horlicks) promoted sleep (Beecham Foods Nutrition Information Centre, 1978), further investigation with comparative groups led to the conclusion that it is not what a person eats or drinks prior to settling for night-time sleep that determines their sleep, but the continuation of habitual patterns of food intake. Volunteers were either given a food drink or an inert capsule at bedtime.

'The subject who normally took a bedtime snack slept better after the food drink, while those who usually had no food in the late evening slept better after the placebo.' (p. 35)

When one considers the sobering findings of malnutrition in hospital (Jung, 1981) the probability of nutrition-related sleep problems seems high.

ASSESSMENT

When assessing the sleep of another person, or our own, we need to consider what exactly we are attempting to assess — a state and a rhythm, the ability to sleep, to stay awake and to alternate these states in synchrony with other circadian rhythms, with the requirements of the individual and with the society in which that person lives. We have, after collecting information, to decide whether a problem and its resolution is primarily one of sleep per se, of scheduling of sleep or both.

Methods of assessing sleep range from high technology objective measurements of physiological changes associated with sleep such as by polysomnography, through medium technology such as the measurement of gross body movement using bed transducers (Crisp et al, 1970) and accelerometers, to low technology observations, such as diaries, interviews and questionnaires. Assessment of waking behaviour similarly may require sophisticated equipment to test, for example, reaction times, or critical flicker fusion threshold (Besser and Duncan, 1967); carefully contrived environments plus EEG monitoring to estimate sleep latency (Carskadon and Dement, 1979); or simply paper and pencil tests (Wilkinson, 1968), questionnaires (Malasanos et al, 1977), rating scales such as the Stanford Sleepiness Scale (Hoddes et al), and observations. On the whole high technology assessment is confined to research or to sleep laboratory studies of people with known or suspected sleep pathologies. Low technology methods of assessment are most easily available to nurses. It is of course a fallacy to equate low technology with ease of administration or ease of interpretation, indeed the converse may be true.

It may be helpful to do a two-level assessment, the first level being a general review of day and night behaviour to determine the existence of or potential for a problem, i.e. insomnia, hypersomnia, phase shift, or parasomnia; the second level to investigate in detail the nature, chronicity and precipitating factors prior to setting realistic goals and appropriate interventions. Information about the existence of a sleep problem may be the spontaneous or elicited views of the patient, co-sleepers and companions such as family, friends or other patients, and day and night nurses. The medical diagnosis, surgical, drug or other treatment, life-style, night and day environment, and nutritional and emotional status should alert us to the likely existence or potential for developing a sleep problem (see Table 3). The following section will be subdivided into assessment of physiological, non-verbal, and verbal responses of sleeping and waking behaviour.

Physiological status

The assessment of physiological status requires either polysomnography or intermittent physical interference. Continuous monitoring may or may not disrupt sleep, but discontinuous measurement of, for example, temperature, pulse and blood pressure is a major cause of sleep disruption (Kavey and Altshiler, 1979) and may grossly alter the very parameters it sets out to measure.

Table 3. Sleep Assessment

Age, sex, medical diagnosis, medical/surgical treatment(s)
Major areas to be assessed Normal pattern of sleep in health Current pattern of sleep Nutritional status Emotional status Daytime and night-time symptoms (awake and asleep) Sleeping environment Sleep-related rituals Wake time behaviour, mental efficiency
Methods of sleep assessment Polysomnography—(EEG, EOG, EMG, ECG, respiratory rate, temperature, oxygen uptake)—sleep status Transducers, accelerometers—bed or patient movement Observation—visual, auditory, touch—abnormal movements, snoring, obstructive apnoea, symptoms Diaries, interviews, questionnaires, rating scales—subjective views
Methods of waking assessment Choice reaction time—fatigue/alertness Critical flicker fusion threshold—alertness/fatigue Multiple sleep latency test—naps, somnolence Observation of waking behaviour—naps, symptoms Oral/written tests—mental efficiency Diaries, interviews, questionnaires, rating scales subjective views

Temperature, pulse, respiration and blood pressure are not direct indices of either sleep or waking states, although all these parameters exhibit rhythmic fluctuations which are synchronised with habitual sleep/wake cycles. A particular physiological finding will be the outcome of at least three influences—the rhythmic fluctuation in that function, the sleep-wake status including sleep stage of the person, and any concurrent pathology. Inaccuracy of recording and/or interindividual differences in accuracy may confound or mask normal variation; nonetheless what is pathologically low or high depends to some extent on *when* it is measured (Delea, 1979).

When deciding whether or not to make physiological measurements we need to ask what will be gained by the knowledge, what action will be taken as a result of the findings and what benefits and costs will accrue to the patient. For example, if the assessment and consequent action will result in a patient who is alive but tired, or if greater understanding will lead to prompt or more rational intervention then it is arguably justified. If, however, the overriding need of the patient is for sleep, then physiological measurement may best be avoided. Given that profound physiological changes are known to be associated with sleep, assessment of sleep problems is primarily looking for changes outside the range of normality, particularly those which may be life threatening, such as arrhythmias and apnoeas, or potentially disruptive to sleep by causing abrupt changes in sleep stages or awakenings.

In summary, intermittent nursing measurements of physiological parameters (a) are limited as assessments of the sleep/wake state, but (b) may reflect circadian variation and (c) are of inestimable importance in the early recognition and monitoring of sleep or time-related symptomatology.

Non-verbal behaviour

The most obvious non-verbal behaviour associated with sleep, apart from normal postural changes (approximately 30–40 times per night) are the parasomnias, especially snoring, bruxism, sleep-talking and sleep-walking, and night terrors. Family and sleeping partners are most likely to identify these, as are communally sleeping patients.

Observation, recording and reporting of non-verbal behaviours by nurses are a central, if contentious, source of information about the sleep/wake behaviour of patients. A major methodological problem is that of activity sampling. Continuous observation is occasionally possible, as in intensive care units. Intermittent sampling of sleep/wake behaviour will inevitably miss some, maybe crucial, changes.

Apart from REM the stage of sleep is not obvious visibly. Sleep apnoea attacks may or may not be visible and/or audible and the leg movements of myoclonus may only be detectable by electromyography, although both conditions can result in multiple micro-arousals and subsequent daytime drowsiness. Symptoms such as pain or a full bladder which are severe enough to awaken the sleeper will be observable only if the person opens his/her eyes and takes action. The occurrence and content of dreams and night-mares will only be known if the patient chooses to share these experiences with others. The recognition and use of dream content in the physically sick is limited so far but is a rich potential source of insight into the anxieties of patients.

Daytime behaviour which may be related to a night-time sleep problem includes sleepiness, frequent napping and symptoms of mental dysfunction (Dement et al, 1982). If someone is sleepy by day this alone does not tell us whether they are suffering from night-time sleep deprivation, from an abnormality of sleep scheduling, or a disorder of excessive somnolence. Twenty-four hour recordings or diaries of sleep/wake behaviour are needed to help us understand the situation, together with consideration of drug, pathology and/or ageing effects on sleep efficiency (Webb, 1982) or circadian control (Shock, 1977).

Verbal behaviour

In so far as there are similarities in the task of constructing valid and reliable assessment tools, whether they be interview schedules, questionnaires, visual analogue scales or categorical scales, the same general problems exist in sleep assessment as are discussed in pain assessment. In addition, there can be serious difficulties of recall when habitual sleep or 'last night's' sleep is assessed (Hauri, 1970). A number of assessment question-naires have been published, Malasanos et al's (1977) assessment of sleep/activity patterns is useful as an initial screening schedule to identify the subjective existence of a sleep problem. It has face validity and includes questions about habitual sleep patterns, sleep environment, nutritional intake and rituals, medication and psychological status.

A more probing investigation of last night's sleep can be achieved by using Webb et al's (1976) post-sleep inventory. This consists of 30 bi-polar anchor phrases, such as frequently awakened at one end, uninterrupted sleep at the other end of a 13-point scale, and elicits recall about 'going to bed', 'during the night' and 'on awakening'.

The construct validity of this tool was demonstrated by the scale's sensitivity in differentiating between subjectively good and bad nights' sleep.

A number of scales have been developed to investigate the consequence of sleep difficulties on waking behaviour. Bipolar visual analogue scales (VAS) such as that developed by Grandjean et al (1971) can be a useful way of investigating subjective sleepiness. The Stanford sleepiness scale (Hoddes et al, 1973) has been used in many sleep researches. Consisting of a seven-statement self-rating scale, it reportedly correlates ($r = 0.68$) with performance tests of vigilance, and addition (Wilkinson, 1968). These performance tests have been found to be independently sensitive to sleep loss. Many scales and questions have been developed for use in specific research studies and are useful to the extent that the research situation was analogous to the patient situation. Porter and Horne (1981) describe a pre- and post-sleep questionnaire used in investigation of the effect of exercise on sleep which includes questions about both day and night. The Leeds sleep evaluation questionnaire (Hindmarch, 1980) has VASs concerning ease and difficulty of sleeping and awakening and extent of 'hangover' following awakening, used to assess the giving and withdrawal of sedatives.

A useful review of methods of assessment of sleep in hospital patients is found in an article by Closs (1988).

PROBLEMS OF ASSESSMENT

Valid, reliable assessment of sleep is not easily achieved. Some of the assessment problems will be discussed (see Table 4).

Table 4. Problems of Assessment

1. Distinction between sleep, coma and simulation
2. Good versus bad sleep
3. Objective versus subjective data

Sleep, simulation and coma

The distinction between sleep and simulation is probably not crucial to the survival or recovery of the sick. We all simulate sleep as a prelude to falling asleep and patients may do so either in attempts to sleep, in their desire to appear comfortable and not in need of the 'busy nurse's' attention (Dodds, 1980), or as a polite way of telling others that they wish to be left alone! The consequence however is that the objective observation of the nurse will not tally with the subjective view of the patient. This constitutes one reason for believing patients' view of their sleep.

Much more seriously we need to be able to distinguish between sleep (a normal altered state of consciousness) and abnormal states of loss of consciousness such as coma. The differences between sleep and coma rest on a number of criteria (Parkes, 1985). The major differences are that it is always possible to arouse someone from sleep, but not from coma, that postural and muscle tone changes occur in sleep, but no spontaneous behavioural changes occur in coma, that EEG cycles of REM and non-REM are evident in sleep, but only monotonous slow-wave EEG activity is present in coma (with rare exceptions), and that pathological conditions such as dorsal pontine tegmental brain lesions or generalised metabolic causes exist in coma. Assessment of patients who have hypersomnolence or low levels of consciousness related to head injury or other pathology requires multi-disciplinary assessment, but nursing neurological observations are crucial in early recognition of problems in patients at risk. Indeed, excessive sleepiness should alert us to thought and action more promptly than complaints of insomnia. Apart from the problem of incipient coma DOES is more frequently a symptom of serious underlying physical pathology than DIMS.

Good versus bad sleep

What is good sleep, and what is bad sleep? This is not a trivial issue. Much of the research findings on prevalence depends on the way in which good/bad is distinguished. There is no clear consensus in the literature. The concepts of quality and quantity are often invoked without operationalising the term quality. Good and bad are relative terms although they are sometimes used as if they were absolute terms.

Monroe (1967) suggested that good sleep is associated with deep sleep and poor sleep with light sleep, but stage 3 and 4 sleep alone is not an adequate criterion of good. Perhaps the concepts of 'obligatory' and 'facultative' help, in that, if a person obtains obligatory sleep—suggested by Horne (1983b) to involve stages 3 and 4 and the first REM episode he/she has 'good enough' sleep. Some researchers (Webb and Bonnet, 1978) classify morning types as good and evening types as bad sleepers, whereas Ishihara et al (1987) suggest that morning types (M) are regular and evening types (E) irregular or flexible sleepers. There are different advantages to M and E types. M can organise the world before E types surface, but Folkard et al (1979) suggest that flexibility of sleeping habit may be an important predictor of tolerance to shift work, so E types might find night duty more bearable. It is estimated that approximately 80% of the population are neither larks nor owls.

The subjective criterion of good/bad sleep depends on the individual and upon the exact question asked. Time taken to fall asleep, overall sleep length, number of awakenings, dreaming recall, and daytime sleepiness all contribute to the picture of good/bad sleep. A typical 'good sleeper' in San Marino (Lugaresi et al, 1983) was characterised as

> 'a person who sleeps 9–10 hours per night if under 15, 7–8 hours if over 15, and does not wake up (or does not recall waking up) during sleep if very young, wakes up one or more times if aged.'

Some good sleepers recall dreams and some take daytime naps. A typical 'poor sleeper' in this study is

> 'over 40 years, usually a woman (housewife), usually falls asleep in more than 10 minutes, has many awakenings during the night, dreams a lot, refrains from drinking coffee, is often "blue" and worried, complains of frequent headaches, is used to sleeping pills and can't do without them.' (pp. 12–13)

As these researchers pointed out, few people consistently sleep well or badly and it is therefore necessary to ask if sleep is good/bad 'always', 'almost always', 'rarely' or 'never' if assessing habitual sleep. Webb et al (1976) stated that 'the measurement problems inherent in subjective responses are formidable' (p. 987). They found that the percentage of subjects who reported sleep as good, fell from 67% when given a dichotomous choice—'Was last night's sleep good or bad?' to 33% when offered more response options—'Was last night's sleep good, bad, both good and bad, neither good nor bad, or I don't know?' The understanding of words poses another bar to accurate assessment. Children in Welstein et al's (1983) study, although reporting early morning awakening, and a long time to get to sleep, were likely to say 'I don't know' when asked 'Would you say you have insomnia?' as it was not a word they used.

There are a number of theories about good and poor sleepers. It has been suggested that good sleepers are those who adapt rapidly to changes in sleep environment. Johnson and Spinweber (1983) hypothesise that poor sleepers have poor coping skills evidenced by persistent sleep problems, reported feelings of anxiety and tension and increased numbers of hospitalisations, as found in a sample of 1,043 men in the USA Navy. Healey et al (1981) theorised that 'the development of insomnia can be seen as a primary manifestation of maladaption to life stresses'. In this context it is interesting to note that Nixon (1976) uses sleep therapy as an initial method of stress reduction following myocardial infarction.

The literature reviewed on good/bad sleep has consistently associated bad sleep with insomnia. Hypersomnia may be classed as sleeping too well rather than badly, although ironically hypersomnia can be far more crippling to a person's life and may indicate serious underlying pathology. Whether or not the mis-scheduling (phase shift) of sleep is regarded as bad sleep depends upon the flexibility of life-style. Some non-working, elderly or socially isolated people may not consider a pattern of sleep/wake which is out of phase with society as bad.

Objective versus subjective data

There have been a number of attempts to compare the intercorrelations between physiological, behavioural and subjective measurements of sleep and waking. As early as 1937 Leomis et al suggested that the depth of sleep as measured by EEG was inversely related to nocturnal motility. Comparisons of subjectively good and bad sleepers have found fairly consistent differences in total sleep length and awakenings as recorded by polysomnography (Adam et al, 1986), although insomniacs tend to underestimate their length of sleep (Carskadon et al, 1976). Monk (1987) did not find a correlation between subjective sleepiness and objective sleepiness as measured by the multiple sleep latency test.

Of particular interest is the relationship between nurses' observations and patients' subjective views of the patients' sleep. Some early studies include Hare (1955) who reported a + 0.70 correlation in estimation of sleep duration. Costello and Selby (1965) found a 0.69 correlation of time spent awake in bed, but a low (0.17) correlation of the nurse/patient estimate of time of awakening. Crisp and Stonehill (1973) mention as one possible cause of discrepancy the observers' reliance of non-movement whereas the patient may be still and be awake or move and remain asleep. Aurell and Elmqvist (1985) found that nurses in an intensive care unit consistently overestimated patients' sleep compared with polysomnographic recordings.

It is possible for nurses' views of patients' sleep to be based on incomplete observation, which is inaccurately interpreted and has a value judgement (good/bad) added, without validating either the estimate or the patients' contentment with their sleep. It is probable that we should be very cautious about stating how patients have slept, without asking for their own views and, where possible, accept an analogy with pain—that good/bad sleep is what the patient says it is and occurs when he/she says it does—(with apologies to McCaffery, 1972).

GOAL SETTING

Goal setting will depend upon the accuracy of assessment, and the nature and likely cause(s) of the sleep problem. Expected or desired outcomes include both sleep and waking behaviour, for example the length and timing of sleep, the subjective satisfaction with sleep, and feeling of refreshment and alert efficient functioning when awake. Realistic goals may be achieved by taking into consideration the medical diagnosis, symptoms and treatment and any conflicting patient problems in the short term, and what is adequate or normal for that person when in health in the long term.

Sleep research findings may help us to set specific goals in terms of how much sleep and what timing of sleep is desirable. Some ideas of what may be needed to achieve 'good enough' sleep include Horne's suggestion that obligatory sleep, perhaps constituting stage 3 and 4 and the first REM sleep, could be adequate. There is a presumption that at least 90 minutes without disturbance is required for one complete sleep cycle (Sanford, 1982). However, the occurrence of a complete cycle seems unlikely in post-operative nights, even if the patient is undisturbed (Aurell and Elmqvist, 1985). Downey and Bonnet (1987) suggest that the accumulation of evidence from studies of sleep disruption support the theory that sleep continuity undisturbed for a period of time in excess of 10 minutes is necessary for the restoration of performance, rather than particular sleep stages or total length of sleep. This is particularly relevant for patients who have repeated arousals due to sleep apnoea attacks. However, without polysomnography it is not possible to know if or when this sleep length has been obtained.

Another aspect of current research concerns the timing and length of naps which will improve performance. Dinges et al (1987) found that a two-hour nap prior to sleep deprivation yielded longer lasting performance benefits (visual reaction time) than a similar nap taken during sleep deprivation in the healthy.

The recognition of temporary sleep disruption following surgery, trauma and serious medical conditions is necessary if planning of recovery sleep is to be realistic. Interdisciplinary discussion and decision taking is vital in planning interventions. Acceptance that the circadian control of sleep/wake cycles may be lost or compromised in some people, or that nocturnal delirium is a feature of severe liver failure can enable carers to adapt rather than expect the patient to change.

INTERVENTIONS

Introduction

If the existence and cause(s) of a sleep problem have been accurately assessed and realistic goals or outcomes set then the relevant interventions may seem obvious. The amelioration of environmental disturbances and symptoms of psychological and physical distress potentially provide ample opportunity to reduce insomnia and facilitate sleep in the sleep-deprived sick. However, improvement in the timing of sleep of patients who are out of phase with society and increase in the alertness of people with excessive somnolence may not be simply achieved. Co-operation and co-intervention by medical, nursing and paramedical staff, patients, families and friends will be necessary to achieve optimal patient outcomes.

To date there is a dearth of research which evaluates the outcome of care and treatment. There is however no lack of suggestions about interventions in the sleep literature (Hayter, 1986; Webster and Thompson, 1986). There are three groups of people for whom interventions are advocated, those with major chronic sleep abnormalities, the general population and the sick with concomitant sleep problems. Norman and Cohn (1985) stressed the need for evaluation of medical interventions for those with serious sleep problems. The treatment of patients in sleep clinics includes medical, surgical, behavioural and sleep schedule hygiene. In a follow-up of 7,783 such people by Coleman (1983) almost 60% reported moderate to much improvement at six months. The outcome of any intervention was reportedly better than that of no intervention.

Oswald and Adam (1983) published a book for the general public which discusses and finally lists 18 'golden rules for better sleep', including advice to lead a regular life, to accept ourselves and the normal variations of life and sleep without becoming overconcerned, to provide the best sleep environment we can afford, and avoid or minimise the use of stimulant and depressant drink and drugs. Media discussion of the deleterious outcome of long-term sedative use has both prompted and supplemented medical research and ensured that the voice of the recipient of medication is heard. Medical dispute about the appropriate use of sedation continues (Oswald, 1986; Glover, 1986). This debate is paralleled by increasing use and understanding of nonpharmacological therapies for stress management and sleep promotion (Lewith, 1985). Johnson and Spinweber (1983) advocated a course in good sleep hygiene and short-term counselling on coping with stress for the majority of poor sleepers in their study of naval personnel.

Welstein et al (1983) asked the subjects of their telephone survey what self-remedies they used for insomnia. In order of the percentage using them the strategies were to: read, use drugs (e.g. marijuana, diazepam, alcohol, aspirin), food/drink (especially milk), exercise (sex or jogging), relaxation (praying, meditating, counting sheep), alter the sleep setting (listen to music, radio, sleep on a hard mattress) watch television, lie in bed, get up and do something, resolve worries, soothing activity (shower, bath), wait until tired, or other. Whether or not these remedies worked was not reported, but it is worth noting that the majority of these strategies require a level of control over the environment and of personal activities which may not be available to sick people, particularly the hospitalised. Amelioration of sleep problems in the sick may require nursing interventions at individual or communal level, and may be undertaken by night or day staff or both. Interventions will be discussed under the same headings as sleep problems (see Table 5). Multiple interventions may be necessary to improve sleep and sustained improvement may take days, weeks, or months to achieve.

Table 5. Nursing Interventions for Sleep Problems

1. *To deal with psychological causes*
    Assessment
    Advocacy
    Teaching
    Counselling
    Relaxation techniques

2. *To deal with physical causes*
    Control or elimination of symptoms,
    e.g. pain, nocturia, asthma, dyspepsia, respiratory and cardiac dysfunction

3. *To deal with drug causes*
    Assessment of drug effects and review with doctors to find optimal/minimal use of
    medications which affect sleep

4. *To deal with environmental causes*
    Personal patient comfort measures
    Control of noise, temperature, light, air movement
    Maintenance of patient's dietary rituals and nutritional intake
    Sleep hygiene measures—activity/exercise/regularity
    Stimulus control therapy

5. *To deal with sleep scheduling difficulties*
    Prolonged assessment to ensure accurate diagnosis
    Progressive postponement of sleeptime until in phase with society then provision
    of strong time cues
    Acceptance of intractable problem in some instances

Amelioration of psychological causes of sleep problems

Assessment, specifically the exploration of patients' subjective views of their sleep and waking states and validation of nursing observations, in itself can be a therapeutic process akin to counselling. In a number of student projects on sleep an incidental finding was that the researcher was the only person who had listened to the patient's sleep description (Williams, 1984; Haynes, 1985; O'Leary, 1987).

Nurse advocacy or patient empowerment can be a sequel to or an aspect of assessment and facilitate co-ordinated interprofessional interventions.

Discussion and teaching about the known relationship between emotional state and sleep pattern can enhance the patient's feeling of control and understanding of the temporary nature of most stress-related sleep disruptions. Teaching of patients, friends, relatives and colleagues may be a crucial intervention. The content of teaching will depend on the nature and causation of the sleep problem. Relaxation techniques (Turton, 1986) including self-hypnosis, meditation and yoga (Lathlean, 1980) have the potential to reduce both psychological and physical tensions and promote sleep. Teaching about life-style changes, including sleep schedule hygiene, relaxation techniques, diet, drinking and drugs (Adam, 1980a; Oswald, 1980a) can be part of discharge planning aimed to overcome temporary sleep disruption occasioned by illness and treatment, and/or to re-educate and reduce long-standing sleep and sleep schedule problems. Interventions for patients with severe neurotic or psychotic disorders are beyond the scope of this chapter.

Amelioration of physical causes of sleep problems

These are primarily interventions to prevent or reduce the occurrence of physical symptoms which cause awakenings and/or shifts to light stages of sleep. The control of pain is obviously important. Paradoxically for some severe persistent pains, 24-hour control may require an analgesic dose in the middle of the night, even if the patient has to be woken rather than wait for the patient to be awakened by the pain. Analgesia will not guarantee sleep. Kavey and Altshiler (1979) cited post-operative pain as a major cause of awakening and poor sleep, but found little difference in the stages of sleep obtained by those who did or did not receive pethidine, or between the recipients of spinal and general anaesthesia. Adequate analgesic dosage (Kavey et al, 1980) can however improve sleep.

The care of patients with 'sleep disordered breathing' consequent to chronic obstructive pulmonary disease (COPD) is well discussed by Parkosewich (1986). It includes all measures to improve respiratory function and, where prescribed, the use of low flow continuous oxygen (Kearley et al, 1980). Oxygen may improve sleep, reducing the number of arousals in 'blue bloaters' (Calverley et al, 1982) though not if it results in carbon dioxide retention (Bone et al, 1978).

Many medical and surgical treatments are advocated for apnoea (Ingbar and Gee, 1985) including tracheostomy, and extensive surgery to tonsils, uvula and soft palate in extreme cases (Kimmelman et al, 1985). Cartwright et al (1985) describe sleep position training for patients with obstructive apnoea. Maintaining a lateral rather than supine position significantly reduced the number of apnoeic attacks. As obstructive apnoea is associated with snoring the sleep of companions would also benefit! Simpler measures, such as weight loss for the obese and avoidance of alcohol and other sedatives may be helpful in reducing the frequency and duration of apnoeas for some patients (Remmers, 1984). The consequences for the patient, apart from improvement in sleep, may include loss of the morning headache and increased efficiency of daytime performance (Yesavage et al, 1985).

The avoidance or reduction of cardiac problems associated with hypoxaemia and apnoea may be achieved by the above measures. The judicious use and gradual withdrawal of REM-suppressant drugs may be important. Although arrhythmias and nocturnal angina are by no means confined to REM sleep (Hemenway, 1980), sudden withdrawal of REM-suppressant drugs resulting in REM rebound might 'precipitate acute episodes of coronary insufficiency in sensitive individuals' (p. 461).

Many serious sleep abnormalities, such as hypersomnolence arising from central nervous system and metabolic abnormalities, seem unlikely to respond unless and until the underlying pathologies are reversed.

The amelioration of drug causes of sleep problems

The use and abuse of drugs which alter sleep, whether as a main or side-effect, is well documented. When sleep is a patient problem the review of self- and medically prescribed drugs would seem essential. The nurses' role in decision making with patients about the use of pro re nata (p.r.n) and optional nocte drugs is a major determinant of actual medication received by the sick. Evaluation of the effect of drugs on mood and efficiency can play an important part in medical choice of drug and optimal dosage.

Particular vigilance is needed regarding sedative (Jovanovic et al, 1980) and stimulant effects on the elderly. It is now widely recognised that

> 'the chronic use of sedatives impairs the already diminished cortical functioning of the elderly, rendering the elderly insomniac patient worse rather than better.' (Regestein, 1982, p. 167)

Recognition and explanation to patients of the effects on sleep of drugs used for the treatment of medical pathologies may be helpful. It has to be admitted that there is no perfect solution in some situations, but that the best compromise between sleep alteration and symptom control is the most logical aim. For example, the use of sedatives to reduce itching, generally induces excessive sleepiness and the treatment of cancers with cytotoxic drugs may result in temporary difficulty in sleeping.

Amelioration of environmental causes of sleep problems

Nurses have a major role in controlling the personal and communal environment of the sick. Improving the physical comfort of patients, reducing noise and light and providing optimal heat and air movements require action by day and night staff. The sleep literature is replete with descriptive studies of environmental disruption of sleep (Carter, 1985; Hopkins, 1980), but there is little research on the outcome of interventions. What research has found is that the cause of poor sleep post-operatively is not simply due to the poor sleep environment and repeated disturbance of the patient.

Kavey and Altshiler (1979) speculated that there might be something intrinsic to operation or trauma which disrupted sleep. Aurell and Elmqvist (1985) in the logically necessary study to investigate further this suggestion, recorded the 24-hour polysomnography of post-operative patients for whom the

> 'presumed optimal conditions for sleep were provided by a concerted effort of staff to offer constant pain relief and reduce environmental disturbance to a minimum.' (p. 1029)

They found that despite their best efforts all nine of their subjects were severely sleep deprived and they too suggest that some fundamental disarrangement of the sleep-wake regulating mechanism occurs as a result of anaesthesia, trauma and surgery. The mechanism is not understood, but should alert us to the likelihood that a sleep debt is incurred during the first days following all surgery. If these people are to recoup their sleep loss we need to ensure that they have the comfort and confidence to sleep in succeeding recovery days.

An entirely different problem is posed by those for whom their usual sleep environment is not a 'sleep promoting stimulus'. Johashahi (1986) describes stimulus control therapy (SCT) as an intervention 'to re-establish the bed and bedroom as descriminative stimuli for sleep alone' (p. 331). This includes advice to avoid non-sleep activities like reading or eating in bed, but to get up and move to another room if unable to fall asleep.

Diet

Interventions to promote sleep include the provision of nutrition at times suited to the individual habit (Beecham Food Information Centre, 1978) and in quantities which maintain or increase body mass. However, a reducing diet may enhance the sleep of some obstructive sleep apnoeics whilst reducing the sleep efficiency of other people (Crisp and Stonehill, 1973). The aims and interventions for one patient problem (sleep) need to be cross-referenced with those of other patient problems (nutrition) so that conflicts are recognised. Resolution may require compromise and the setting of priorities in the short and long term.

Exercise

There are two aspects of the relationship between activity and sleep which need to be clearly distinguished when planning exercise as part of sleep intervention. One is the promotion of sleep hygiene by advocating regular timing of sleep/wake activities. The other is the use of exercise per se as a promoter of sleep. It is not evident from the literature that physical exercise does any more towards promoting sleep than act as a relaxation technique (Horne, 1981). Exercise has surprisingly little effect on the sleep of the healthy (Porter and Horne, 1981) and acute sickness and ageing generally preclude strenuous exercise.

Sleep scheduling and phase shifting

The most thorny problem posed to nurses and families is the patient who sleeps and wakes out of phase with society, other patients and hospital routine. Before planning interventions we need to ask why this mistiming of sleep exists and whether it is amenable to change. For some patients, such as those with degenerative changes in the central nervous system, the probability of returning to a normal sleep pattern is minimal (Armstrong-Esther and Hawkins, 1982). Understanding and acceptance of this fact by colleagues and relatives can result in changes in attitude and behaviour toward the patient and reduce the sense of failure and frustration. Many patients are elderly and therefore may have reduced sleep efficiency (time in bed/total sleep time) requiring prolonged opportunities to sleep if they are to avoid sleep deprivation. They may have poor circadian control and reversion to polyphasic sleep (Webb, 1982) in which some daytime sleep is essential, and in addition they may have sleep/wake cycles which are more easily disrupted than those of younger people (Preston, 1973), and therefore need time to adapt to a changed regime.

Many human sleep/wake cycles if left to free-run are found to be longer than 24 hours (around 25 hours) and it is easier for a person progressively to postpone sleep time than to sleep earlier. Czeisler et al (1983) describe the success of this strategy in a group of people who have a disorder of sleep timing in which they cannot make the necessary phase advance (of one hour for a 25-hour rhythm) every 24 hours. Winfree (1982) describes the sleep of

'some sightless individuals, some recluses and some older people living indoors with little social contact (who) sometimes retire and rise later and later every day like the tides—eventually pursuing their solitary interests by night and sleeping by day 180° out of phase with surrounding society, they drift still later into synchrony again after another two weeks or so.' (p. 200)

Such people may require nursing care or be admitted to hospital at any stage of their sleep/wake pattern. Enabling them to shift into synchrony with society could take days or weeks, and as with Czeisler et al's subjects it would then be important to provide strong time cues to maintain that person's rhythm in harmony with conventional day/night behaviour. Wessler et al (1976) found that institutionalised elderly patients had a high order of circadian regularity and synchronisation, and they concluded that the strict institutional regime was probably beneficial.

It may be apt when considering the problem of patients' sleep to recall the ideas expressed in the prayer for serenity: ·

'to accept the things I cannot change, courage to change the things I can, and wisdom to know the difference.'

CONCLUSION

There are large areas of sleep literature which have scarcely been mentioned in this chapter, including dreams and nightmares (Kales et al, 1980) shift work and time zone displacements (Colquohoun, 1971 and 1972; Minors and Waterhouse, 1981). All nurses have experience of sleep disruption and deprivation arising from shift work schedules which may increase understanding of patients' sleep problems. The hospital can be an amazing place in which the sleep deprived staff (Folkard et al, 1978; Friedman et al, 1971) are caring for the sleep deprived sick. A more paradoxical state of affairs can exist in hospital, institution or private home where the sleep deprived staff or family are looking after the well-rested sick and might mutually benefit from a role reversal! In addition the carers may be suffering as much if not more than the sick from de-synchronisation of their circadian rhythms, resulting in all the sequelae of anxiety, depression, restlessness, irritability and decreased accuracy in task performance characteristic of phase shifts (Taub, 1974; Taub and Berger, 1976). The good idea that patients might benefit from being nursed night and day by the same group of nurses is not such a good idea when some of those nurses find rotating shifts intolerable (Eaves, 1980).

Sleep is a burgeoning research area and its importance to nursing is reflected in the increasing number of reviews appearing in nursing literature (Closs, 1988; Fordham, 1986; Webster, 1986). Some differences in the credence placed on findings and theories are evident in this literature. Our task is to remain open to changing ideas and new research findings, to apply what knowledge we have to the benefit of patients and to evaluate the outcome. There seems to be a greater need for practical action and evaluation of nursing interventions than for further descriptive studies of the sleep environment. If as seems probable from the prevalence in research, 20% of people have sleep problems before they become acutely sick, what percentage have sleep problems during and following illness and operation? Longitudinal studies crossing the hospital/community boundary could elucidate this issue.

Finally, the understanding and alleviation of sleep problems in the sick requires a uniquely high level of co-operation between day and night staff in the assessment, planning, intervention and evaluation of care. Someone who is well nursed will have optimal sleep, even if this is a compromise in the particular circumstances, and not as good as it would be in full health.

FUTURE RESEARCH

In common with many areas of research there are few longitudinal studies or studies undertaken by multi-disciplinary teams of researchers. Both types of investigation are expensive and difficult to set up, but have the potential to produce rich data essential for the fuller understanding of the phenomena of sleep.

Suggestions for future nursing research include:

1. Longitudinal studies, for example of patients' sleep before, during and after illness or operation in both community and hospital.
2. Descriptive studies, for example of the concurrent effect of the multiple variables which affect the sleep of the sick including drugs, operation, anxiety, change in nutrition and activity, and systematic description and analysis of the dreams or nightmares of the physically ill patient.
3. Evaluation studies of the effectiveness of interventions in maintaining or promoting sleep, for example by changes in the communal environment, reduction of sleep disrupting symptoms, and teaching and practice of sleep schedule hygiene.
4. Comparative studies, for example comparison of nurses' and patients' views of what is normal or good sleep in various situations and in different age groups.
5. Cross cultural studies of the sleep of different ethnic groups in one society and of sleep in different societies, for example high and low technological societies. The development and refining of assessment and evaluation tools may be a prerequisite of many of these studies.

REFERENCES

Adam K (1980a) A time for rest and a time for play. *Nursing Mirror* **Mar 6**, 17–18.

Adam K (1980b) Sleep as a restorative process and a theory to explain why. *Progress in Brain Research* **53**, 289–306.

Adam K, Oswald I (1977) Sleep is for tissue restoration. *Journal of Royal College of Physicians* **11**, 376–388.

Adam K, Tomeny M, Oswald I (1986) Physiological and psychological differences between good and poor sleepers. *Journal of Psychiatric Research* **20**(4), 301–306.

Armstrong-Esther CA, Hawkins CH (1982) Day for night. Circadian rhythms in the elderly. *Nursing Times* **July 28**, 78(30), 1263–1266.

Aurell V, Elmqvist D (1985) Sleep in the surgical intensive care unit: continuous polygraphic recording of sleep in nine patients receiving post-operative care. *British Medical Journal* **290**, 1029–1032.

Beck U, Brezinova V, Hunter W and Oswald I (1975) Plasma growth hormone and slow wave sleep increase after interruption of sleep. *Journal of Clinical Endocrinology and Metabolism* **40**(5), 812–815.

Beecham Foods Nutrition Information Centre (1978) How diet affects sleep. *Nursing Mirror* **147**(20), 32–35.

Bennot O, Foret J, Bouard G, Merle B, Landau J, Marc ME (1980) Habitual sleep length and patterns of recovery sleep after 24 hours and 36 hours sleep deprivation. *Electro-encephalography and Clinical Neurophysiology* **50**, 477–485.

Berger RJ, Oswald I (1962) Effects of sleep deprivation on behaviour, subsequent sleep, and dreaming. *Journal of Mental Science* **108**, 457–465.

Besser GM, Duncan C (1967) The time course of action of single doses of diazepam, chlorpromazine and some barbiturates as measured by auditory flutter fusion and visual flicker fusion thresholds in man. *British Journal of Pharmacology* **30**, 341–348.

Bone RC, Pierce AK, Johnson RL (1978) Controlled oxygen administration in acute respiratory failure in chronic obstructive pulmonary disease. *American Journal of Medicine* **65**, 896–902.

Bonnet MH (1986) Auditory thresholds during continuous sleep. *Biological Psychology* **22**, 3–10.

Calverley PMA, Brezinova V, Douglas NJ, Catterall JR, Fenley DC (1982) The effects of sleep quality in chronic bronchitis and emphysema. *American Review of Respiratory Disease* **126**(2), 206–210.

Carpenito LJ (1983) *Nursing Diagnoses. Application to Clinical Practice*. JB Lippincott Co, Philadelphia.

Carskadon M, Dement WG, Mitler MM, Guilleminault C, Zarcone VP, Spiegel R (1976) Self-reports versus sleep laboratory findings in 122 drug free subjects with complaints of chronic insomnia. *American Journal of Psychiatry* **133**, 1382–1388.

Carskadon M, Dement W (1979) Effects of total sleep loss on sleep tendency. *Perceptual and Motor Skills* **48**, 495–506.

Carskadon MA, Van Den Hoed J, Dement WC (1980) Sleep and daytime sleepiness in the elderly. *Journal of Geriatric Psychiatry* **13**(2), 135–151.

Carskadon MA (1982) The second decade. In: Guilleminault C (ed) *Sleeping and Waking Disorders: Indications and Techniques*, pp. 99–125. Addison-Wesley, Menlo Park, California.

Carskadon MA, Orav EJ, Dement WC (1983) Evolution of sleep and daytime sleepiness in adolescents. In: Guilleminault C, Lugaresi E (eds) *Sleep/Wake Disorders Natural History, Epidemiology and Long Term Evolution*, pp. 201–215. Raven Press, New York.

Carter D (1985) In need of a good night's sleep. *Nursing Times* **Nov 13**, 24–26.

Cartwright RD, Lloyd S, Lilie J, Kravitz H (1985) Sleep position training as treatment for sleep apnoea syndrome: a preliminary study. *Sleep* **8**(2), 87–94.

Chen CN, Kalucy RS, Hartmann MK, Lacy JH, Crisp AH, Bailey JE, Eccleston EG, Coppen A (1974) Plasma, trypotophan and sleep. *British Medical Journal* **4**, 564–466.

Closs SJ (1988) Assessment of sleep in hospital patients. A review of methods. Occasional paper. *Nursing Times* **84**(1), 48–50 and (2), 54–55.

Clugston GA, Garlick PJ (1982) The response of protein and energy metabolism to food intake in lean and obese man. *Human Nutrition: Clinical Nutrition* **36C**, 57–70.

Coleman R, Mile SL, Guilleminault C (1981) Sleep-wake disorders in the elderly: a polysomnographic analysis. *Journal of the American Geriatric Society* **29**, 289.

Coleman RM (1983) Diagnosis, treatment and follow-up of about 8,000 sleep/wake disorder patients. In: Guilleminault C, Lugaresi E (eds) *Sleep/Wake Disorders: Natural History Epidemiology and Long Term Evolution*, pp. 87–97. Raven Press, New York.

Colquhoun WP (ed) (1971) *Biological Rhythms and Human Performance*. Academic Press, London and New York.

Colquhoun WP (ed) (1972) *Aspects of Human Efficiency. Diurnal rhythm and sleep loss*. English University Press, London.

Costello CG, Selby MM (1965) The relationship between sleep patterns and reactive and endogenous depression. *British Journal of Psychiatry* **111**, 497–501.

Crisp AH, Stonehill E, Eversden ID (1970) The design of a motility bed including its calibration for the subjects' weight. *Medical and Biological Engineering* **8**, 455–463.

Crisp AH, Stonehill E (1973) Aspects of the relationship between sleep and nutrition. A study of 375 psychiatric outpatients. *British Journal of Psychiatry* **122**, 379–394.

Crisp AH, Stonehill E (1976) *Sleep, Nutrition and Mood*. John Wiley and Sons Ltd, Chichester.

Czeisler CA, Moore-Ede MC, Coleman RM (1983) Resetting circadian clocks: application to sleep disorders medicine and occupational health. In: Guilleminault C, Lugaresi E (eds) *Sleep/Wake Disorders: Natural History, Epidemiology and Long Term Evolution*, pp. 243–260. Raven Press, New York.

Delea CS (1979) Chronobiology of blood pressure. *Nephron* **23**, 91–97.

Dement WC, Kleitman N (1957) The relationship of eye movements during sleep to dream activity: an objective method for the study of dreaming. *Journal of Experimental Psychology* **53**, 339–346.

Dement WC, Miles LE, Carskadon MA (1982) 'White Paper' on sleep and ageing. *American Geriatric Society Journal* **30**(1), 25–50.

Dinges DF, Orne MT, Whitehouse WG, Orne EC (1987) Temporal placement of a nap for alertness: contributions of circadian phase and prior wakefulness. *Sleep* **10**(4), 313–329.

Dobbs ME (1972) *Behavioural responses during sleep of men and women to aircraft noises.* Paper presented at the 12th Annual Meeting of the Association for the Psychological Study of Sleep, 4–7 May. Lake-Minnewaska, New York.

Dodds EJ (1980) *Slept Well? A Study of Ward Activity and Nurse–Patient Interaction at Night.* Unpublished MSc Thesis, University of Surrey, Guildford.

Downey R, Bonnet MH (1987) Performance during frequent sleep disruption. *Sleep* **10**(4), 354–363.

Eaves D (1980) Time for a change (night-duty). *Nursing Mirror* **Feb 7**, 22–24.

Feinberg I, Hiatt JF (1978) Sleep patterns in schizophrenia: a selective review. In: Williams RL, Karacan I (eds) *Sleep Disorders: Diagnosis and Treatment*, pp. 205–231. Wiley, New York.

Folkard S, Monk TH, Lobban MC (1978) Short and long term adjustment of circadian rhythms in 'permanent' night nurses. *Ergonomics* **21**, 785–799.

Folkard S, Monk TH, Lobban MC (1979) Towards a predictive test of adjustment to shiftwork. *Ergonomics* **22**, 79–91.

Fordham M (1986) Sleep and rest. In: Redfern SJ (ed) *Nursing Elderly People*, pp. 202–220. Churchill Livingstone, Edinburgh and London.

Friedman RC, Bigger JT, Corfield DS (1971) The intern and sleep loss. *New England Journal of Medicine* **285**, 201–203.

Glover M (1986) Drugs for poor sleepers? Letter. *British Medical Journal* **292**, 1200.

Glyn CL, Lloyd JW, Folkard S (1976) The diurnal variation in perception of pain. *Proceedings of the Royal Society of Medicine* **69**, 369–372.

Grandjean EP, Wotzka G, Schaad R, Gilgen A (1971) Fatigue and stress in air traffic controllers. *Ergonomics* **14**, 159–165.

Guilleminault C, Dement W (1974) Pathologies of excessive sleep. In: Weitzman ED (ed) *Advances in Sleep Research* vol. 1, pp. 345–390. Spectrum Publications, New York.

Guilleminault C, Dement WC (1978) Sleep apnoea syndromes and related sleep disorders. In: Williams RL, Karacan I (eds) *Sleep Disorders: Diagnosis and Treatment*, pp. 9–28. John Wiley, New York.

Guilleminault C, Cummiskey J, Dement WC (1980) Sleep apnoea syndrome: recent advances. *Advances in Internal Medicine* **26**, 347–372.

Guilleminault C (1983) Natural history, cardiac impact and long-term follow-up of sleep apnoea syndrome. In: Guilleminault C, Lugaresi E (eds) *Sleep/Wake Disorders: Natural History, Epidemology and Long-Term Evolution*, pp. 107–125. Raven Press, New York.

Hare EH (1955) Comparative efficiency of hypnotics: a self-controlled self-recorded clinical trial of neurotic patients. *British Journal of Preventative and Social Medicine* **9**, 140–141.

Hartmann E (1973) *The Functions of Sleep.* Yale University Press, New Haven.

Hauri P (1970) What is good sleep? In: Hartmann E (ed) *Sleep and Dreaming International Psychiatric Clinics* Series vol. 7, pp. 70–77. Little Brown and Co, Boston, Mass.

Haynes YM (1985) *An Investigation into the Occurrence of Unpleasant Dreams in Patients who have undergone Open or Closed Heart Surgery.* Unpublished BSc thesis. King's College, University of London, London.

Hayter J (1986) Advances in sleep research: implications for nursing practice. In: Tierney AJ (ed) *Clinical Nursing Practice* Vol 14. Churchill Livingstone, Edinburgh pp. 21–45.

Healey ES, Kales A, Monroe LJ, Bixler EO, Chamberlain K, Soldatos CR (1981) Onset of insomnia: role of life-stress events. *Psychosomatic Medicine* **43**, 439–451.

Helton MC, Gordon SH, Nunnery SL (1980) The correlation between sleep deprivation and the intensive care syndrome. *Heart and Lung* **9**, 465–468.

Hemenway JA (1980) Sleep and the cardiac patient. *Heart and Lung* **9**, 453–463.

Henderson V, Nite G (1978) *Principles and Practice of Nursing*. Macmillan, New York.

Hindmarch I (1980) Calling time on hypnotic drugs. *Nursing Mirror* **Mar 13**,37–40.

Hoddes E, Zarcone V, Smythe H, Phillips R, Dement WC (1973) Quantification of sleepiness: a new approach. *Psychophysiology* **10**, 431–434.

Hopkins S (1980) Silent night? Sleep and comfort. *Nursing* **20**, 870–873.

Horne JA, Ostberg O (1976) A self assessment questionnaire to determine morningness – eveningness in human circadian rhythm. *International Journal of Chronobiology* **4**, 97–110.

Horne JA (1978) A review of the biological effects of total sleep deprivation in man. *Biological Psychology* **7**, 55–102.

Horne JA (1980) Sleep and body restitution. *Experientia* **36**, 11–13.

Horne JA (1981) The effects of exercise upon sleep: a critical review. *Biological Psychology* **12**(4), 241–90.

Horne J (1983a) Sleep and tissue repair. *Psychiatry in Practice* **2**(18), 9–12.

Horne JA (1983b) Mammalian sleep function with particular reference to man. In: Mayes A (ed) *Sleep Mechanisms and Functions in Humans and Animals: an evolutionary perspective*, pp. 262–312. Von Nostrand Reinhold (UK), Wokingham.

Ingbar DH, Gee JBL (1985) Pathophysiology and treatment of sleep apnoea. *Annual Review of Medicine* **36**, 369–395.

Ishihara K, Miyasita A, Inugami M, Fukuda K, Miyata Y (1987) Differences in sleep wake habits and EEG sleep variables between active morning and evening subjects. *Sleep* **10**(4), 330–342.

Jefferson LS (1980) Role of insulin in the regulation of protein synthesis. *Diabetes* **29**, 487–496.

Johashahi M (1986) Insomnia. In: sleep and comfort. *Nursing* **3**(9), 328–339.

Johnson LC, Spinweber CL (1983) Quality of sleep and performance in the Navy: a longitudinal study of good and poor sleepers. In: Guilleminault C, Lugaresi E (eds) *Sleep/Wake Disorders. Natural History, Epidemiology and Long Term Evolution*. Raven Press, New York.

Jovanovic VJ, Ott H, Heidrich I, Stephan K, Schratzer M (1980) Age-specific doses of Lormetazepam as a night sedative in cases of chronic sleep disturbance. *Waking and Sleeping* **4**, 223–235.

Jung R (1981) Nutrition. *Hospital Update* **7**, 883–898.

Kales A, Soldatos CR, Caldwell AB (1980) Nightmares: clinical characterisation and personality patterns. *American Journal of Psychiatry* **137**(10), 1197–1201.

Karacan I, Heine W, Agnew HW, Williams RL, Webb WB, Ross TJ (1968) Characteristics of sleep patterns during late pregnancy and the post-partum periods. *American Journal of Obstetrics and Gynecology* **101**, 579–586.

Karacan I, Thornby JI, Anch M, Holzer L, Warleit GJ, Williams RL (1976a) Prevalence of sleep disturbances in a primarily urban Florida county. *Social Science and Medicine* **10**, 239–244.

Kavey NB, Altschiler KZ, Woodward AC (1980) The effects of meperidine on sleep in the clinical situation. In: Chase MH et al (eds) *Sleep Research*. Brain Research Institute, University of California, Los Angeles.

Kavey NB, Altshiler KZ (1979) Sleep in herniorrhaphy patients. *American Journal of Surgery* **138**, 683–687.

Kearley R, Wynne JW, Block AJ, Bousen PG, Lindsey S, Martin C (1980) The effect of low flow oxygen on sleep-disordered breathing and oxygen de-saturation. *Chest* **78**, 682–685.

Kimmelman CP, Levine SB, Shore ET, Millman RP (1985) Uvulopalatopharyngoplasty: a comparison of two techniques. *Laryngoscope* **95**, 1488–1490.

Kleitman N (1972) Implications of the rest-activity cycle. In: Hartman E (ed) Sleeping and Dreaming. *International Psychiatric Clinics* **7**, 13–14, Little Brown & Co, Boston.

Koreorgos J (1980) Sleep and sleep disorders. *Practitioner* **224**(1345), 717–721.

Lathlean J (1980) Relaxation using yoga. Sleep and Comfort. *Nursing* **1**(20), 882–884.

Leomis AL, Harvey EN, Hobart GA (1937) Cerebral states during sleep as studied by human brain potentials. *Journal of Experimental Psychology* **21**, 127–144.

Lewith GA (1985) *Alternative Therapies*. Heinemann, London.

Lobban M, Tredre B (1964) Diurnal rhythms of renal excretion and of body temperature in aged subjects. *Journal of Physiology* **170**, 29.

Lugaresi E, Cirignotta F, Zucconi M, Mondini S, Lenzi PL, Coccagna G (1983) Good and poor sleepers: an epidemiological survey of the San Marino population. In: Guilleminault C, Lugaresi

E (eds) *Sleep/Wake Disorders: Natural History, Epidemiology and Long Term Evolution.*, Raven Press, New York.

McCaffery M (1972) *Nursing Management of the Patient in Pain.* J.B. Lippincott, Philadelphia.

McGhie A, Russell S (1962) Subjective sleep disturbances in the normal population. *Journal of Mental Science* **108**, 642–654.

Malasanos L, Barkauskas V, Moss M, Stoltenberg-Allen K (1977) *Health Assessment.* CV Mosby Co, St. Louis.

Martin BJ (1981) Effect of sleep deprivation on tolerance of prolonged exercise. *European Journal of Applied Physiology* **47**, 345–354.

Minors DS, Waterhouse JM (1981) *Circadian Rhythms and the Human.* John Wright, Bristol.

Monk T (1987) Subjective ratings of sleepiness—the underlying circadian mechanisms. *Sleep* **10**(4), 343–353.

Monroe LJ (1967) Psychological and physiological differences between good and poor sleepers. *Journal of Abnormal Psychology* **72**, 255–264.

Nightingale F (1969) *Notes on Nursing: What it is and What it is Not.* Dover, New York.

Nixon PG (1976) The human function curve. With special reference to cardiovascular disorders. Part I & II. *Practitioner* **217**(1301), 765–770, 935–944.

Norman SE, Cohn MA (1985) Follow-up care at sleep disorders centers: a commitment beyond diagnosis. Letter. *Sleep* **8**(1), 71–73.

Ogilvie AJ (1980) Sources and levels of noise on the ward at night. *Nursing Times* **July 31**, 1363–1366.

O'Leary K (1987) *Hospitalized Patients' Sleep: an investigation of the effect of a sleep information package for nurses on hospitalised patients' sleep.* Unpublished BSc Thesis, King's College, University of London, London.

Oswald I, Taylor AM, Triesman M (1960) Discriminative responses to stimulation during human sleep. *Brain* **83**, 440–453.

Oswald I (1969) Human brain protein, drugs and dreams. *Nature* **223**, 893–897.

Oswald I (1980a) No peace for the worried. *Nursing Mirror* **Mar 13**, 34–35.

Oswald I (1980b) Sleep as a restorative process: human clues. *Progress in Brain Research* **53**, 279–288.

Oswald I, Adam K (1983) *Get a Better Night's Sleep. Positive Health Guide.* Prentice Hall, Canada Inc; Martin Dunitz Ltd, London.

Oswald I (1986) Drugs for poor sleepers? *British Medical Journal* **292**(1), 715.

Pacini CM, Fitzpatrick J (1982) Sleep patterns of hospitalised and non-hospitalised aged individuals. *Journal of Gerontological Nursing* **8**(6), 327–332.

Parker DC, Rossman LG, Kripke DF, Hershman JM, Gibson W, Davis D, Wilson K, Pekary E (1980) Endocrine rhythms across sleep-wake cycles in normal young men under basal state conditions. In: Orem J, Barnes CD (eds) *Physiology of Sleep*, pp. 145–179. Academic Press, New York.

Parkes JD (1981) Day-time drowsiness. *Lancet* **ii**, 1213–1218.

Parkes JD (1985) *Sleep and its Disorders (Major Problems in Neurology*: volume 14). WB Saunders Co, London.

Parkosewich JA (1986) Sleep-disordered breathing: a common problem in chronic obstructive pulmonary disease. *Critical Care Nurse* **6**(6), 60–64.

Poitras A, Thorkildsen A, Gagnon M, Norman J (1973) Auditory discrimination during REM and non-REM sleep in women before and after delivery. *Canadian Psychiatric Association Journal* **8**, 519–526.

Porter JM, Horne JA (1981) Exercise and sleep behaviour. A questionnaire approach. *Ergonomics* **24**(7), 511–521.

Preston F (1973) Further sleep problems in airline pilots on world-wide schedules. *Aerospace Medicine* **44**, 775.

Price VA, Coates TJ, Thoresen CE, Grinstead OA (1978) Prevalence and correlates of poor sleep among adolescents. *American Journal of Diseases of Children* **132**, 583–586.

Rechtschaffen A, Hauri P, Zeitlin M (1966) Auditory awakening threshold in REM and non-REM sleep stages. *Perceptual and Motor Skills* **22**, 927–942.

Regestein QR (1982) Insomnia and sleep disturbances in the aged. Sleep and insomnia in the elderly. *Journal of Geriatric Psychiatry* **13**(2), 153–171.

Reinberg A (1966) Circadian rhythms. *Journal of the American Medical Association* **196**, 108 (letter).

Remmers JE (1984) Obstructive sleep apnoea: a common disorder exacerbated by alcohol. *American Review of Respiratory Diseases* **130**, 153–155.

Roffwarg HP (ed) (1979) Diagnostic classification of sleep and arousal disorders. *Sleep* **2**, 1–137.

Roper N, Logan WW, Tierney AJ (1985) *The Elements of Nursing* 2nd edition. Churchill Livingstone, Edinburgh.

Roth B (1978) Narcolepsy and hypersomnia. In: Williams RL, Karacan I (eds) *Sleep Disorders: Diagnosis and Treatment*, pp. 29–60. John Wiley, New York.

Roth T, Kramer M, Trinder J (1972) The effect of noise during sleep on the sleep patterns of different age groups. *Canadian Psychiatric Association Journal* **17**(Supplement 2), 197–201.

Russell Davis D (1951) Studies in malnutrition, Wuppertal 1946–49 viii. *Emotional Disturbances and Behavioural Reactions*, pp. 147–164. MRC Special Report Series No. 275. HMSO, London.

Samis HV, Capobianco S (1978) Ageing and biological rhythms. *Advances in Experimental Medicine and Biology*. Volume 108. Plenum Press, New York.

Sanford S (1982) Sleep and its implications for intensive care nursing. *International Intensive Care Nursing Conference Proceedings*, 73–77.

Sassin JF, Parker DC, Mace JW Gotlin RW, Johnson LC and Rossman LG (1969) Human growth hormone release: relation to slow-wave sleep and sleep-waking cycles. *Science* **165**, 513–515, 1299.

Scheving LE (1959) Mitotic rhythm in the human epidermis. *Anatomical Record* **135**, 7–20.

Serio M, Romano M, DeMagistris L et al (1970) The circadian rhythm of plasma cortisol in subjects over 70 years of age. *Journal of Gerontology* **25**, 95.

Shock N (1977) Biological theories of ageing. In: Birren J, Schaie K (eds) *Handbook of the Psychology of Ageing*. Van Nostrand Reinhold, New York.

Smirne S, Franceschi M, Zamproni P, Crippa D, Ferini-Strambi L (1983) Prevalence of sleep disorders in an unselected in-patient population. In Guilleminault C, Lugaresi E (eds) *Sleep/Wake Disorders: Natural History, Epidemiology and Long Term Evolution*, pp. 61–71. Raven Press, New York.

Stahl ML, Orr WC, Bollinger C (1983) Postprandial sleepiness: objective documentation via polysomnography. *Sleep* **6**, 29–35.

Stonehill E, Crisp AH, Koval J (1976) The relationship of reported sleep characteristics to psychiatric diagnosis and mood. *British Journal of Medical Psychology* **49**, 381–391.

Takahashi Y (1979) Growth hormone secretion related to the sleep and waking rhythms. In: Drucker-Colin R et al (eds) *The Functions of Sleep*, pp. 113–145. Academic Press, New York.

Taub JM and Berger RJ (1974) Acute shifts in the sleep-wakefulness cycle: effects on performance and moods. *Psychosomatic Medicine* **36**(2), 164–173.

Taub JM, Berger RJ (1976) The effects of changing the phase and duration of sleep. *Journal of Experimental Psychology: Human Perception and Performance* **2**, 30–41.

Thomas D (1952) 'I fellowed sleep' in *Collected Poems 1934–1952*. Dent & Sons Ltd, London.

Tirlapur VG, Mir MA (1982) (letter) *Lancet* i, 163–164.

Turton P (1986) Relaxation techniques. In: Sleep and Comfort. *Nursing* **3**(9), 348–351.

Usdin G (ed) (1973) *Sleep Research and Clinical Practice*. Brunner/Mazel, New York; Butterworths, London.

Webb WB (1971) Sleep as a biorhythm. In: Colquhoun WP (ed) *Biological Rhythms and Human Performance*. Academic Press, London.

Webb WB (ed) (1973) *Sleep: an active process. Research and Commentary*. Brighton Scott Foreman, Glenview, Illinois.

Webb WB, Agnew HW (1973) *Sleep and Dreams*. William C Brown, Dubuque, Iowa.

Webb WB (1975) Current sleep research: methods and findings. Abstract in the J S A S Catalogue of Selected Documents in Psychology **6**(4), 93. *American Psychological Association* MS, 1332.

Webb WB, Bonnet MH, Blume G (1976) A post-sleep inventory. *Perceptual and Motor Skills* **43**, 987–993.

Webb WB, Bonnet AH (1978) The sleep of 'morning' and 'evening' types. *Biological Psychology* **7**, 29–35.

Webb WB (1982) Sleep in older persons: sleep structures in 50 to 60-year old men and women. *Journal of Gerontology* **37**, 581–586.

Webb WB (1983) Theories of modern sleep research. In: Mayes A (ed) *Sleep Mechanisms and Functions in Humans and Animals: an evolutionary perspective*, pp. 1–16. Van Nostrand Reinhold Ltd, Wokingham.

Webster RA, Thompson DR (1986) Sleep in hospital. *Journal of Advanced Nursing* **11**(4), 447–457.

Weitzman ED, Czeisler CA, Zimmerman JC, Moore-Ede MC, Ronda JM (1983), Biological rhythms in man. In: Chase MH, Weitzman ED (eds) *Sleep Disorders: Basic and Clinical Research*. Spectrum, New York.

Welstein L, Dement WC, Redington D, Guilleminault C, Mitler MM (1983) Insomnia in the San Francisco Bay Area: a telephone survey. In: Guilleminault C, Lugaresi E (eds) *Sleep/Wake Disorders: Natural History Epidemiology and Long Term Evolution*, pp. 73–85. Raven Press, New York.

Wessler R, Rubin M, Sollberger A (1976) Circadian rhythm of activity and sleep-wakefulness in elderly institutionalised patients. *Journal of Interdisciplinary Cycle Research* **7**, 333.

White L, Hahn P, Mitler M (1980) Sleep questionnaire in adolescents. In: Chase MH, Kripke DF, Walter PL (eds) *Sleep Research vol 9*, p. 108. UCLA Brain Information Service/Brain Research Institute, University of California, Los Angeles.

Wilkinson RT (1968) Sleep deprivation: performance tests for partial and selective sleep deprivation. In: Abt LA, Riess BF (eds) *Progress in Clinical Psychology 8*, pp. 28–34. Grune and Stratton, New York.

Williams J (1984) Hypnotics or Nursing Care? Unpublished BSc thesis. King's College, University of London, London.

Williams RL, Karacan I (1973) Clinical disorders of sleep. In: Usdin G (ed) *Sleep Research and Clinical Practice*. Brunner/Mazel, New York; Butterworths, London.

Winfree AT (1982) Circadian timing of sleepiness in man and woman. *American Journal of Physiology*, Sept **243**(3), 193–204.

Wordsworth W (1896) 'To Sleep' Sonnet in *The Poetical Works of Wordsworth*. F. Warne & Co, London.

Yesavage J, Bliwise D, Guilleminault C, Carskadon M, Dement W (1985) Preliminary communication: intellectual deficit and sleep-related respiratory disturbance in the elderly. *Sleep* **8**(1), 30–33.

Chapter 10

Mobility Problems

INTRODUCTION

A literature search over the 20 year period between 1963 and 1983 revealed fewer than 20 articles which could be classified as reporting nursing research on some aspect relevant to mobility or impaired mobility (Creason et al, 1985). This review of over 70 articles which dealt with mobility/immobility showed that the majority were anectdotal in nature, including care studies, reports of experiences, or reviews of a problem.

On the whole able-bodied people tend to take mobility for granted. The ability to get out of bed, wash and dress yourself, feed yourself, and go to work are all carried out without a thought until some problem makes this difficult or impossible.

'Impaired physical mobility' is one of the most frequently identified nursing diagnoses with the closely related diagnosis of 'activity intolerance' ranked as the fourth most frequently identified diagnosis (Kim et al, 1984). A study by Creason et al (1985) attempted to identify what nurses defined as 'impaired physical mobility'. This was carried out by examining problem statements and their aetiologies which were made by nurses on patients' care plans. The aetiologies most frequently stated by nurses for the problem of impaired physical mobility were neuromuscular impairment and musculo-skeletal impairment. These two causes comprised over 50% of the aetiologies. The aetiology 'perceptual cognitive impairment' made up 10% of the total. The researchers also identified the patient behaviours that were related to each aetiology. The most frequently observed behaviour for the diagnosis of impaired physical mobility was the inability to perform self care. This means that patients had difficulty washing, dressing, eating, and moving between bed and chair, or·bed and toilet. The remaining causes related to this diagnosis included decreased muscle strength, control and mass, limited range of joint movement, impaired co-ordination, imposed restriction (for example bedrest for fracture healing), and cognitive impairment such as mental confusion. The data also revealed an average of two aetiologies per diagnostic statement, which suggests that a problem statement with a single cause is probably unrealistic. The diagnosis of 'activity intolerance' is useful in relation to impaired physical mobility and may be of relevance in acute situations. For example where patients with impaired gas exchange as in acute/chronic bronchitis have difficulty with physical mobility; or cardiac patients with haemodynamic problems who are intolerant of activity because of poor tissue perfusion. Therefore in most settings the concept of mobility would include the ability to move purposefully within the physical environment including bed mobility, transfer and ambulation, and the ability to provide one's self care, which would include upper limb movements.

The major disease categories leading to limitation of physical activity have not changed significantly in the last 20 years (Kottke, 1982), so that data from the National Centre for Health Statistics in the USA (1972, cited by Kottke et al, 1982) provide a reasonable representation of the current picture. Limitation of activity is defined as significant impairment of ability for self care, ambulation, or ability to carry out usual daily activities. Data from the Center for Health Statistics showed that one-third of all disabilities were due to conditions of the musculoskeletal system especially disabilities of the joints; stroke and heart disease were responsible for 21% of significant disabilities; and disabilities due to diseases of the nervous system and sense organs constituted 12% of all limitation of activity. Disabilities in these three categories of disease constitute two-thirds of all of the disability as measured by limitation of physical activity. Current European epidemiological data support these findings. In Scotland it has been estimated that the acute care of patients with stroke accounts for approximately 5% of the national health budget (Carstairs, 1976). A recent review showed that in the UK there were approximately 200 hospital admissions for stroke a year per 100,000 of the population and an estimated prevalence of disabled survivors of 250 per 100,000 (Jennett, 1982).

Arthritis is a major cause of limitation of physical ability. English populations have a high prevalence of osteoarthritis, with an overall incidence of radiological change in approximately 70% of those over the age of 35 (Huskisson, 1985).

Recent epidemiological data appear to show that the incidence rate of rheumatoid arthritis in the UK is falling, with a decline in new episodes of rheumatoid arthritis from 136 to 74 per 100,000 of the population per year between 1980 and 1985 (Silman, 1986). No likely explanation for this decline is forthcoming.

Multiple sclerosis is a disease of the central nervous system which causes widespread disability and limitation to activity, both ambulatory and self care. It is generally accepted that the UK has a relatively high prevalence usually recorded as over 30–40 per 100,000 of the population, but a recent survey in southern England using accurate sources of data estimate that the prevalence for south east England may well be in the region of 100 per 100,000 of the population (Edwards and McKeran, 1986). Therefore it can be seen that these three chronic conditions, stroke, arthritis, and multiple sclerosis, represent between them, a large percentage of the disease-related mobility impairment and self-care limitation to be found in acute and continuing care hospitals, and in patients at home. However, the effects these disease processes have on the patient's mobility differs with each condition. For example muscle tone abnormalities such as spasticity will demonstrate different patterns and effects depending on whether the underlying cause is multiple sclerosis or cerebrovascular accident. The differing functional consequences of these conditions on mobility means that few interventions are common to them all. Therefore, for this reason and because stroke illness has received recent and increasing attention from researchers, this chapter will concentrate on the mobility consequences of stroke.

STROKE: DEFINITION

A stroke has been defined by the World Health Organisation as

> 'rapidly developed clinical signs of focal (or global) disturbance of cerebral functions, lasting more than 24 hours or leading to death, with no apparent cause other than vascular origin.' (Aho et al, 1980)

The syndrome of stroke results from different pathological processes, including haemorrhage, thrombosis and embolus, and the range of neurological dysfunction that is found in stroke patients is extremely wide ranging. A summary of the most frequently found neurological disturbances (Table 1) following stroke is derived from the following studies: Wade et al, 1986; Ebrahim et al, 1985; Kotila et al, 1984; the National Survey of Stroke (Walker et al, 1981); and the WHO survey (Aho et al, 1980; Herman et al, 1982).

Table 1. The Most Frequently Found Neurological Disturbances Following Stroke

Neurological disturbance	Frequency
Hemiplegia and hemiparesis	50–80%
Difficulty in swallowing	20–30%
Sensory disturbance	25%
Level of consciousness	30–40%
Cognitive impairment	10–40%
Dysphasia/aphasia	25–30%
Slurred speech	30–40%

PREVALENCE OF MOBILITY-RELATED IMPAIRMENT FOLLOWING ACUTE STROKE

Paralysis and weakness of muscles

Paralysis of limbs and trunk of varying degree of severity is the dysfunction most commonly associated with a stroke. It is usually immediately obvious to the patient and relative. The limb paralysis usually occurs on the side of the body which is opposite to the side of the brain which has received the damage. Hemiplegia and hemiparesis is seen to occur in 50–80% of all patients who have an acute stroke. Wade et al (1985a) found that 76% of patients in a community study had some degree of muscle weakness as measured by the motoricity index (Demeurisse et al, 1980).

Disturbances in muscle tone, and joint contractures

Early studies found the prevalence of joint contracture to be variable. Drake et al (1973) found that only four of 455 stroke patients had contractures, while Moskowitz et al (1972) found that 50% of 518 patients had contractures of the shoulder at one year, and 10–15% had contractures around other joints. These differences may have more to do with the way that contractures were defined rather than their actual presence.

Observations in a large stroke unit in southern England more recently (Wade et al, 1985b), has led to the impression that contractures are now notable by their rarity. The reason proposed for the observed decline is a more general appreciation of the import- ance of maintaining a full range of passive movements in the paralysed limbs from the early stage. The picture may not be so optimistic in general medical wards, or in wards for the elderly.

Few studies consider the prevalence of disturbance in muscle tone in stroke patients. However, disturbance in tone is closely associated with the paralysis and weakness of muscles. Strokes not only disturb direct voluntary control over muscles, but also affect the many subcortical control mechanisms that maintain posture, balance, and co- ordination. So that, associated with paralysis, is a disturbance of spinal reflex activity which can result in an increase in muscle tone and spasticity, or a decrease in tone. Spasticity is usually more prevalent than flaccidity, although a flaccid upper limb may be seen to persist in a significant number of patients. Because tone disturbances are so closely associated with muscle paralysis their prevalence can be estimated to be similar to that of hemiplegia or hemiparesis, that is disturbances may be seen in about 50–80% of stroke patients.

Impairment of walking ability

Prevalence of walking disability following acute stroke is difficult to estimate. Stroke recovery studies record levels of disability at different time periods. It appears that around 40–70% of patients have problems with walking immediately after the stroke (Andrews et al, 1981; Skilbeck et al, 1983).

Problems with carrying out activities of daily living (ADL), arm dysfunction

Activities of daily living which are seen as most relevant to stroke patients include feeding, dressing, washing and bathing, transferring in or out of bed or chair, and using the toilet. The ability to carry out these activities relies on normal control and function of muscles and joints. A study of stroke patient recovery by Wade et al (1985b) showed that immediately after the stroke 82% of patients needed help with feeding, 91% with dressing and 82% with transfers, and 37% were incontinent. More commonly ADL ability is reflected as a total score of dependence on a measuring scale. Kotila et al (1984) measured ADL as (1) fully independent, (2) needs some help, (3) needs much help, and (4) totally disabled. Activities measured included walking, feeding, dressing, and personal hygiene. Immediately after the stroke 68% of patients needed some help, or a lot of help with these activities. Arm function has a large influence on the perform- ance of ADL, but there have been few studies which have specifically focused on this aspect of stroke. The loss of function of the arm is associated with the loss of function of all the other limbs so the prevalence could be expected to be the same.

ASSESSMENT FOR STROKE-RELATED MOBILITY PROBLEMS

Voluntary muscle power

The assessment of muscle power in stroke recovery is not by itself of great importance because the brain damage specifically affects the central control of muscle groups, and loss of strength is only a small part of the motor disability (Wade et al, 1985b). However, taken as part of a mobility assessment, evaluation of muscle power is a useful indicator of return of voluntary movement. It does not give information on the patient's ability to use the muscle strength for functional purposes, that is to carry out activities. Nurses could be satisfied with simply assessing in a fairly global way whether or not patients were able to move specific limbs voluntarily on command. But there are assessment tools available, which although in the main used by doctors, could be used effectively by nurses as well. This would encourage a common language about function of paralysed muscles, and may facilitate communication. The most widely used general measure of voluntary muscle power is that devised by the Medical Research Council (1976). This scale grades power at 6 levels, and relies on an experienced tester (Table 2). As with other crude grading schemes it is insensitive at the upper range of function. The use of such a grading scheme at regular periods during recovery can provide an initial assessment of voluntary muscle power loss, and then regular assessments of recovery as time progresses.

Table 2. Muscle Power Grading (Medical Research Council, 1976)

Grade	Strength
0	No movement or contraction seen.
1	Able to feel a contraction, but no movement observed.
2	Movement seen at the joint, with gravity removed.
3	Able to move the joint against gravity.
4	Able to move the joint against resistance, but not the same as the normal side.
5	Full usual power.

Demeurisse et al (1980) adapted the MRC scales specifically for use with stroke patients and called it the motoricity index. Following repeated measurements over time of the power of many groups of muscles in 100 stroke patients, they found that the strength of any one movement about a joint is similar to the strength of all other movements at the same joint. Therefore it is necessary to measure the strength of only one movement at each joint. They also calculated the proportion of total recovery represented by each change of grade, and so were able to give some quantitative value to the recovery process. Other scales have been devised by researchers to measure muscle strength after stroke (Fugl-Meyer et al, 1975). On the whole these are lengthy and time-consuming procedures which produce more information than the MRC scale or the motoricity index, and are probably more appropriate as research tools than clinical tools. For the purposes of quick ward-based assessment on the extent and recovery of motor loss following stroke, the motoricity index or the MRC scale would appear to be of most use. It is only by nurses trying out such tools in their usual practice, that they will be evaluated in relation to their clinical usefulness in different settings.

Disturbance in muscle tone

Normal tone is defined as the resistance developed in a muscle as a result of an outside examiner applying passive stretch to the muscle (De Lateur, 1982). This is usually

Table 3. Assessment Criteria for Muscle Power Loss

Muscle power	
Upper limb	
The ability to move on request, with or without assistance:	
1. Raise the arm out from the side of the body.	Abduction of the shoulder.
Bring the arm across the front of the body.	Adduction of the shoulder.
2. Bend or straighten elbow.	Flexion/extension of the elbow.
3. Bend or straighten fingers.	Flexion/extension of the fingers.
Lower limb	
1. Bend the hip.	Flexion of the hip.
2. Bend or straighten knee.	Flexion/extension of the knee.
3. Flex the foot towards the patient.	Ankle dorsiflexion.

assessed by the examiner bending or straightening the joint whilst the patient relaxes. The degree of tone present in the muscle reflects to some extent the sensitivity or level of firing of the motor neurones in the spinal cord. Tone must be high enough to resist gravity but low enough to allow for movement. Spasticity is a state of increased excitability of the motor neurones in the spinal cord, and is seen in the patient as a resistance to stretch of a muscle. For example a flexed elbow joint may prove difficult or impossible to straighten. Conversely a decrease or lack of tone may be seen. In this case the limb is floppy, and movement around the joint is loose and unstable. In stroke patients these disturbances in tone are due to the damage in the brain 'releasing' other mechanisms in other parts of the brain and spinal column which usually maintain posture, movement balance, and co-ordination. The result is that the spasticity is frequently associated with abnormal patterns of movement (Johnson and Olson, 1980; Bobath, 1978). Spasticity is evident in large numbers of hemiplegic stroke patients and can vary in both quality and quantity from individual to individual over time. The assessment of muscle tone is difficult and unreliable. In stroke patients spasticity can vary in intensity during activity, and during periods of stress and fear. However it does have profound effects upon movement of limbs and walking, and can predispose to the development of unwanted joint contractures. Therefore a basic assessment of the level of tone present at various joints as part of a mobility assessment of stroke patients is appropriate. For clinical purposes disturbances of tone can be assessed by an examiner applying passive movement to a joint and noting the resistance to that movement. Therefore assessing and stating which parts of the limbs have increased, normal, or decreased tone using this procedure would provide sufficient information to identify the problem, and be able to set appropriate outcomes and interventions.

Table 4. Assessment Criteria for Muscle Tone Disturbance

Upper limb
1. Resistance felt to shoulder flexion.
2. Resistance felt to elbow extension.
3. Resistance felt to finger extension.
Lower limb
1. Resistance felt to hip flexion.
2. Resistance felt to knee flexion/extension.
3. Resistance felt to ankle dorsiflexion/plantar flexion.

Walking ability

The ability to walk depends on normal motor power sensation and proprioception, balance control and co-ordination. Following stroke most of these functions are disturbed. There are many detailed and complex methods available for measuring walking ability (Grieve, 1980). Most are unsuitable for routine clinical use in wards. Walking ability is most frequently assessed as part of an ADL assessment. Commonly it involves a decision as to the amount of assistance required for the patient to be able to walk. For example, (1) can walk independently, (2) can walk with the help of an aid, (3) can walk with help of another person, or (4) cannot walk at all (Skilbeck et al, 1983). Walking ability is assessed as part of the Barthel index of ADL (Mahoney and Barthel, 1965). This index has received widespread use for stroke patient assessment both in research and in practical settings (Gresham et al, 1980; Wade et al, 1983a; Myco, 1984; Wade et al, 1985a). Among ADL indices it has proved to be fairly valid and reliable as a measure of stroke patients' independence. Walking is assessed in relation to the amount of help required, (1) independent, (2) can walk with an aid, (3) needs help: verbal or physical supervision required, (4) independent in a wheelchair, and (5) immobile. In addition to this fairly superficial information it should be possible to assess some aspects of the quality of the walking. For example whether weight is being taken on the affected leg, whether the length of the step taken is equal, whether the pelvis is being hitched forward, and whether the heel is being put to the ground first, or the toe being dragged along the floor (Wall and Ashburn, 1979). More detailed assessment of quality of gait is usually undertaken by the physiotherapist.

Table 5. Assessment Criteria for Walking Ability

Degree of dependence/independence
1. Ability to walk unsupported without personal or other help.
2. The degree of help required to walk.
The quality of walking pattern
1. Ability to stand in a controlled and balanced posture.
2. Ability to extend the knee on standing upright (without hyperextension).
3. Ability to take weight on the affected limb.
4. Ability to put the heel to the floor first.
5. Ability to put the foot flat on the floor.
6. Ability to keep the hips level when walking forward.

Assessment of self-care activities (ADL)

The ability to look after yourself and carry out all the normal activities of daily living is central to the question of mobility in stroke illness. In the recent rehabilitation literature there is considerable agreement that self care related to usual daily activities and mobility, is central to rehabilitation and management of chronic disease (Keith, 1984). There is also agreement on the range of activities which are most important for stroke patients. These include personal hygiene and grooming, bathing, dressing, feeding, using the toilet, continence, transfer ability, and walking on the level, and up and down stairs (Mahoney and Barthel, 1965; Katz et al, 1963; Sheikh et al, 1979). The ADL measurement scales devised by these authors have been used to assess the patient's ability to carry out the activities in relation to the amount of help required. Independence as measured by these scales only gives the indication that the patient should be able to manage in the home to look after himself and get around it. It does not imply that he is independent outside of this environment. The Barthel index of ADL has been referred to in the section related to walking assessment. This assessment can be carried out quickly and efficiently on the ward by nursing staff. In its original form it measures 10 activities (see Table 6). The activities are scored in increments of 5 points, with a total possible score of 100 representing fairly full independence in the home. Recently the scale has been modified and tested on 400 consecutive stroke patients by Wade et al (1985b) and was found to be easy, quick, and reliable to use. Patients should be assessed immediately following the stroke and at regular intervals during the recovery process. This would serve to motivate the patient, relatives, and professional carers, and provide a more objective record of the patient's progress. Where possible the assessment of individual patients should be carried out by the same person on subsequent occasions thus reducing the problem of observer variability.

Table 6. Activities Measured by Barthel's Index of ADL

Self Care	Mobility
Feeding	Chair-bed transfers
Grooming	Use of the toilet
Continence	Walking or wheelchair
Dressing	Stairs
Bathing	
Washing	

Table 7. Assessment Criteria for Self-Care Activities

Self-care activities
1. Ability to carry out the activity without personal help.
   The degree of help required: Personal help from another person. Provision of a physical aid. Help from a person may be physical or verbal.
   Amount of time taken to carry out the activity.
   Any special method used to help carry out the activity.

Mobility
1. Ability to get in and out of bed and transfer to chair without personal help.
   If not, the degree of help required.
   The method required for helping.
2. Ability to use the toilet independently.
   If not, the degree of help for getting there, managing clothing, cleaning self, flushing toilet

IDENTIFICATION OF PROBLEMS; DIAGNOSES, SETTING OUTCOME GOALS

Voluntary movement and muscle power

The return of muscle power and control is necessary before the patient is able to carry out functional activity such as using the arms for dressing or washing. The problem may be complete loss of movement in the limb or limbs, or there may be partial or incomplete movement left (Bard and Hirschberg, 1965; Newman, 1972). In order to set realistic outcome goals for the patient it is necessary to review the research which has documented the return of voluntary movement and muscle power in stroke patients. A summary has been made based on the following studies: Smith et al (1983); Wade et al (1985a); Wade et al (1983a); Andrews et al (1981); Newman (1972); Bard and Hirshberg (1965).

Table 8. Diagnosis: Impaired Voluntary Movements of Upper and Lower Limbs Related to Damage to Central Control of Muscle Power and Movement

Unable to move arm or leg, or can only move part of the limb, for example bend the elbow but not move fingers.
Outcome goals 1. Arm: First voluntary movements within 4 weeks. 　　　　Full recovery within 4 weeks. 　　　　Partial recovery within 3 months. 　　　　If no recovery by 3 months, then adaptation to one-sided function to take 　　　　place. 2. Leg: Full recovery within 2–4 weeks, up to 3 months. 　　　　After 6 months and no further recovery, adaptation to limited function.

General recovery pattern of upper and lower limbs

1. Most recovery occurs in the first 6 months after the stroke.
2. A small number of patients may show slow recovery after this period.
3. Approximately 20–25% of patients will demonstrate no weakness at any time.
4. Arm and leg usually recover at the same rate; however the leg may be a week or so in front of the arm.
5. Some patients (10–20%) will demonstrate no recovery.

The upper limb

a. If a full recovery is going to take place, then the first movements will usually return in the first 4 weeks.
b. If full recovery is going to take place, this usually occurs in the first 3 months, and usually in the first 4 weeks.
c. If no movement is seen within the first 4 weeks, then only partial recovery may be seen to occur.
d. Partial recovery can take up to 6 months.
e. If partial recovery takes place it is usually the elbow segment which recovers first, and makes the best recovery.
f. Recovery of shoulder or finger function may take place last.
g. In some patients with partial recovery, the function of the arm may fluctuate over time. This probably relates to muscle tone disturbance (spasticity).

The leg

a. Most full recovery takes place in the first 3 months, and usually in first 2 weeks.
b. Little recovery may take place after 6 months.

Disturbance in muscle tone

Spasticity is a major problem mainly because of its close relationship with motor control and movement, and if left untreated can prevent normal movement patterns, and predispose to joint contracture which may be irreversible (Twitchell, 1951; Bobath, 1978). Current theories on the physiological mechanisms underlying spasticity suggest that it is due to a disinhibition of spinal reflex pathways, and at present there is no evidence of increased fusimotor drive (Musa, 1986). The tonic stretch reflex is a poly-synaptic spinal reflex and in a normal relaxed subject is not evident on passive movement or stretch of a muscle. In spasticity there is a hyperactivity of the dynamic component of the tonic stretch reflex, so that it can be elicited by passive stretching of the muscle. Neilson (1972) studied the tonic stretch reflex in normal subjects and in patients with spasticity due to cerebral palsy and found that in the spastic patients the reflex was fully 'switched on' or hyperactive at all times.

Table 9. Diagnosis: Paralysed Limbs Aggravated by Spasticity in Specified Muscle Groups

Spasticity caused by loss of central inhibition of tonic spinal reflexes.

Outcome goals
1. Patient's limbs in a resting posture which opposes the dominant spastic pattern; for example:
    Raised shoulder.
    Extended elbow, wrist, and fingers, or hands clasped in front supported on a suitable table.
    Hip slightly flexed.
    Knee slightly flexed. Or if sitting, at 90°.
    Foot in neutral position, or flat on the floor.
    Leg in neutral position.
2. Handling and moving that does not increase spasticity.
3. Mobile joints following return of voluntary movements.

Following careful observation of hemiplegic stroke patients, it can be suggested that in a significant number of these patients spasticity can be seen to affect the muscles and joints in a predictable pattern in the upper and lower limbs. This makes problem identification somewhat less speculative. The following studies and empirical obser-vations by some authors have been summarised to provide a guide to problem identifi-cation in this area (Twitchell, 1951; Bard and Hirschberg, 1965; Bobath, 1978). It is emphasised that this is a general guide and that some patients will present with patterns of spasticity which do not follow the stereotyped pattern.

The upper limb

In general spasticity is most evident in the muscles that affect flexion (flexors) in the upper limb, so that there is a tendency for increased flexion of fingers, wrist, and elbow, the shoulder adducted, internally rotated, and the shoulder girdle depressed and retracted. The picture presents as clenched fingers, bent wrist and elbow, with the shoulder pulled backward and downwards. Not every patient will have this full clinical picture, some may have only the fingers or shoulder involved.

The lower limb

In the lower limb the spasticity is most evident in the muscles that affect extension or straightening so that the hip tends to extend and become adducted, with extension of the knee, plantar flexion of the ankle, with the foot slightly inverted. The picture that this presents is a straight hip and knee, foot pointing towards the floor and turned inwards with a tendency of the whole limb to move towards the centre of the body. Again this full-blown pattern may not be seen in all patients.

If the fully developed 'hemiplegic pattern' was not evident then the most frequently found patterns were flexion of fingers and wrist, and plantar flexion of the ankle (Twitchell, 1951).

The onset of spasticity in relation to timing is variable among patients and limbs involved. The first limbs to be involved were the hand and foot. This was seen to develop 45 hours to 10 days after the stroke. Patients who had 'typical' patterns in both upper and lower limbs developed this between 48 hours and 2 months after the stroke. Some patients did not appear to develop spasticity for up to three weeks after the stroke.

Almost all patients demonstrated some degree of spasticity in at least one joint at some time following the stroke. Assessment and problem identification for spasticity following stroke will therefore have to occur on a regular basis throughout the immediate recovery period.

In order to set realistic outcome goals for these patients, it is necessary to have knowledge of the resolution and effects of spasticity on function.

Spasticity develops and then decreases concurrently with the recovery of voluntary movement in the limbs concerned (Twitchell, 1951) and where only partial recovery of active movement occurs these patients may be seen to have some continuing degree of spasticity (Bard and Hirschberg, 1965). The return of voluntary movement in the upper and lower limbs may be seen to follow the pattern observed by Twitchell (1951) and others. Flexion movements of the shoulder were first observed, followed by flexion of the elbow and then some time later flexion of the fingers and wrist. In the leg, movement was first observed at the hip followed by the knee and ankle. It takes some time before movements of the limb become smooth and rapid. Jerky slow clumsy movements will be seen to occur throughout the period that the spasticity is decreasing. Before the start of return of voluntary movement immobile limbs will lead to fibrosis and shortening of muscle tissue, and to joint contracture. These contractures may become permanent and any degree of functional independence is at risk (Newman, 1985).

Walking ability

The act of walking is complex and its disruption following stroke follows damage to many areas of the brain and spinal cord. The ability to walk for stroke patients is closely dependent upon the recovery of normal muscular activity, normal reflex and balance mechanisms, and normal sensation and proprioception.

Stroke patients may not have the ability to remember how to walk due to damage to specific areas on the right side of the brain. According to a review of studies by Wall and Ashburn (1979) the inability of the hemiplegic stroke patient to walk in a normal fashion appears to be related to:

Table 10. Diagnosis: Impaired Walking Ability Related to Damage to Motor Pathways Following Cerebrovascular Accident.

The characteristics of a typical hemiplegic gait have been described.
Outcome goals 1. Normal symmetrical walking pattern. 2. Weight bearing on both sides. 3. Confident and safe walking both inside and outside the home. 4. Wheelchair independence if walking is not possible.

1. Abnormal muscular activity, which results in the patient being unable to use groups of muscles in the normal way. When voluntary movements start to return, and the patient can start to weight bear and walk, he/she cannot use muscles selectively, but only in mass patterns of flexion and extension. This abnormal way of using limbs is exacerbated by the presence of spasticity in groups of muscles.

2. A disorder of the normal balance and righting reactions. These patients are seen to be off balanced easily, to be unable to balance sitting or standing without support from a helper, and may not take action to protect themselves when falling, for example stretching out the arms to break a fall (Clemesson, 1951; Bobath, 1978).

3. A sensory deficit may mean that these patients have reduced sensation in the affected limbs, and have difficulty in being aware of the position of their limbs in relation to the other parts of their body and the environment. Several studies have identified some common problems that hemiplegic patients have with walking ability following stroke (Brunstromm, 1964; Colasso and Joshi, 1971; Wall and Ashburn, 1979):

    (a) The amount of weight that can be taken on the affected leg is reduced, and the patient spends more time taking weight through the unaffected side.

    (b) The step lengths are unequal. In short, the gait is not symmetrical. Steps taken are also shorter than normal.

    (c) The patient may not be able to put the heel to the floor first when taking a step forward. Instead the toe goes down first. This is a result of plantar flexion of the foot. The toe may be dragged along the ground.

    (d) The patient may not be able to control the knee movements adequately, so bending and then straightening the leg to take weight is difficult. The knee may be hyperextended.

    (e) Where there is a reduction in tone, and a flaccid limb, the patient is unable to take weight on it.

    (f) Where the patient is unable to lift the leg to take a step forward, he/she may resort to throwing or 'hitching' the pelvis forward from the hip. The result is a one-sided staggering type of walk, with the patient being easily unbalanced and nervous.

What outcomes can be expected for these patients? By three months, 64% of patients who could not walk following a stroke had regained independence (Wade et al, 1985a). Most walking ability returns in the first two weeks to three months (Andrews et al, 1981; Wade et al, 1985a). At the present level of development of stroke rehabilitation, patients should expect that the walking ability recovered should be of the highest quality possible. It is not sufficient that a patient should struggle in an uncontrolled fashion from one object of support to another. However some patients may have too much residual dysfunction to allow for a gait pattern which is entirely normal, and in these cases the aim may not be to return to a normal gait, but to establish safety and confidence in walking, or a wheelchair independence (Capildeo and Clifford Rose, 1979).

Interventions by physiotherapists and nurses are aimed to help the patient to achieve the following outcomes:

1. Equal weight bearing on both limbs.
2. Correct body position that aids the transmission of weight symmetrically.
3. Pelvis level, not leaning on the affected side.
4. Feet flat on the floor not resting on the ball of the foot when step taken.
5. Stable controlled knee.

In summary, walking in a symmetrical pattern with weight bearing on the affected leg (Parry and Eales, 1976; Bobath, 1978).

Activities of daily living (ADL)

The performance of ADL is dependent upon functional recovery, that is the patient's returning ability to carry out purposeful voluntary movements, such as rolling over and sitting up in bed, getting in and out of bed, and moving between chair and bed. This involves the return of voluntary muscle control, and recovery of sensation and perception to some degree. Most of these gross functional activities are required for dressing, carrying out personal hygiene, feeding oneself, and moving about a restricted environment. Sheikh et al (1980) found a significant association between these gross body movements, and ability to carry out ADL.

Table 11. Diagnosis: Limited Ability to Carry Out Usual Self-care Activities

The assessment will have identified which activities are impaired. For example:
Problem   Impaired ability to feed self due to paralysed right arm (patient is right handed).
Outcome goal: 1. Comfortable adaptation to using left hand to feed self.   2. Adequate intake of food/nutrition (specific amount, timing, etc.).
General outcome goals for ADL problems: 1. Before function returns: safe and comfortable adaptation to performing the activity without feeling anxious or stressed.   2. As function returns: gradual use of affected limbs in a symmetrical fashion to carry out the activity successfully.   3. If function is not going to return (in for example the arm): safe and comfortable performance of the activity with the degree of help that is appropriate.

Problem identification can be made more systematic if the nurse has some idea of what functional ability a patient will regain. This can be predicted to some extent. Work done at Rivenmead Rehabilitation Centre (Lincoln and Leadbitter, 1979) appears to show that these movements recover in a hierarchical pattern summarised as:

1. Ability to sit unsupported. Wade et al (1983a) found that the ability to sit unsup-

ported on the side of the bed meant that the patient usually recovered a good degree of ADL function).

2. Sitting up from lying, first with a little help, then alone.
3. Ability to stand and transfer to the chair.
4. Ability to walk first with help then alone.
5. Ability to climb stairs.

Arm function has a large influence upon the performance of ADL. Patients with useless arms have difficulty in dressing themselves and carrying out personal hygiene. Studies show that large numbers of stroke patients do not recover arm function. It appears that 30–50% of patients may not recover functional movement in the arm and hand (Wade et al, 1983b; Newman, 1972). Most recovery takes place in the first 3 months, but some more improvement might take place for up to a year later (Skilbeck et al, 1983).

As recovery in the ability to carry out ADL mirrors the recovery of motor function, most research that has studied recovery of ADL ability has found that most recovery occurs within the first 3 months (Skilbeck et al, 1983; Wade et al, 1985a). A few patients make a late recovery, 9% in Katz et al's (1966) study, and 2 out of 92 found by Skilbeck et al (1983).

The rate of recovery of different activities may be predicted from the research. The activities mainly concerned with lower limb function recover more rapidly. For example the ability to transfer in and out of bed, or on and off the toilet. Wade et al (1985a) found that for independence in transferring, there was an initial rapid recovery so that 50% of patients were independent within two weeks, with a slower recovery after this (80% by 47 days). However, at the end of 3 months a small number of patients still needed help from two people. Most people can feed themselves with either right or left hand, so that it is not surprising that this ability recovers rapidly, while those activities that need skilled arm and hand function such as dressing, recover more slowly (Wade et al, 1985a). A number of patients will not regain significant ADL function and will require help to carry out these activities. Andrews et al (1981) found that 27% of patients needed some help with ADL, and 13% were severely dependent one year after the stroke, whilst Kotila et al (1984) found that 18% needed some help, 8% needed a lot of help, and 7% were totally disabled, one year after the stroke. This should be kept in mind when planning for discharge.

In summary, ability to carry out ADL relies on the return of functional limb and trunk movements. Mobility and balance is also crucial. If full recovery is going to take place, this will usually happen in the first 2 weeks to 3 months. A few patients will continue to recover ability for longer periods (up to one year, maybe more). Activities which require complex arm and hand movements, including dressing and washing all over the body, may recover later than those needing lower limb function such as sitting and transferring. Approximately half of the survivors will regain total independence in ADL, 30–40% will require varying degrees of help, and about 10% will be totally dependent.

INTERVENTIONS AND RATIONALE FOR THE PROBLEMS IDENTIFIED

After a stroke almost all patients will show some recovery of function independent of any treatment or therapy that may have been given. This spontaneous or natural recovery can be improved upon by therapy and interventions from various health providers including nurses.

The methods and techniques that nurses use to help patients with problems related to mobility after hemiplegic stroke, are largely influenced by the techniques that are practised by physiotherapists. If popularity is used as an indicator, a survey of techniques used in 30 physical therapy departments in the north of England, and in several centres in North America and Europe, shows that in this country more than 90% of the centres surveyed use a combination of conventional functionally orientated exercises, and facilitation techniques (Chin et al, 1980). Of the latter the Bobath technique was one of the two most widely used. As seen by this approach to stroke treatment, the main problems are abnormal patterns of movement exacerbated by abnormal muscle tone. Three primary techniques are used to encourage normal movement and to normalise muscle tone on the involved side: weight bearing, counter rotation, and protraction of the shoulder.

Weight bearing

Use of a limb to support weight causes muscles to contract in a normal fashion.

Counter rotation

Rotation of the shoulder girdle upon the pelvis relaxes spasticity, 'counter rotation' in which the shoulder girdle rotates in one direction and the pelvis in the opposite direction has the greatest effect for normalising tone (Bobath, 1978).

Protraction

The spasticity tends to retract or pull back the pelvis and shoulder girdle, which is caused by constant contraction of the scapular retractors and low back extensors. Bringing the shoulder girdle and pelvis of the affected side forward has the effect of relaxing the spasticity (Johnson and Olson, 1980). The Bobath approach does not claim to make spasticity 'go away'. It is designed to give normal input into a hemiplegic side, encourage normal movement and reduce spasticity. To date few studies have been carried out which evaluate the so called 'facilitation' methods of therapeutic exercise. Stern et al (1970) reported on a controlled trial of the effectiveness of facilitation techniques in stroke rehabilitation. The facilitation techniques did not significantly influence mobility and leg strength. According to Inaba et al (1973) facilitation techniques were no more effective in helping to improve activities of daily living than two other methods, but they achieved the result in half the time. It is clear that such methods require systematic study and evaluation to determine their effectiveness as they are heavily reliant on therapists' time and involvement, and carry over by the nurses. Some early studies comparing physical therapy given by trained therapists with functional therapy given by nurses appear to show that nurses produced as effective results as the trained therapists (Gordon and Kohn, 1966; Feldman et al, 1962). It has to be said that the nurses were trained rehabilitation nurses. It is evident that to provide continuity of care in the management of stroke patient mobility, nurses will have to become familiar with the techniques for moving and handling patients that are currently being practised by physiotherapists. Such techniques for moving and handling patients are described in specialist texts (Bobath, 1978) but communication with physiotherapy staff is essential.

The return of voluntary movement to paralysed limbs is probably wholly dependent upon recovery of the damaged nervous system and there are various theories as to how and why this recovery takes place (Rothi and Horner, 1983). Interventions based on the techniques just described may promote a better functional outcome by preventing complications.

There appear to be no studies which evaluate care and handling of paralysed limbs, but clinical experience would suggest that careful handling and positioning and full range of passive movements to all joints are necessary to ensure patients can recover well and are not limited by contractures and painful joints.

Spasticity

As previously stated spasticity is seen to be a major deterrent to patients moving their limbs in a normal fashion. Despite this contention by physiotherapists and others there is little empirical evidence to support it. McLellan (1977) in a study to test the effect of a drug to reduce spasticity, using electrophysiological techniques, showed that the problem in the use of a group of spastic muscles was an abnormal pattern of muscle contraction with a heightened stretch reflex, but correcting this did not alter the abnormal co-contraction. Miller and Hammond (1981) in a study of stroke patients showed a similar disturbance in control of muscles of arm movement. Their explanation was that there was a disorder of reciprocal inhibition between antagonistic muscle groups. This would increase resistance to voluntary movement but the underlying cause would not arise from an abnormal stretch reflex alone. However techniques for inhibiting spasticity based on Bobath (1978) have received widespread recognition in British nursing literature (Newman, 1985; Myco, 1983; Batehup, 1983; Parry and Eales, 1976). Until the time that careful study gives guidance for intervention for spastic stroke patients (that can be used by nurses) there is no reason why these techniques should not be used, and although the neurophysiological theories underpinning them may be disputed by some, they are supported by others. The basic principle is that patients should be moved and their limbs positioned to reduce spasticity and oppose the dominant patterns of flexion or extension. The techniques are described in the texts already referred to and will not be described further. Patients should be handled and positioned in this way from immediately after the stroke, and this is better facilitated if the patient and relatives can be taught how to position the limbs correctly. The use of position charts that are large enough to be seen and used by patients and relatives, will help to ensure continuity and help communication. Where spasticity is present and inhibiting movement of the joint, the application of local cooling may be effective in reducing it. Studies have shown that local cooling (for example by icepack) for 20–30 minutes may reduce spasticity for one to two hours so that exercises and movements can be carried out (Arlien-Soborg et al, 1976).

Contractures

Interventions to prevent contractures at joints should be started immediately after the stroke. Contractures are a phenomenon of disuse and therefore should be completely preventable. As contractures arise from a combination of spasticity and immobility around the joint it is proposed that regular passive and active movements may prevent this happening although this is unsupported by empirical studies. A combination of measures was proposed by Newman (1985) following a small scale study:

1. Correct positioning—this has been referred to in the section on spasticity.
2. Exercise, passive, assisted or active.
3. Early weight bearing.

The timing of this application of passive or assisted movements for joints is arbitrary as little or no evidence exists for guidance. Most authors suggest joints should be put through their full range of movements two to four times a day (Newman, 1985; Kottke, 1982). Where possible the patient and relative should be taught how to perform the exercises safely. Care should be taken when manipulating paralysed joints as inexperienced helpers can cause damage. The shoulder joint is particularly vulnerable following a stroke, as the stability of the normal shoulder depends mainly on the support of the surrounding muscle cuff (Fitzgerald-Finch and Gibson, 1975). A prospective study by Smith et al (1982) found that 46% of stroke patients had radiological evidence of shoulder malalignment, 75% of these showing it immediately following the stroke. It probably occurs during the initial period of reduced muscle tone and may be related to faulty lifting and positioning of the patient (Fitzgerald-Finch and Gibson, 1975). Before joints are moved through their range of movement (ROM) helpers should be aware of the normal physiological range of all joints, and the technique to be used to perform the exercise safely and comfortably. According to McNeil (1975), a stroke victim, ROM exercises 'relieved muscle ache, promoted circulation and relieved tension, more than turning'.

Walking

Interventions for walking stroke patients are aimed to promote a safe, symmetrical walking pattern. Again full details of such techniques are available in the nursing and physiotherapy literature (Bobath, 1978; Johnson and Olson, 1980; Parry and Eales, 1976). The patient may start to move from the correct sitting position which has been previously learned and practised. Suitable shoes should be worn which should be supporting and non-slip. Slippers are usually unsuitable. Standing is achieved in a controlled way with the patient taking weight on both limbs. The nurse can support the patient from behind whilst keeping the pelvis level and preventing pelvic hitching. The use of aids is debatable, and currently there is little agreement as to whether or not a stick should be used (Wade et al, 1985b). When the stroke patient starts to walk again this will be closely supervised by the physiotherapist. A danger is that the physiotherapist may become protective of the patient's walking and movement retraining in an effort that other staff do not induce the patient to carry out activities too early or inappropriately. A consequence is that nursing staff present on wards all day are not continuing the walking training, and the patient is confined to a chair following 20–30 minutes of therapy in a physiotherapy department. More communication is required between physiotherapy and nursing staff to ensure practice and continuity of appropriate training.

Walking practice can be carried out when functional activities are required such as going to the toilet, or bathroom. Nurses should ensure (Parry and Eales, 1976) that before this happens the patient is capable of:

1. Getting out of the chair.
2. Standing correctly.
3. Moving forwards with controlled weight transfer.
4. Negotiating the confines of the bathroom.
5. Sitting down in a controlled manner.

Activities of daily living (ADL)

Nurses are concerned in a major way with helping disabled patients to carry out the usual activities of daily living. The major goal of these interventions is usually the promotion of the patient's independence. Unfortunately several studies of stroke patient recovery have shown that nurses do not promote independence, but rather appeared to promote dependence in most patients. Myco (1986) studied nurses' promotion of independence in elimination, mobility, nutrition and personal hygiene; all activities that are crucial to functioning at home. Results revealed that over 50% of patients were not receiving care which would promote independence in elimination. Some attempt was made to promote mobility in 66% of patients, but between 63% and 97% of patients were inactive at any point in the day. These stroke patients were not doing anything, having anything done for them, or communicating with anyone. Nurses did attempt to promote independent eating in 87% of patients. In summary, patients who have the greatest need to relearn how to carry out these activities (those who are most disabled by the stroke), tend to be given care rather than encouraged to help themselves. No doubt nurses would say that lack of time prevents them allowing patients to try to carry out the activity. This is probably not the only reason. Nurses need to be aware that patients can increase their independence to carry out the activities if they are given guidance and time to do it. This is sometimes a lengthy process, and it may be more effective to let relatives come into hospital at the relevant times (in the mornings and evenings) to help the patient, whilst also gaining some knowledge about the patient's ability which would be helpful to them when the patient gets home.

An earlier study by Patrick (1972) demonstrated similar problems. Few nurses seemed to provide conditions under which stroke patients could perform activities unaided. Food and fluids were fed to patients who could have fed themselves. Bowel and bladder training was not seen as important. At all times patients should be encouraged to use both arms in order to promote bilateral function. However aids may have to be used when it has been established without doubt that functional return is unlikely.

Nurses can help patients regain independence in ADL by:

1. Providing the optimum environment for the patient to carry out the activity.
2. Providing the level of help which promotes independence but does not cause stress and anxiety. This relies on a careful assessment.

3. Teaching the patient techniques which will make the task easier.
4. Giving the patient time to carry out the activity before helping.

EVALUATION

The evaluation concerns what outcomes, in terms of recovery and functional ability, the patient has achieved. Outcome criteria in the form of patient goals have been identified in previous sections. The tools used for measurement during assessment will continue to be used for the assessment and evaluation during recovery. It is possible to develop non-specific tools for various parts of the recovery process. For example Myco (1983) describes a chart for assessing the patient's ability to wash the upper part of the body. This identifies 21 steps in the procedure, and could be used by the patient as a guide to carrying out the activity, as well as for the nurse assessing learning and performance of the activity.

In previous sections on problem identification and outcome setting, research was identified which gave general guidelines for timing and patterns of recovery in muscle movements, functional movements including walking, and the carrying out of self-care activities. Therefore there are some basic data on which acquisition of skills and return of function can be predicted. It is important that nurses document interventions and relate them to the patient's predicted and actual outcomes. In this way data may be made available which can provide clues to successful interventions, and realistic outcomes for patients.

In summary evaluation may be concerned with:

1. Rate of progress of recovery of voluntary movement, functional movements, return of self-care skills—levels of independence.
2. Patterns of recovery of voluntary movements, functional movements and self-care skills.
3. Quality of walking and movements.

IMPLICATIONS FOR NURSING PRACTICE

It is evident that large numbers of people suffer a stroke, especially among those who are elderly or very elderly. Most of these stroke victims will have some degree of mobility impairment. The assessment of this impairment can be carried out by nurses using observation and simple assessment tools. In practice this rarely happens. Stroke patients are not seen to recover rapidly, and are regarded by many nurses as boring long-term problems. This need not be so. Many patients do recover function. Nurses have a major role to play in rehabilitation involving mobility and self-care. Problems can be identified in a more systematic and scientific fashion; outcome goals can be set which are based on studies of stroke recovery, and interventions can be carried out which will help patients to achieve these goals. Systematic evaluation in the light of the research already done, will highlight similarities and differences in individual patients' rate and quality of progress.

FUTURE RESEARCH

1. Studies to evaluate methods and strategies that nurses can use to promote independence in stroke patients.
2. Evaluative studies to establish the optimum frequency and type of exercise which prevents joint immobility in paralysed limbs.
3. Studies to evaluate assessment and teaching guides for specific self-care activities such as dressing, washing, and feeding.
4. Evaluative studies on the effect of more systematic stroke nursing education for nurses.
5. Evaluative studies on more planned and systematic participation by relatives in stroke rehabilitation.
6. Evaluative studies of using a 'stroke unit approach' in general medical wards.

REFERENCES

Aho K, Harmsen P, Hatano S, Marquardsen J, Smirnov VE, Strasser T (1980) Cerebrovascular disease in the community: results of a WHO collaborative study. *Bulletin WHO* **58**, 113–130.

Andrews K, Brocklehurst JC, Richards B, Laycock PJ (1981) The rate of recovery from stroke and its measurement. *International Rehabilitation Medicine* **3**, 155–61.

Arlien-Soborg P, Mai J, Pedersen E (1976) Changes in motor response during cooling. In: Komi PV (ed) *International Series on Biomechanics, Biomechanics VA Vols 1A*. University Press, Baltimore.

Bard G, Hirschberg GG (1965) Recovery of voluntary motion in upper extremity following hemiplegia. *Archives of Physical Medicine and Rehabilitation* **46**, 567–572.

Batehup L (1983) How teaching can help the stroke patient's recovery. In: Wilson-Barnett J (ed) *Patient Teaching*. Churchill Livingstone, Edinburgh.

Bobath B (1978) *Adult Hemiplegia: Evaluation and Treatment*. 2nd edition. William Heinemann Medical Books, London.

Brunstromm S (1964) Recording gait patterns of adult hemiplegia patients. *Journal of the American Physical Therapy Association* **44**(1), 11–18.

Capildeo R, Clifford Rose F (1979) The assessment of neurological disability. In: Greenhalgh RM, Clifford Rose F (eds) *Progress in Stroke Research*. Pittman Medical, London.

Carstairs V (1976) Stroke: resource consumption and the cost to the community. In: Gillingham G, Maudsley C, Williams AE (eds) *Stroke*. Churchill Livingstone, Edinburgh.

Chin PL, Rosie A, Irving M, Smith R (1980) *Final Report on Hemiplegic Gait Studies* to the Research Department Northern Regional Health Authority.

Clemesson S (1951) Some studies on muscle tone. *Proceedings of the Royal Society of Medicine* **47**, 593–594.

Colasso H, Joshi J (1971) Variations of gait patterns in adult hemiplegia. *Neurology India* (Bombay) **19**(4), 212–216.

Creason NS, Pogue NJ, Nelson AA, Hoyt CA (1985) Validating the nursing diagnosis of impaired physical mobility. *Nursing Clinics of North America* **20**(4), 669–683.

De Lateur B (1982) Therapeutic exercise to develop strength and endurance. In: Kottke TJ, Stillwell GK, Lehman JF (eds) *Krusens Handbook of Physical Medicine and Rehabilitation*. WB Saunders, Philadelphia.

Demeurisse G, Demol O, Robaye E (1980) Motor evaluation in vascular hemiplegia. *European Neurology* **19**, 382–389.

Drake WE, Hamilton MJ, Carlsson M, Blumenkrantz J (1973) Acute stroke management and patient outcomes: the value of neurovascular care units. *Stroke* **4**, 933–945.

Ebrahim S, Nourv R, Baker D (1985) Cognitive impairment after stroke. *Age and Aging* **14**, 345–350.

Edwards ES, McKeran RO (1986) Prevalence of multiple sclerosis in a south London borough. *British Medical Journal* **293**, 237–239.

Feldman DJ, Lee PR, Unterecker J, Lloyd K, Rusk HA, Toole A (1962) A comparison of functionally orientated medical care and formal rehabilitation in the management of patients with hemiplegia due to cerebrovascular accident. *Journal of Chronic Disease* **15**, 297–310.

Fitzgerald-Finch OP, Gibson IIJM (1975) Subluxation of the shoulder in hemiplegia. *Age and Aging* **4**, 16–18.

Fugl-Meyer AR, Jasko L, Leyman L, Olsson S, Steglind S (1975) The post-stroke hemiplegic patient. 1. A method for evaluation of physical performance. *Scandinavian Journal of Rehabilitation Medicine* **7**, 13–31.

Gordon EE, Kohn KH (1966) Evaluation of rehabilitation methods in the hemiplegic patient. *Journal of Chronic Disease* **19**, 3–16.

Gresham GE, Phillips TF, Labi HLL (1980) ADL status in stroke: relative merits of three-standard indexes. *Archives of Physical Medicine and Rehabilitation* **61**, 355–359.

Grieve DW (1980) Monitoring gait. *British Journal of Hospital Medicine* **24**, 198–204.

Herman B, Leyten ACM, Van Luijk JH, Frenken CWGM, Opde Cool AAW, Schulte BPM (1982) Epidemiology of Stroke in Tilberg the Netherlands. *Stroke* **13**, 629–634.

Huskisson EC (1985) *Osteoarthritis: Pathogenesis and Management*. The Update Group Ltd, London.

Inaba M, Edberg E, Montgomery J, Gillis MK (1973) Effectiveness of functional training, active exercise, and resistive exercises for patients with hemiplegia. *Physical Therapy* **53**, 28–35.

Isaacs B (1971) Identification of disability in the stroke patient *Modern Geriatrics* **1**, 390–402.

Jennett B (1982) Research aspects of rehabilitation after acute brain damage in adults. *Lancet* **ii** 1034–1036.

Johnson K, Olson E (1980) Application of Bobath principles for nursing care of the hemiplegic patient. *Journal of the Association of Rehabilitation Nurses* **31**(Mar/Apr), 8–11.

Katz S, Ford AB, Chinn AB, Newill VA (1966) Prognosis after stroke. 2. Long term course of 159 patients. *Medicine* **45**, 236–246.

Katz S, Ford AB, Moscowitz RW, Jackson BF, Jaffe MW (1963) The Index of ADL: standardised measure of biological and psychosocial function. *Journal of the American Medical Association* **185**, 914–919.

Keith RA (1984) Functional assessment measures in medical rehabilitation: current status. *Archives of Physical Medicine and Rehabilitation* **65**, 74–78.

Kim MJ, McFarland GK, McLane AM (eds) (1984) *Classification of Nursing Diagnosis: Proceedings of the Fifth National Conference*. CV Mosby, St Louis.

Kotila M, Waltimo O, Niemi ML, Laaksonen R, Lempinen M (1984) The profile of recovery from stroke, and factors influencing outcome. *Stroke* **15**(6), 1039–1044.

Kottke FJ (1982) The neurophysiology of motor function. In: Kottke FJ, Stillwell GK, Lehman JF (eds) *Krusens Handbook of Physical Medicine and Rehabilitation*. WB Saunders, Philadelphia.

Lincoln N, Leadbitter D (1979) Assessment of motor function in stroke patients. *Physiotherapy* **65**, 48–51.

McLellan DL (1977) Co-contraction and stretch reflexes in spasticity during treatment with Baclofen. *Journal of Neurology, Neurosurgery, and Psychiatry* **40**, 50–58.

McNeil F (1975) Stroke — nursing insights from a stroke-nurse victim. *Registered Nurse* **38**, 75–81.

Mahoney FI, Barthel DW (1965) Functional evaluation: the Barthel index. *Maryland State Medical Journal* **14**, 61–65.

Medical Research Council (1976) *Aids to the Examination of the Peripheral Nervous System*. HMSO, London.

Miller S, Hammond GR (1981) Neural control of arm movement in patients following stroke. In: Van Hof MW, Mohn G (eds) *Functional Recovery from Brain Damage*. Elsevier, Amsterdam.

Moskowitz E, Lightbody FEH, Freitag NS (1972) Longterm follow up of the post-stroke patient. *Archives of Physical Medicine and Rehabilitation* **53**, 167–172.

Musa IM (1986) The role of afferent input in the reduction of spasticity: an hypothesis. *Physiotherapy* **72**(4), 179–182.

Myco F (1986) A new way of living. *Nursing Times* **Apr 2**, 24–27.

Myco F (1984) *Nursing Care of the Hemiplegic Stroke Patient in General Medical Wards in Hospitals in Northern Ireland.* Submitted for PhD, New University of Ulster.

Myco F (1983) *Nursing Care of the Hemiplegic Stroke Patient.* Harper and Row, London.

Neilson PD (1972) Interaction between voluntary contraction and tonic stretch reflex: transmission in normal and spastic patients. *Journal of Neurosurgery and Psychiatry* **35**, 853–860.

Newman D (1985) Essential physical therapy for stroke patients. *Nursing Times* **Feb 6**, 16–18.

Newman M (1972) The process of recovery after hemiplegic stroke. *Stroke* **3**, 702–710.

Parry A, Eales C (1976) Hemiplegia 1–5 *Nursing Times* **Oct 14**, 1590–1592, **Oct 21**, 1640–1641, **Oct 28**, 1681–1683, **Nov 4**, 1762–1767, **Nov 11**, 1767–1769.

Patrick G (1972) Forgotten patients on medical wards. *The Canadian Nurse* **Mar**, 27–31.

Rothi LJ, Horner J (1983) Restitution and substitution: two theories of recovery with application to neurobehavioural treatment. *Journal of Clinical Neuropsychology* **5**(1), 73–81.

Sheikh K, Smith AS, Meade TW, Brennan PT, Ide L (1980) Assessment of motor function in studies of chronic disability. *Rheumatology and Rehabilitation* **19**, 83–90.

Sheikh K, Smith DS, Meade TW, Goldenberg E, Brennan PJ, Kinsella G (1979) Dependability and validity of a modified activity of daily living index. ADL in studies of chronic disability. *International Rehabilitation Medicine* **1**, 51–58.

Silman AJ (1986) Recent trends in rheumatoid arthritis. *British Journal of Rheumatology* **25**(4), 328–330.

Skilbeck CE, Wade DT, Wood VE (1983) Recovery after stroke. *Journal of Neurology, Neurosurgery and Psychiatry* **46**, 5–8.

Smith DL, Akhtar AJ, Garaway WM (1983) Proprioception and spatial neglect after stroke. *Age and Aging* **12**, 63–69.

Smith RG, Cruikshank JG, Dunbar S, Akhtar AJ (1982) Malalignment of the shoulder after stroke. *British Medical Journal* **284**, 1224–1226.

Stern PH, McDowell T, Miller JM, Robinson M (1970) Effects of facilitation exercise techniques in stroke rehabilitation. *Archives of Physical Medicine and Rehabilitation* **51**, 526–531.

Twitchell T (1951) The restoration of motor function following hemiplegia in man. *Brain* **74**, 443–480.

Wade DT, Langton Hewer R, David RM, Enderby PM (1986) Aphasia after stroke: natural history and associated deficits. *Journal of Neurology, Neurosurgery and Psychiatry* **49**, 11–16.

Wade DT, Wood PA, Langton Hewer R (1985a) Recovery after stroke—the first three months. *Journal of Neurology, Neurosurgery and Psychiatry* **48**, 7–13.

Wade DT, Langton Hewer R, Skilbeck CE, David RM (1985b) *Stroke: a critical approach to diagnosis treatment and management.* Chapman and Hall, London.

Wade DT, Skilbeck CE, Langton Hewer R (1983a) Predicting Barthel ADL score at six months after an acute stroke. *Archives of Physical Medicine and Rehabilitation* **64**, 24–28.

Wade DT, Langton Hewer R, Wood VA, Skilbeck CE, Ismail HM (1983b) The hemiplegic arm after stroke: measurement and recovery. *Journal of Neurology, Neurosurgery and Psychiatry* **46**, 521–524.

Walker AE, Robins M, Weinfeld FD (1981) Clinical findings in the national survey of stroke. Weinfeld FD (ed) *Stroke* **12**(Suppl 1), 13–44.

Wall JC, Ashburn A (1979) Assessment of gait disability in hemiplegics. *Scandinavian Journal of Rehabilitation Medicine* **11**, 95–103.

Chapter 11
Problems with Wound Healing

INTRODUCTION

A wound involves a disruption of the integrity and function of tissues in the body, and wound healing is the complex process of repair that is triggered into a sequence of events by the presence of the wound itself.

Healing by primary intention occurs when full thickness wound edges are closely approximated shortly after the wound has been created. Examples of wounds that heal in this way are surgical incisions and clean lacerations without tissue loss.

Healing by secondary intention occurs in wounds usually associated with tissue loss, including decubitus ulcers and venous ulcers.

Wound healing

Wound healing has been conveniently described as four closely connected and overlapping stages (Westaby, 1985; Torrance, 1986):

1. The acute inflammatory phase.
2. The destructive phase.
3. The proliferative phase.
4. The maturation phase.

The inflammatory phase of wound healing is characterised by recognisable signs of inflammation, local increase in heat, redness and oedema. The inflammatory response is essential if healing is to proceed (Torrance, 1986). During this phase dead cells and bacteria are cleared away and the healing process is stimulated by substances released from such cells as platelets. Prolonging the inflammatory phase for any reason will delay healing and may result in excessive granulation tissue at a later date. The presence of necrotic devitalised tissue, or blood clots, and even the presence of sutures, can prolong the inflammatory phase.

During the destructive phase the wound macrophages are the important cells. Macrophages are responsible for debridement of necrotic tissue, and for removal of bacteria from the wound. They are also important in the process of growth of new blood vessels (angiogenesis) and for attracting the fibroblasts via a series of hormone messengers (Hunt and Halliday, 1980).

The proliferative phase is characterised by proliferation of endothelial cells and fibroblasts. Collagen synthesis begins and is randomly organised in the wound. The new granulation tissue consists of new capillary loops, supporting collagen, and a glycoprotein ground substance. In wounds healing by secondary intention, such as ulcers, the formation of granulation tissue is a disorderly process, and may be disrupted with further tissue damage. Granulation tissue contains many new blood vessels which are delicate and easily damaged. The process proceeds with the maturation of the granulation tissue, including reorientation of the collagen fibres, and regaining of strength in the wounded tissues. In open wounds and with good healing conditions, the granulation tissue fills the space. In wounds such as ulcers closure is due mainly to a process of contraction. In the early phase of healing the wound area may increase when the edges of the wound retract to some extent. But as the wound heals the edges begin to move inwards probably mediated by a form of fibroblast called a myofibroblast (Forrest, 1983).

Epithelialisation

Epithelialisation, the migration of epithelial cells across a wound, ensures protection against dehydration and contamination by providing a watertight seal (Edlich et al, 1979). Wounds with only skin loss will begin epithelialisation within 12 hours of the injury, and sutured wounds should have a watertight seal within 24 hours. Deeper wounds require collagen formation and granulation before epithelial cell migration (Hunt et al, 1984). Factors which affect wound healing are not confined to the wound in isolation, but concern the patient's general health state, and also his environment. Local factors which can affect wound healing include the oxygen and nutrient supply to the wound, the wound temperature, infection, and inadequate and inappropriate use of topical applications and dressings. The patient's physical health is also important in relation to the healing wound. Level of nutrition, the presence of other conditions such as diabetes and cardiovascular problems and therapies which affect the patient's immunocompetence, are all relevant when considering problems with healing wounds. Chronic wounds such as venous leg ulcers and decubitus ulcers invariably are accompanied by adverse factors that delay healing (Leaper, 1986a).

Venous leg ulcers rarely heal without compression bandages to help the failing calf pump; diabetic ulcers on the heels need debridement of necrotic tissue and good diabetic control; pressure sores are unlikely to heal without attention to adequate pressure relief and good nutrition (Leaper, 1986a).

THE PREVALENCE OF THE PROBLEM OF DELAYED WOUND HEALING

In this chapter the problem of delayed wound healing has been divided into the problem of infected wounds, which may either be incisional wounds or open wounds; and wounds with delayed healing because of the presence of necrotic or sloughing tissue in the wound. These will be confined to chronic wounds such as venous and decubitus ulcers.

Wound infection—post-operative

In general a wound can be considered infected if purulent material drains from it, even without the confirmation of a positive wound culture (Howard et al, 1964). Positive culture does not always indicate infection since many wounds, infected or not, are colonised by bacteria, and some wounds may not yield pathogens by culture because the pathogens require special techniques for their detection, or the patient has been taking antibiotics (Garner, 1986; Meers et al, 1981).

A national study of the prevalence of surgical wound infection in England and Wales (Meers et al, 1981) revealed that depending on the type of surgery, the prevalence of wound infections was between 3.5 and 12.8% Studies of incidence of surgical wound infections in hospitals have found that overall clean wounds have a 1–5% risk of infection, and contaminated wounds involving surgery on the large bowel, have a 10–17% risk of becoming infected (Cruse and Foord, 1980). The complications of surgical wound infections can be confined locally to the wound area and near tissues, or may be systemic. Local complications include destruction of tissues and wound dehiscence, incisional hernias, pain, and disfiguring scars. Wound infections place an increased metabolic demand on the patient, and may result in spread of infection to other parts of the body. Any infection involving an implanted prosthesis such as heart valves, or artificial hip joint, can have catastrophic effects. Gram-negative bacteria make up approximately 40% of pathogens isolated from surgical wounds (Garner, 1986); *Staphylococcus aureus* is the most frequently isolated species (Meers et al, 1981).

Chronic wounds with tissue loss

Ulceration of the leg, especially the lower leg is very common. A recent survey has shown that between 1 and 2% of the population may be suffering from venous ulceration (Cornwall and Lewis, 1983). Of the patients identified in the Lothian and Forth Valley survey of leg ulcer prevalence (Dale et al, 1983), females outnumbered males by a ratio of 2.8:1. For patients in their 70s the ratio was 4:1, rising to 7:1 after the age of 80.

Prevalence studies related to the presence of pressure sores report a prevalence of pressure sores in the range 4–8.8% (David, 1983; Clark et al, 1978; Lowthian, 1978). The survey by David (1983) showed that the majority of patients with pressure sores were to be found in geriatric, general medicine, and orthopaedic wards, and were mostly over the age of 65 years confirming previous studies (Clark et al, 1978) that the incidence of pressure sores rises with increasing age. The study by Clark et al (1978) found that the most common site for sores was the sacrum, followed by ischial tuberosities, hips, heels, ankles, elbows, and knees. David (1983) found that more sores were reported on the sacrum followed closely by buttocks and heels.

It is probably rare to find a sterile chronic wound. Most leg ulcers, and probably decubitus ulcers support a mixed flora of common commensals such as *Staphylococcus aureus*, *Pseudomonas aeruginosa* and *Proteus bacilli* (Morgan, 1987). There is little consensus on the relative importance of the presence of these bacteria to the healing process. The mere presence of micro-organisms does not necessarily mean they are interfering with healing (Morgan, 1987), and according to Leaper (1986a) organisms which are usual skin commensals may even be enhancing wound healing by pulling host defence mechanisms, bacterial substances, lysozymes, and complement systems to the wound surface. There is some experimental animal research which supports these concepts (Tenorio et al, 1976). Wound swabs from such chronic wounds should be treated with caution. However the presence in the wound of a beta-haemolytic Streptococci group A, should always be treated seriously (Morgan, 1987).

It is difficult to make a statement about the prevalence of sloughing or necrotic ulcers. It is probably true that most leg ulcers at some time have sloughing or necrotic tissue present. In a survey of pressure sores by David (1983), in those sores classified as having broken skin, 27% had necrotic tissue, and 10% appeared infected.

Delayed wound healing presents a considerable problem both in hospital and the community. Early diagnosis of the problem, and effective management could save considerable patient and economic costs.

ASSESSMENT AND PROBLEM IDENTIFICATION

The assessment of wound problems does not concern the wound in isolation, nor is assessment confined to the time after the wound has occurred, but also concerns the time before wounding. This may be especially relevant for surgical wounds, and chronic wounds such as pressure ulcers. Assessment will focus on the patient's physical and emotional health, the wound itself, and the environment (see Table 1).

Table 1. Assessment of Wound Healing

Criteria	Methods
Endogenous—wound	
1. *Type of wound*:	
Open wounds	
Wounds with tissue loss e.g. pressure sores, leg ulcers, fungating wounds, minor abrasions, donor and recipient skin graft sites.	
Surgically closed wounds	
(classification by surgical operation)	
Wounds without tissue loss	
2. *State of wound*:	
Surface area of open wound	Physical examination
Depth of wound	Patient report
Base of wound	Physiological responses
Edges	Chart wound progress
Discharge	Laboratory findings
Pain	
Inflammation	
Drains	
Sutures	
Endogenous—patient	
Physical state	Physical health assessment
Associated conditions e.g. diabetes	Nutritional assessment
Other therapies, e.g. chemotherapy, radiation	Laboratory findings
Exogenous—environment	
Hospitalisation	Patient self-report
Topical applications and dressings	Physical examination
Wound management	Systematic recording of wound assessment and management
	Observation

The patient's physical and emotional health

Nutrition

Protein energy malnutrition (PEM) in hospitalised patients is estimated to be as high as 50% of adults (Bistrian et al, 1974; Butterworth and Blackburn, 1975). The causes of PEM are complex. Some patients may be malnourished on admission while others become so during their stay. Patients who may be at risk include the elderly with restricted mobility and purchasing power; patients who have had gastrointestinal surgery, and other major surgical patients with increased metabolic requirements and are fasting post-operatively; stroke patients are also at risk because of impairments in swallowing, or in feeding themselves. Cancer patients are also in a high risk group because of anorexia, nausea and vomiting. The influence of the nutritional state on the healing process is well documented (Dickerson, 1986; Caldwell and Kennedy-Caldwell, 1981). Patients who are overweight are also at risk for delayed healing. Cruse and Foord (1973) found that obese patients had a 'clean' wound infection rate of 13.5%, compared to 1.8% overall for 'clean' operations. Apart from an increased risk of infection, obese patients have a tendency to form incisional hernias (Mason, 1981). Wound dehiscence is also more common in obese patients when strain causes the sutures to break (Hunt, 1976). Finally seromas are likely to develop in wounds of obese patients because there is a large potential for dead space (Groszek, 1982).

According to Goodinson (1987a) nutritional assessment is a collegiate responsibility involving nurse, doctor, dietitian, pharmacist and catering services. This author reviews methods of nutritional assessment including anthropometry, biochemical indices, and dietary assessment (Goodinson, 1987b). Nutritional assessment may include measurements of body weight, limb skinfold thickness, and skeletal muscle mass. These can give a guide to changes in fat and protein stores. Such techniques are inexpensive and non-invasive. It should be noted that these measures are prone to measurement error and interpretive problems (Goodinson, 1987c).

Biochemical tests include measurement of serum proteins: albumin, transferrin, retinol binding protein, thyroxine and binding prealbumin, fibronectin, creatinine, and 3-methyl histidine. None of these biochemical markers is totally satisfactory as an index of nutritional state, but some may be useful in monitoring some patients who are not in an acute catabolic state (Goodinson, 1987a).

Dietary assessment

Certain patients may be predisposed towards poor wound healing as a consequence of nutritional depletions arising as the result of increased nutrient requirements or inability to maintain an adequate intake. Haider (1984) suggests that the subjective methods of nutritional assessment including a dietary history and physical examination of the patient should be used to identify high risk patients. Detsky (1984), in comparing more objective methods of assessment with subjective methods (which include a dietary history) for predicting the possibility of infection in a group of surgical patients, found that the subjective methods produced a good contribution of sensitivity and specificity in predicting outcome. Nurses have the responsibility for feeding patients, and are best placed to be aware of what patients are eating, and whether or not such symptoms as dysphagia, nausea, vomiting, anorexia, diarrhoea or constipation are present. Awareness is also required regarding the increased metabolic demand imposed by an infected, or chronic wound. It should be remembered that even well-nourished patients lose considerable amounts of body protein and fat during the early post-operative period when 5% dextrose may be the only form of nutritional support.

Associated conditions and therapies that have adverse effects on wound healing

Diabetes

An assessment to identify potential wound healing problems should take into account other disease states and therapies that patients may have or be lacking, which may influence wound repair.

Complications in wound healing are common for many diabetic patients. In a review of 23,649 patients, Cruse and Foord (1973) found that in clean surgical wounds, diabetics had a five-fold increase in the incidence of wound infection. Wounds in diabetic patients have been found to have a tendency to become infected with organisms such as *Staphylococcus aureus*, *Staphylococcus epidermidis*, *Escherichia coli* and *Candida* species (Feigin and Shearer, 1975), organisms commonly found on the skin of most individuals. A summary of experimental research on diabetic wound healing by Goodson et al (1980) shows a variety of causes for delayed wound healing, including:

1. Ischaemia caused by large and small vessel occlusive disease causing wound hypoxia and malnourishment of the tissues of the wound area.
2. Decreased inflammatory response caused by both hyperglycaemia resulting in white cells with depressed chemotactic responses and phagocytosis, and intracellular killing of ingested bacteria.
3. Possible effects of insulin deficiency on fibroblasts resulting in production of defective collagen.

The result of these impairments means that diabetic wounds may take longer to heal, incisions can break down, infection rates are higher, and in addition, impaired sensation of diabetic neuropathy can result in mechanical trauma which also impairs healing (Carrico et al, 1984).

Nurses should be aware of these potential problems with diabetic wounds. Stability of diabetic control should be assessed regularly by blood glucose estimation and the condition of the wound assessed for a delayed inflammatory response, and adequate blood supply.

Radiation therapy

There are some unavoidable effects of radiation on tissues which will be important for patients with wounds. Tissue changes are directly related to dose increments, frequency, and total dose received (Bloomer and Hellman, 1975). Usually, less than 4,000 rads produces cellular and tissue effects which are transient. More than 4,000 rads results in permanent effects such as endarteritis obliterans causing vessel narrowing and reduced blood flow, and fibrosis in the muscular layers (Bloomer and Hellman, 1975). Poor wound healing is manifested as fistulas, dehiscence, or more commonly, by a prolonged period of delayed healing. Infection is also a common problem (Dirksen et al, 1977).

Immunosuppression in delay of wound healing

The components of the immune system that contribute to wound healing include the inflammatory response, phagocytosis, and hormonal and cell-mediated immunity. Patients at risk include:

1. Those who have congenital or acquired immunological diseases which may compromise phagocytosis (leukaemia), or cell-mediated immunity (Hodgkin's disease).
2. Older people may have impaired immunological functions (Chvapil and Koopman, 1982), and in addition have decreased function of essential organs as well as nutritional influences which may delay healing.
3. Patients with underlying conditions that may delay healing. Diabetes and malnutrition have already been mentioned in this respect. Cancer patients have been shown by some authors to have an increased incidence and severity of wound complications (Finn et al, 1980; White et al, 1977).
4. Patients taking drugs which compromise wound healing. The effects of steroids on wound healing have been under debate for many years. Experimental studies have shown that anti-inflammatory steroids decrease the tensile strength of closed wounds, slow the rate of epithelialisation, and new vessel proliferation and inhibit wound contraction (Ehrlich and Hunt, 1969; Stephens et al, 1971). Steroids will suppress the repair process if administered before the injury or within 2 or 3 days afterwards. Delayed healing will be as a consequence of reduced contraction and epithelialisation in open wounds, and of infection in both open and closed wounds.

Cytotoxic chemotherapy

The effect of chemotherapeutic agents on wound healing has been summarised by Ferguson (1982). A review of experimental animal studies examining wound healing and cytoxic drugs showed that these drugs, by interfering with cell proliferation, produce a variety of wound healing problems including decreasing wound strength, inhibiting contraction, reducing collagen production, reducing inflammatory response and neovascularisation. This has resulted in increased rate of wound dehiscence and wound infection, and in granulating wounds, less exudate and granulation tissue, and a slower rate of wound contraction. A review of clinical studies however by the same author (Ferguson, 1982) failed to support the experimental work. Reasons for this may include, reporting of complications in the clinical studies was usually secondary to testing the chemotherapeutic agents, the chemotherapy was usually delayed until wound healing was well under way, and methods for assessing healing differed greatly. Westaby (1981) reported that the use of cytotoxic drugs in the pre-operative treatment of long term cancer patients resulted in the absence of healing in thoracotomy wounds when sutures were removed. It is obvious that timing of therapy and wounding is important.

Environmental factors relevant for predicting wound complications

During the assessment stage, it is necessary to take into account environmental factors which may predispose to delayed wound healing.

The hospital environment itself may predispose the surgical patient to an increased risk of infection after the operation. Cruse and Foord (1980) reported that with a one-day pre-operative stay the infection rate was 1.2%, with a 1 week stay it was 2.1% and for a pre-operative stay of more than 2 weeks, 3.4%. It is likely that patients' skin becomes colonised with bacteria to which they are not resistant, and which may be more virulent than the 'community' bacteria.

The proximity of an infected patient to uninfected patients should be assessed. Transmission of infection by contact between people or via equipment is the most common method of spreading infection. Transient organisms can be picked up during contact with an infected patient or his equipment including bedpans, urinals, wound dressings and catheter bags. These can then be carried to uninfected patients.

Wound management itself may be a factor in delayed wound healing. Inappropriate topical applications, frequent changes of wound dressing materials and methods may all contribute to delayed healing, and these factors should be considered when assessing for wound healing problems.

Assessment of the wound itself

In surgical wounds the risk of infection in the post-operative period can be assessed in relation to the type of surgical operation carried out.

Table 2. Wound Classification

Clean wounds These are operative wounds in which no inflammation is encountered and the respiratory, alimentary, genital or uninfected urinary tract are not entered. This would include hernia repair, varicose vein operations, orthopaedic operations (not traumatic), and cardiac surgery (excluding leg vein incisions). Clean wounds have a 1–5% risk of infection (Cruse and Foord, 1980; Olson et al, 1984).
Clean-contaminated wounds These are operative wounds in which the respiratory, alimentary, genital or urinary tract are entered but without significant contamination. This would include hysterectomy, appendicectomy (without evidence of inflammation) and cholecystectomy. Clean-contaminated wounds have a 3–11% risk of infection (Cruse and Foord, 1980; Olson et al, 1984).
Contaminated wounds These are operation wounds where there has been gross spillage from the gastrointestinal tract, or where inflammation is encountered without evidence of frank pus. Recent traumatic wounds are also considered contaminated. Contaminated wounds have a 10–17% risk of infection (Cruse and Foord, 1980; Olson et al, 1984).
Dirty or infected wounds These include old traumatic wounds which contain devitalised or nectrotic tissue, and those that involve existing infection or perforated viscera. Dirty wounds have an infection rate over 27% (Cruse and Foord, 1980; Olson et al, 1984).
Being aware of the possible level of risk of infection after particular operations can help alert nurses to early identification of the problem.

Assessment of the wound state

Wounds without tissue loss

Wound edges (margins)

1. *Apposition*: A wound in which skin edges are brought into apposition usually heals quickly. Assessing the skin edges is useful in predicting the development of a potential scar. There should be even gathering of tissues with no gaps or spaces or lumps and bumps.
2. *Capillary fill*: To determine if blood supply to the area is adequate following pressure to the area the blanching should be followed by normal pigmentation in 4–5 seconds in healthy tissue. Slow or poor capillary filling may highlight future problems in wound healing, such as a prolonged healing time. This may be evident for diabetic patients.
3. *Colour*: Following wounding and for some days the inflammatory response will result in reddening of the immediate wound margins. Suture puncture areas may become increasingly more red the longer the suture remains in the skin. For about the first three days after wounding the redness will be accompanied by oedema and warmth (Westaby, 1981). Prolonged redness, increase in oedema, and warmth should alert observers to the possibility of reasons for delayed healing. This may include infection, haematoma or sutures in for too long.
4. *Discharge*: The normal inflammatory reaction with exudation or transudation of serum from dilated vessels contributes to oedema, cellular infiltration and swelling. Therefore some drainage is normal. Prolonged and heavy drainage or exudate from wounds is indicative of an irritating toxin, or perhaps bacteria. Its colour, amount and odour should be noted.
5. *Drains and sutures*: The presence of drains and sutures can predispose to infection (Cruse and Foord, 1980), so these should be removed at the earliest possible time.
6. *Pain*: Tissue injury is an adequate stimulus for pain, caused by the release of chemicals which may mediate pain. Pain should be assessed in relation to the time after wounding, and other accompanying indicators such as increased and prolonged inflammation. Local incisional pain should be differentiated from pain in other parts of the body.

Wounds with tissue loss

Wound measurement
Direct measurement of wound size is commonly used in wound assessment. Changes in size and shape may be interpreted as being the result of healing (Forrest and Gamborg-Nielsen, 1983). For clinical use one of two methods have been used:

1. Measurement with ruler or dividers, of one or more diameters of the wound: usually the length and breadth. It is essential that the skin is marked in such a way that measurements of the same axes are taken at each observation. It is also important that the same observer carry out the measurement on all occasions, so that inter-observer variability is limited (Anthony, 1985). The posture of the patient can also

influence wound size, and care should be taken to ensure that the patient is in the same position at each measurement.

2. Wound mapping is considered to be more reproducible than direct measurement but is subject to some of the difficulties associated with direct measurement (Forrester and Gamborg-Nielson, 1983; Anthony, 1985). This is carried out by making a tracing of the wound through some transparent medium such as a polythene bag. This can be compared visually with previous tracings to assess relative change, or can be placed over squared graph paper of known dimensions, and squares counted to give the value of the area. The same conditions for reproducibility in direct measurement apply to wound mapping. Change in the surface area of the wound is a useful reflection of healing or regression, and should be carried out at weekly intervals.

   Wound measurement of this type should be carried out on all wounds with tissue loss including venous and decubitus ulcers.

3. Wound casting may be used to make models of a wound that allow accurate measurement of its volume and visualisation of its shape (Pories et al, 1966). Silicone polymer foam can be used to make casts (Wood et al, 1977). This is an expensive practice, but if the wound is being treated with this material then saving the serial casts can allow for observing relative changes in shape and volume.

Wound base

Assessment of the base of the wound cavity should be carried out to identify the presence of necrotic or devitalised tissue. This may be adherent, or loose and partially adherent to the wound base. The presence and amount of slough and exudate should be noted. Production of exudate from a wound is normal and accompanies the inflammatory phase of healing. Some wounds produce copious slough which is a yellowish creamy colour, infected wounds with sloughing usually produce greenish slough with pus, and an offensive odour.

Most wounds with tissue loss are colonised by bacteria (Ryan, 1985). Caution should be used in interpreting wound swabs. Infected wounds will usually display erythema and swelling of the wound margins extending in excess of 1 cm (Siddall, 1983). Accurate wound assessment is necessary for accurate diagnosis of wound progress and complications. Wound measurements should be recorded at weekly intervals, but other parameters should be assessed at dressing change. Several assessment tools have been described in the literature (Morison, 1987a; Ziegler Cuzzell, 1986; Jaber, 1986). Their use could make wound assessment and management more precise and systematic. A holistic assessment taking account of the patient's physical state, presence of conditions and therapies which impair healing, environmental factors, and local wound condition, will enable identification of causes and contributing factors for delayed wound healing in individual patients. Two wound diagnostic categories have been defined: delayed healing because of infection, and delayed healing because the wound contains necrotic or sloughing material.

Table 3. Diagnosis of Wound Problems: Incisional Wound

Criteria	Identification of different causes of delayed wound healing
Endogenous—Incisional Wound	Findings and Measures
	Tool: wound classification: Potential risk for wound infection according to type of surgery: Gastric, gall bladder, gynaecological surgery—medium risk. Colon surgery—high risk.
State of wound	Tool: wound assessment
Wound edges	Red, warm swollen along the length of the incision, prolonged inflammation. Approximation at risk.
Discharge	Discoloured, green, brown, bloodstained leaking out of suture line.
Pain	Tender, painful.
Sutures	If present, may be red around suture area, but this is not indicative of infection.
Drains	Drain holes may be adjacent to the incision.
Culture	There may be a heavy growth of organisms, but this is not necessary before diagnosis is made.
Endogenous—Patient Physical state	Tool: nutritional assessment Anorexic Loss of weight Feels unwell May be obese Temperature elevated On intravenous fluids only
Associated conditions	Diabetes may be present with erratic control
Associated therapies	Radiation—wound acquired more than six weeks after treatment Cytotoxic—neutropenia. Chemotherapy.
Exogenous—Environment	Lengthy pre-operative hospitalisation Standard pre-operative skin preparation
Diagnosis: delayed wound healing related to infection	

GOALS/OUTCOMES

In general, the expected outcome for wounds with delayed healing, irrespective of aetiology, is a healed wound with intact skin. In chronic wounds such as venous or pressure ulcers, or traumatic wounds such as open fractures, healing will be slow and protracted with both regression and progression throughout the healing process. Short-term goals will depend upon the state of the wound, for example infection eliminated, or necrotic or sloughing tissue removed. In some circumstances goals may not include healing, but will relate to needs of comfort and aesthetics such as odour reduction. This may include fungating wounds of breast cancer in a terminally ill patient.

Table 4. Diagnosis of Wound Problems: Open Wound

Criteria	Identification of different causes of delayed wound healing
Endogenous—Open Wound	*Findings and Measures*
State of wound:	Tool: wound assessment (Morison, 1987a; Jaber, 1986)
Surface area	Static or increasing (by tracing/measuring)
Depth	Static or increasing
Base	Presence of pus, slough, or necrotic tissue
Edges	Tender, red, warm. Cellulitis present
Pain	Present all the time
Culture	May have a heavy growth of organisms, but this is not necessary for diagnosis. Beta-haemolytic streptococci are of note. Malodour
Endogenous—Patient	
Physical state	Tool: nutritional assessment
	The following may be relevant:
	Weight loss
	Reduction in muscle mass
	Anorexia
	Fasting
	Temperature elevation
Associated conditions	May or may not be diabetic. Blood sugars may be unstable indicating erratic control
Exogenous—Environment	Lengthy period of hospitalisation
	Proximity of infected patient
Diagnosis: delayed healing related to infection	

RATIONALE AND INTERVENTIONS

Nutrition

Many patients experience lengthy periods of illness before admission which may cause malabsorption or dietary restriction resulting in nutritional depletion and weight loss. In some cases periods of nausea, vomiting, or diarrhoea may also have contributed to a decline in nutritional status. Patients at risk may include those with large bowel and rectal cancer, patients with ulcerative colitis or Crohn's disease, or indeed any patient with gastrointestinal problems. In addition patients are being subjected to numerous diagnostic tests which require them to fast or take only clear liquids. If the patient is admitted in less than optimal nutritional state then this type of investigation can only compound the problem. The exact relationship between protein calorie malnutrition and susceptibility to infection is still unclear. However, experimental research provides some evidence that malnutrition induces defects in specific and non-specific host resistance which renders the malnourished patient more susceptible to infection (Kahan, 1981). Studley (1936) found that in patients having operations for peptic ulcer, there

Table 5. Diagnosis of Wound Problems: Open Leg Wound

Criteria	*Identification of different causes of delayed wound healing*
Endogenous—Open Wound Type of wound:	*Findings and Measures* Tool: leg ulcer assessment (Dale and Gibson, 1986) to aid diagnosis of ulcer aetiology
State of wound:	Tool: wound assessment (Morison, 1987a, Jaber, 1986)
Surface area	Static or increasing
Depth	Static or increasing
Base	Blackened eschar or yellow slough
Edges	May or may not be tender or red
Culture	Wound colonised by organisms but usually insignificantly
Exudate	Varying degrees
Endogenous—Patient Physical state	Tool: nutritional assessment, dietary history Inadequate nourishment Weight: normal, obese, underweight Hydration may be inadequate Temperature normal Oedema of legs
Pain	Rule out arterial ulcer of leg
Associated conditions	Diabetes may be present
Exogenous—Environment	Frequent changes of topical applications and dressings Uncertainty as to appropriate treatment
Depending on the type of open wound:	Unrelieved pressure on the wound Inappropriate position of the limb
Diagnosis: delayed wound healing related to presence of either necrotic or sloughing tissue	

was a 33% mortality rate in those with a pre-operative weight loss of more than 20% body weight, compared with the 3.5% mortality rate in those with better nutritional status. Many of these fatalities were attributable to infection. Rhoads and Alexander (1955) reported increased incidence of post-operative infection in patients with hypoproteinaemia. Chandra (1983) reported an infection rate of 23.5% in malnourished patients following major surgery compared with 5.6% for well-nourished patients. Although infections may be more common and have more serious consequences in the malnourished patient, it is important to recognise that infection can precipitate negative nitrogen balance (Beisel, 1977), and can convert a borderline nutritional status into one of malnutrition.

However, nutritional defects and depletion can also have a marked effect on rate and quality of the healing process, especially in wounds with tissue loss. Experimental research has documented that protein deficiency can result in prolonging the inflammatory phase of healing and lead to reduced fibroblast proliferation and collagen synthesis. Adequate carbohydrates and fats are needed to supply energy for successful white cell activity including phagocytosis and intracellular killing of bacteria (Ruberg, 1984).

Minerals such as zinc have a major role as cofactors in a variety of enzyme systems responsible for cell proliferation. Proliferation of cells is essential for wound healing.

For example adequate numbers of inflammatory cells are needed during the inflammatory stage, and multiplication of fibroblasts is essential for synthesis of sufficient amounts of collagen (Ruberg, 1984).

Zinc deficiency impairs healing, and restoration of levels to normal can restore the healing process to normal (Chvapil, 1980). Vitamin C has a dominant role in wound healing being an essential cofactor in collagen synthesis (Ruberg, 1984).

Malnutrition will not be recognised unless it is looked for. Assessment has been discussed, and intervention will depend on the findings. Doubtless this will involve other professionals including dietitian and doctor, and the dietitian will usually be responsible for setting the level of nutritional requirements for the patient. Holmes (1986) proposes several indicators for nutritional support, including patients who:

1. show a loss of 10% or more of usual body weight;
2. a lymphocyte count less than 1200/mm³;
3. a serum albumin less than 30 g/l;
4. show muscle wasting;
5. report impaired nutritional intake for one week or more;
6. after surgery have had more than five days inadequate feeding; and
7. pre-operatively have had fluid or foods restricted.

When possible, normal oral feeding is the method of choice (Dickerson, 1986). Weak and anorexic patients should be encouraged to drink a supplementary enteral diet. Three packets of Build-up (Carnation), each mixed with 300 ml of milk, will provide an extra 1000 Kcals and additional protein. Some patients may have neither the motivation nor strength to carry out these interventions and in this case use of a fine bore soft feeding tube can be used to supplement what the patient is taking normally.

The research that identifies the effects of malnutrition on healing and infection is evidence that vigorous support for malnourished patients will reduce the risk of wound complications such as infection and prolonged healing. An awareness of these facts should alert nurses to possible complications, and enable them to request early specialist dietary advice for such patients, so maximising their response to treatment.

Patients with open wounds also have a need for increased nutritional support. Wounds such as venous and pressure ulcers can lose large amounts of exudate high in protein content. Such wounds are also commonly colonised with bacteria causing an increased catabolic state in the patient.

Indications for nutritional support would include:

1. wounds with medium to high exudate,
2. wounds with severe infection,
3. draining fistulas.

Pre-operative preparation to reduce risk of infection

If patients are to be shaved before operation this should be done as near to the time of operation as possible, just before anaesthetic is optimum. Studies have shown that shaving 18–24 hours before operation increases the rate of post-operative infection (Seropian and Reynolds, 1971; Court-Brown, 1981; Alexander et al, 1983). This is probably related to the damage to the skin, both microscopic and macroscopic, which is evident after a razor shave (Hamiliton et al, 1977). Lowest infection rates are evident if hair is left intact (Cruse and Foord, 1973), but the use of a depilatory cream will produce lower rates than for shaving (Court-Brown, 1981). The superiority of no shave, or depilatory cream in reducing risk of post-operative infection is most evident in clean or clean-contaminated operations where the patient's own skin flora are most frequently implicated in post-operative wound infections (Nichols, 1981).

Pre-operative bathing or showering

Pre-operative bathing is a routine procedure usually carried out on surgical patients. Research indicates that total body washing with non-medicated soap shows an increase in the numbers of viable bacteria (Brandberg and Anderson, 1980). However the use of an antiseptic solution has been shown to reduce superficial skin bacteria (Nielsen et al, 1975). However, there is some indication that one bath or shower with chlorhexidene is insufficient to reduce post-operative wound infection (Ayliffe et al, 1983). Brandberg and Anderson (1980) showed that three showers, one on the morning of the pre-operative day, one the night of the pre-operative evening, and one on the day of the operation, reduced the infection rates in groin wounds from 17.5% to 8% (p<0.05).

Wound management

Many surgical wounds closed primarily will not require dressing. Forty-eight hours following closure of the wound, epithelialisation will have resulted in sealing the edges of the incision. Exceptions to this would include patients who have had surgery later than six weeks after radiotherapy (Krizek, 1979), where a compromised local wound circulation can predispose the patient to suture line failure and infection. Other at-risk patients are those compromised by cytotoxic chemotherapy, or steroid therapy (Kottra, 1982). With appropriate identification of high risk patients and an understanding of the effects of these therapies on wound healing, nurses can intervene by ensuring adequate nutrition, and using meticulous wound care.

Obesity affects the wound both directly and indirectly. Obese patients may hypoventilate because the thick chest wall and abdominal adiposity restrict the descent of the diaphragm. Shallow respiration means inhalation of smaller lung volumes. Vaughan et al (1976, 1974) found that obese patients were hypoxaemic before and during surgery. These alterations in physiology mean that pre-operative interventions in the form of breathing exercises should be given priority. Techniques that promote expectoration of secretions but do not create excessive wound tension should be taught. For example extending the tongue when coughing, and splinting the abdomen (Schumann, 1979). A double cough has also been found to be more effective than a single cough, the first clears the major airways, and the second clears the smaller channels (Macklem, 1973). Inappropriate encouragement of vigorous inefficient coughing can impair wound healing by causing an increase in intrathoracic pressure and undue stress on the abdominal wall.

Prevention of respiratory complications is important in satisfactory oxygenation for collagen formulation at the wound edges.

Vomiting also increases intra-abdominal pressure producing stretching of the local musculature and inhibiting migration of epithelial cells to the wound edges for reunion (Groszek, 1982). Interventions would include positioning of the patient for adequate gastric drainage, withholding oral fluid, and the use of appropriate anti-emetics.

Although these factors and interventions are crucial for obese and very obese patients, they are also important for all patients with incisional wounds, particularly of the abdomen.

Pain control as a factor in wound healing is a complex phenomenon. With the stress of pain a series of metabolic events are initiated that end in the production of cortisol, a hormone implicated in delayed wound healing (Cooper and Schuman, 1979). Because of the characteristics and extent of surgical procedures today, post-operative patients may be in an unsuitable condition for decision making with respect to pain control. Pain has haemodynamic outcomes that can lead to blood pressure instability, increased heart rate and metabolic activity which are detrimental to recovery and wound repair. Meticulous, adequate pain control by nurses can result in stabilising vital signs and help to make patients willing to participate in post-operative breathing and circulatory exercises, including ambulation.

Local wound management

The optimum environment for wound healing has been described as allowing for maximum enzymatic and cellular activity, cell migration, granulation, proliferation of endothelial cells and epithelialisation (Turner, 1983). Local conditions at the wound site which delay healing are numerous.

Oxygen and blood supply to the wound

Decreased circulation around a wound site may be a direct result of surgery (sutures which are too tight, damage to blood vessels), or may be a secondary effect (vasoconstriction, shock, haemorrhage). Hypovolaemia causes underperfusion of the edges of the wound, which may lead to underperfusion of the wound for several days after restoration of blood volume (Silver, 1980). This seriously impairs the healing process. Monitoring of vital signs and wound state following surgery will help to identify this problem promptly, and should lead to rapid correction of fluid state. Hypoxia can influence many aspects of wound healing including collagen formation, leucocyte activity, and new vessel formation (Ninikoski, 1977). Wounds in ischaemic tissues become infected more frequently than wounds in well-vascularised tissues (Hunt et al, 1975). In addition, the presence of aerobic bacteria in the wound consuming high levels of oxygen, can cause a large fall in the wound's oxygen tension (Torrance, 1986). Management includes the removal of devitalised tissue by debridement, and prevention or alleviation of infection in wounds. Increasing the oxygen supply to the tissues causes only a small rise in oxygen tension at the wound site (Hunt et al, 1969), and in addition can result in peripheral vasoconstriction owing to the direct effect of high oxygen tension on capillary vessels (Silver, 1980). Blowing oxygen on the wound will dry and cool the wound retarding epithelialisation (Winter, 1971), and delaying the healing process.

Wound temperature

A fall in the wound temperature can delay the healing process by retarding cell division (Lock, 1980) and reducing leucocyte function to zero (Lawrence, 1982). The recovery of these processes once the wound returns to body core temperature takes several hours. A ritualistic dressing practice which takes time to perform, and the over-use of cold topical applications to the wound are contributing factors, which are easily rectified.

Necrotic tissue and sloughing at wound site

The presence of necrotic tissue such as a blackened eschar in a pressure sore, or necrotic debris, dead cells and bacteria in the wound, delays healing and promotes infection (Haury et al, 1980). Necrotic tissue acts as a culture medium promoting bacterial growth, and in addition inhibits leucocyte phagocytosis of bacteria and subsequent intracellular killing. If there is blackened necrotic tissue present then debridement is the intervention of choice. The most rapid method of debridement is by surgical removal, and this may be appropriate for some patients. For example, to get a patient with a necrotic pressure sore mobile and well quickly, surgical debridement would be the method of choice. Debridement may also be carried out with enzymatic preparations such as Varidase (Lederle). It can be injected under dried eschar or applied on the surface of the scab which has been scored with a sterile scalpel. Dressings need to be applied once or twice a day (Morgan, 1987). Auto-debridement should be considered as an alternative to the use of chemicals. Wound macrophages are the primary agents which break down dead tissue and cells (Silver, 1985). Wound fluid has also been found to have potent antibacterial properties against bacteria such as *Staphylococcus aureus* and *Escherichia coli* (Hohn et al, 1977). A suitable environment for auto-debridement can be provided by a hydrocolloid dressing such as Granuflex (Squibb Surgicare). Maintenance of the wound cavity should allow for the wound fluid and its constituents such as macrophages and proteolytic enzymes to operate at their optimum physiological level, whilst preventing the collection in the wound cavity of excessive exudate. This type of dressing can provide this environment (Turner, 1985; Mani et al, 1985). It should be noted that the process of auto-debridement may cause an ulcer to appear to become larger before granulation tissue starts to form (Leaper, 1986a). There is still evidence that the use of hypochlorite agents for the purpose of debridement and cleansing is still prevalent (Anthony, 1987). According to Brennan and Leaper (1985) the effects of hypochlorite solutions on healing tissues may be sufficiently toxic to preclude their clinical value. Experimental research by these workers has found that Eusol caused blood flow in capillaries to stop, production of collagen to be delayed, and the inflammatory response to be delayed in wounds healing by secondary intention. There is now sufficient evidence to deter use of this agent (Morgan, 1987) and sufficient alternatives with which to replace it.

Wounds with heavy slough and exudate

Management of wounds with slough and exudate should aim to maintain a moist healing environment whilst removing excess exudate from the wound surface. Research by Winter (1971) and Hinman et al (1963), demonstrated that wounds kept moist show more rapid epithelialisation than wounds allowed to dry. A balance needs to be maintained between presence of wound fluid containing active macrophages, enzymes, and other chemotactic factors, and exudate containing dead cells, bacteria, and other debris which will retard cleansing and subsequent promotion of granulation tissue. This decision must be made by the nurse examining the type and quantity of exudate, and providing a dressing that satisfies the local wound conditions. Absorbent dressings such as hydrogels and hydrocolloids are suitable for wounds with moderate exudate. A polymeric bead dressing such as Debrisan (Pharmacia) is suitable for heavily exudative and infected wounds with tissue loss (Johnson, 1986). Some research indicates that bacteria from wounds can be cleansed in a matter of one or two days by the use of Debrisan (Chambers, 1984).

Wound dressings

No one dressing is suitable for all wounds (Turner, 1983), and it is obvious that the state of the wound, for example the need for debridement or desloughing, or presence of infection, or presence of healthy granulation tissue, will determine the use of a particular dressing at a particular time in the healing process. An expansion in the number of products available for wound management (Morrison, 1987a) has been preceded by lengthy research which resulted in the performance parameters necessary for a dressing to maintain a suitable wound environment during the various stages of healing (Turner, 1986). For a dressing to provide the optimum environment for healing it should:

1. Remove exudate and toxic components. This factor has been discussed previously. The ideal dressing should have absorption properties relative to the amount of exudate present. The presence in the wound of large numbers of dead cells and bacteria can retard healing. The dressing also needs to be absorbent enough to prevent 'strike-through' of the exudate to the upper surface of the dressing. Owens (1943) demonstrated that bacteria could pass through 64 thicknesses of gauze. Cotton wool, tulle gras as well as gauze show 'strike-through' of exudates (Morgan, 1987). Absorbent products with low strike-through properties are shown in Table 6.

Table 6. Absorbent Products with Low Strike-through Properties

Product	Manufacturer
Actisorb Plus	Johnson and Johnson
Debrisan	Pharmacia
Granuflex	Squibb Surgicare
Iodosorb	Stuart Pharmaceuticals
Lyofoam	Ultra Laboratories
Melolin	Smith and Nephew
Scherisorb	Smith and Nephew
Silastic Foam	Dow Corning
Sorbsan	Steriseal Ltd

2. Maintain high humidity at wound/dressing interface. There should be a delicate balance between humidity and absorption (Turner, 1983). A high humidity will

encourage granulation and assist epithelialisation (Winter, 1971; Turner, 1983). Traditional dressings such as gauze and lint do not restrict the evaporation of water from the wound and a scab is formed (Winter, 1971). A semi-occlusive dressing such as semi-permeable film (for example, Opsite, Smith-Nephew) allows fluid to be lost by water vapour transmission but maintains a moist wound interface (Morgan, 1987).

3. Allow for gaseous exchange of oxygen, carbon dioxide and water vapour. The importance of oxygen to the healing process has been discussed previously. Hydrocolloids are impermeable occlusive dressings (for example, Granuflex). They appear to stimulate angiogenesis by maintaining wound hypoxia (Cherry and Ryan, 1985). Therefore there is some controversy as to the precise role of oxygen levels and gradients in healing wounds.

4. To provide thermal insulation. This parameter has been previously discussed. By preventing evaporation of exudate, dressings protect the wound bed from cooling and provide optimum temperature for cellular activity.

5. To be impermeable to micro-organisms. The impermeability of the dressing to bacteria is important in preventing airborne organisms from contaminating a clean wound, resulting in infection, and in preventing bacteria from the wound passing into the environment and infecting others. The 'strike-through' properties of the dressing are important in this respect.

   The use of occlusive or semi-occlusive dressings has produced fear of increased wound infection. Several research studies have indicated that this is not a problem, and that bacteria present in venous leg ulcers treated with occlusive dressings, did not influence significantly the healing process (Easmon, 1985; Eriksson, 1985).

6. To be free from particulate contaminants. According to Lawrence (1982) dressings such as cotton wool and gauze are unlikely to have toxic effects on the wound. The hydrocolloids release polysaccharides in a gel form to the cell interface, and the release of monomers subsequent to biodegradation is a possibility (Turner, 1986). These advantages or disadvantages to the healing process are undergoing consideration. Products which separate into the wound usually require irrigation when the dressing is changed.

7. To allow removal without trauma at dressing change. Secondary trauma is often caused by dressings adhering to the wound surface which, when removed forcibly, can induce an inflammatory response and delay healing (Turner, 1983). Dry exudate which glues the dressing to the wound is often responsible (Scales and Winter, 1961). Dressings are often removed unnecessarily from wounds. If there are no indications such as pain, exudate or discharge it may be more sensible to leave the dressing in place until keratinisation of new epithelium allows it to fall away (Lawrence, 1982).

   Little practical information about the adherence of dressings is available. Gentle (1970) compared tulle gras, dry gauze, and a perforated plastic film dressing for adhesion to minor wounds, and found adhesion was less with plastic films (e.g. Melolin). Winter (1965) showed that perforated plastic film dressings adhered at the site of perforation. Perforated film dressings are most appropriate for light exuding wounds, and need to be covered with a secondary dressing (Morgan, 1987).

In addition to these seven performance parameters proposed by Turner (1986), Morgan (1987) proposes a further 13, including:

1. to be safe to use,
2. acceptable to the patient,
3. cost-effective,
4. carrier for medicaments,
5. to be capable of standardisation and evaluation,
6. to allow monitoring of the wound,
7. to provide mechanical protection,
8. to have properties which remain constant,
9. to be non-inflammable,
10. to be sterilisable,
11. to be conformable,
12. to be available, and
13. to be changed infrequently. A study by Williams et al (1985) showed that frequent dressing changes adversely affected the rate of wound healing in experimental deep wounds.

There is at present no ideal dressing, because no dressing has all the ideal characteristics, but with the availability of a wide variety of wound dressings, it should be possible to select the right dressing for nearly every situation. Product formularies are available (Morgan, 1987; Morrison, 1987a), and should be readily accessible for nurses involved with wound management. Without such information it is impossible for nurses to treat wounds with appropriate products.

Wound cleansing and topical applications

It seems apparent that for a large number of wounds, cleaning is inappropriate and may be detrimental (Leaper, 1986a). Brennan and Leaper (1985) demonstrated that most antiseptic agents exert some effect on the local wound micro-environment, and in some cases this will retard healing. Chlorhexidine does not appear to delay healing nor does it prolong the inflammatory response, but should be kept for the topical treatment of heavily infected chronic ulcers (Leaper, 1986a). Normal saline has no apparently adverse effects on healing, and as ward dressing changes do not probably give enough time for antiseptics to work (Ayliffe et al, 1982), the use of normal saline for removing debris and particulate food sources for bacteria would seem to be satisfactory. The appropriateness of cleaning a wound should be considered at every occasion it is proposed. Incisional wounds without indications of infection or exudate should not need disturbing. Research already referred to (Easmon, 1985; Eriksson, 1985) with occlusive dressing used for treating ulcers has shown that surface colonisation of healthy granulation tissue by saprophytes and even some pathogens (including *Staphylococcus aureus*) has little effect on the healing process.

In addition the wound exudate over healthy granulation tissue is antimicrobial and contains many substances which aid the healing process, and disturbing this and the delicate granulation tissue for unnecessary cleansing, can delay wound healing (Leaper, 1986b). The toxic effects of hypochlorite solutions such as Eusol on the wound and surrounding intact tissues have previously been described, their use as cleansing agents is to be deprecated (Leaper, 1986a). The importance of aseptic wound dressing management is emphasised during nurse training and beyond and it is reasonable to expect that careless and inadequate handling may lead to infection and so to delayed wound healing. However, research on occlusive dressings (Ryan, 1985) is leading to the conclusion that wounds and ulcers healing by secondary intention may be dressed by a clean technique alone. On the one hand they are colonised by saprophytes and some pathogens which do not appear to detract from healing, and on the other hand there is evidence that the wound exudate is the host defence mechanism (Leaper and Stewart, 1986). Scrupulous handwashing technique is the single most important procedure for preventing spread of infection (Garner and Farero, 1985), and is especially relevant to the management of open wounds colonised with bacteria.

Additional interventions for specific wounds

Venous ulcers

Chronic ulcers of the leg invariably have adverse factors which delay healing. For example venous ulcers at the ankle rarely heal without adequate compression therapy to aid the failing calf pump (Leaper, 1986a).

Interventions should follow assessment of the ulcer to distinguish between venous ulcers, and those in which ischaemia is involved (Dale and Gibson, 1986; Cherry and Ryan, 1987). Treating ischaemic ulcers with compression bandaging is contraindicated whereas one of the main components in the management of venous ulcers in ambulant patients is compression therapy (Cherry and Ryan, 1987). Venous ulcers cannot be healed by dressings alone, without at the same time correcting the abnormally high blood pressure in the superficial veins of the lower leg (Dale and Gibson, 1987), caused by incompetent valves in the deep and perforating veins of the leg. The pathological process resulting in venous ulceration has been reviewed by Browse and Burnand (1982). Compression improves the function of the calf muscle pump and reduces venous hypertension (Cherry and Ryan, 1987). The exact pressure needed to provide good compression therapy is controversial. Shull et al (1979) found that in limbs with ambulatory venous pressures greater than 60 mmHg the incidence of ulceration was 60%, dropping to 26% with pressures of 40–60 mmHg, and with pressures below 40 mmHg ulceration was absent. Therefore pressures of 20–30 mmHg at the ankle graduating to the knee by about 50% should be adequate. The bandage should provide adequate support without compromising blood supply, so should therefore be applied when the leg is at its least oedematous in the early morning or after a period of elevation. The technique of applying bandages with graduated compression is a skilled one, and it is imperative that the operator is aware of its rationale and is skilled in its application (Dale and Gibson, 1987). Healing rate of venous ulcers can be increased by elevation of the legs above the level of the heart so improving the return of blood from the leg. This may be contraindicated in patients with decompensated heart failure.

Although bacteria in leg ulcers have not been shown to adversely affect healing, signs of gross infection such as cellulitis with pain, tenderness, and inflammation, will usually require treatment with appropriate systemic antibiotics (Cherry and Ryan, 1987).

Pressure sores

Sacral sores, or sores in dependent areas are unlikely to heal without attention to pressure relief. Nutritional state is also important, and has been previously discussed. If the patient cannot move independently then consideration should be given to relief systems such as Clinitron Air Fluidized Bed and Mediscus Air Support Bed, which both provide low pressure, decrease shear and prevent moisture build-up (Fowler, 1987).

IMPLICATIONS FOR PRACTICE

Nurses as managers of wound care

It is increasingly evident that wound management has become and will continue to be a complex process. New wound management products become available daily, and the selection of the appropriate product for a particular wound has to be based on a knowledge of the healing process, and the characteristics of the product. There is evidence that nurses are continuing to treat wounds with inappropriate and possibly toxic agents (Anthony, 1987) despite the growing body of research that indicates the damage that may be being caused by such practices.

The process of wound management and healing cannot be treated wholly in relation to the state of the wound itself, but must encompass other factors such as nutrition, and other states and diseases which have important consequences for wound healing. Research indicates that nutrition probably plays a crucial role in the healing process, but inadequate training in nutrition received by doctors and nurses (Dickerson, 1986) resulting in lack of awareness of the implications of malnourishment, leaves patients at a disadvantage.

With the increasing complexities of wound management in view, it is appropriate for some nurses to become expert specialists in the field, acting as consultants and a resource and undertaking relevant research.

FUTURE RESEARCH

1. Studies to standardise and validate wound assessment parameters and methods.
2. Clinical product evaluation studies.
3. Evaluative studies on the effect of more systematic wound management education for nurses.
4. Evaluative studies of the effects of specialist wound care nurses on wound management practices and outcomes.
5. Comparative studies in the use of aseptic and clean techniques in the care of colonised open wounds.
6. Studies to develop less complicated aseptic dressing procedures, and evaluate them.

REFERENCES

Alexander JW, Fischer JE, Boyajian M, Palmquist J, Morris MJ (1983) The influences of hair removal methods on wound infection. *Archives of Surgery* 118, 347–352.

Anthony D (1985) Measuring pressure sores. *Nursing Times* **May 29**, 57–61.

Anthony D (1987) Are you in the dark? *Nursing Times* 83(34), 24–26.

Ayliffe GAJ, Noy MF, Babb JR, Davies JG, Jackson J (1983) A comparison of pre-operative bathing with chlorhexidine detergent and non-medicated soap in the prevention of wound infection. *Journal of Hospital Infection* 4, 237–244.

Ayliffe GAJ, Collins BJ, Taylor LJ (1982) *Hospital Acquired Infection. Principles and Prevention.* Wright, PSG, Bristol.

Beisel WR (1977) Magnitude of the host nutritional responses to infection. *American Journal of Clinical Nutrition* 30, 1236–1247.

Bistrian BR, Blackburn GL, Hallowell E, Heddle R (1974) Protein status of general surgical patients. *Journal of American Medical Association* 230, 858–860.

Bloomer WD, Hellman S (1975) Normal tissue responses to radiation therapy. *New England Journal of Medicine* 293, 80–83.

Brandberg A, Anderson I (1980) Whole body disinfection by shower bath with chlorhexidine soap. In: *Problems in the Control of Hospital Infection.* Royal Society of Medicine International Congress and Symposium Series 23, 65–70. Academic Press and RSM, London.

Brennan SS, Leaper DJ (1985) The effect of antiseptics on the healing wound: a study using the rabbit ear chamber. *British Journal of Surgery* 72, 780–782.

Browse NL, Burnand KG (1982) The cause of venous ulceration. *Lancet* i, 243–245.

Butterworth GE, Blackburn GL (1975) Hospital malnutrition and how to assess the nutritional status of a patient. *Nutrition Today* 10, 8–18.

Caldwell MD, Kennedy-Caldwell C (1981) Normal Nutritional Requirements. *Surgical Clinics of North America* 61(3), 489–507.

Carrico TJ, Mehrhof AI, Cohen K (1984) Biology of wound healing. *Surgical Clinics of North America* 64(4), 721–733.

Chambers A (1984) Microbiological studies on Debrisan, a wound healing agent. Unpublished, on file. *Pharmacia.*

Chandra RK (1983) Nutrition, immunity and infection: present knowledge and future directions. *Lancet* i, 688–691.

Cherry GW, Ryan TJ (1987) *Blueprint for the treatment of leg ulcers and the prevention of neuresence.* Squibb Surgicare, Hounslow.

Cherry GW, Ryan TJ (1985) Enhanced wound angiogenesis with a new hydrocolloid dressing. In: Ryan TJ (ed) *An Environment for Healing: the Role of Occlusion.* Royal Society of Medicine, London.

Chvapil M (1980) Zinc and other factors of the pharmacology of wound healing. In: Hunt TK (ed) *Wound Healing and Wound Infection.* Appleton Century Crofts, New York.

Chvapil M, Koopman CF (1982) Age and other factors regulating wound healing. *Otolaryngologic Clinics of North America* 15(2), 259–270.

Clark MO, Barbenel JC, Jordan HM, Nicol SM (1978) Pressure sores. *Nursing Times* **Mar 2**, 363–366.

Cooper DM, Schumann D (1979) Post-surgical nursing intervention as an adjunct to wound healing. *Nursing Clinics of North America* 11(4), 713–725.

Cornwall JV, Lewis JD (1983) Leg ulcers revisited. *British Journal of Surgery* 10, 681–683.

Court-Brown CM (1981) Pre-operative skin depilation and its effect on post-operative wound infection. *Journal of the Royal College of Surgeons of Edinburgh* 26(4), 238–241.

Cruse PJE, Foord R (1980) The epidemiology of wound infection. *Surgical Clinics of North America* 60(1), 27–40.

Cruse PJE, Foord R (1973) A prospective study of 23,649 surgical wounds. *Archives of Surgery* 107, 206–208.

Dale JJ, Callan MJ, Ruckley CV, Harper DR, Berry PN (1983) Chronic ulcers of the leg: a study of prevalence in a Scottish community. *Health Bulletin* (Edinburgh) 41, 310–314.

Dale J, Gibson B (1986) Leg ulcers: the nursing assessment. *Professional Nurse* **June**, 236–238.

Dale J, Gibson B (1987) Compression bandages for various ulcers. *Professional Nurse* **Apr**, 211–214.

David J (1983) *An Investigation of the Current Methods Used in Nursing for the Care of Patients with Established Pressure Sores*. Nursing Practice Research Unit, Northwick Park Hospital and Clinical Research Centre, Harrow.

Detsky AS (1984) Evaluating the accuracy of nutritional assessment techniques. *Journal of Parenteral and Enteral Nutrition* **8**(2), 153.

Dickerson JWT (1986) Hospital induced malnutrition: prevention and treatment. *Professional Nurse* **Sept**, 314–316.

Dirksen PK, Matolo NM, Trelford JD (1977) Complications following operation in the previously irradiated abdominopelvic cavity. *The American Surgeon* **Apr**, 234–241.

Easmon CSF (1985) Skin flora under chest dressings. In: Ryan TJ (ed) *An Environment for Healing: the Role of Occlusion*. Royal Society of Medicine, London.

Edlich RF, Rodeheaver O, Thacken JG (1979) Technical factors in wound management. In: Hunt TK, Dunphy JE (eds) *Fundamentals of Wound Management*. Appleton Century Crofts, New York.

Ehrlich HP, Hunt TK (1969) The effect of cortisone and anabolic steroids on the tensile strength of healing wounds. *Annals of Surgery* **170**, 203–206.

Eriksson G (1985) Bacterial growth in venous leg ulcers—its clinical significance in the healing process. In: Ryan TJ (ed) *An Environment for Healing: the Role of Occlusion*. Royal Society of Medicine, London.

Feigin RD, Shearer WT (1975) Opportunistic infections in children: II In the compromised host. *Journal of Paediatrics* **87**, 677.

Ferguson MK (1982) The effect of antineoplastic agents on wound healing. *Surgery Gynecology and Obstetrics* **154**, 421–429.

Finn D, Steele G, Osteen RJ, Wilson RE (1980) Morbidity and mortality after surgery in patients with disseminated or locally advanced cancer receiving systemic chemotherapy. *Journal of Surgery and Oncology* **13**, 237.

Forrest L (1983) Current concepts in soft connective tissue wound healing. *British Journal of Surgery* **70**, 133–140.

Forrest RD, Gamborg-Nielsen P (1983) Wound assessment in clinical practice. A critical review of methods and their application. *Acta Medica Scandinavica Suppl* **687**, 9–14.

Fowler EM (1987) Equipment and products used in management and treatment of pressure ulcers. *Nursing Clinics of North America* **22**(2), 449–461.

Garner J (1986) C D C Guidelines for prevention of surgical wound infections, 1985. *Infection Control* **7**(3), 193–200.

Garner J, Farero MS (1985) Guidelines for handwashing and hospital environmental control. *American Journal of Infection Control* **14**(3), 110–129.

Gentle M (1970) Melolin trial. *Nursing Mirror* **131**, 36.

Goodinson SM (1987) Assessment of nutritional status. *Professional Nurse* **Aug**, 367–369.

Goodinson SM (1987a) Biochemical assessment of nutritional status. *Professional Nurse* **Oct**, 8–12.

Goodinson SM (1987b) Anthropometric assessment of nutritional status. *Professional Nurse* **Sept**, 388–393.

Goodinson SM (1987c) Assessing nutritional status. Subjective methods. *Professional Nurse* **Nov**, 48–51.

Goodson WH, Radolf J, Hunt TK (1980) Wound healing and diabetes. In: Hunt TK (ed) *Wound Healing and Wound Infection*. Appleton Century Crofts, New York.

Groszek DM (1982) Promoting wound healing in the obese patient. *AORN Journal* **35**(6), 1138.

Haider M (1984) Assessment of protein-calorie malnutrition. *Clinical Chemistry* **30**, 1286.

Hamilton HW, Hamilton KR, Lone FJ (1977) Pre-operative hair removal. *Canadian Journal of Surgery* **20**(3), 269–275.

Haury B, Rodeheaver G, Vensko J, Edgerton MT, Edlich RF (1980) Debridement: an essential component of traumatic wound care. In: Hunt TK (ed) *Wound Healing and Wound Infection*. Appleton Century Crofts, New York.

Hinman CD, Maiback H, Winter JD (1963) Effect of air exposure and occlusion on experimental human skin wounds. *Nature* **200**, 377–379.

Hohn DC, Granelli SG, Burton RW, Hunt TK (1977) Antimicrobial systems of the surgical wound. *American Journal of Surgery* **133**, 601–606.

Holmes S (1986) Nutritional needs of surgical patients. *Nursing Times* **May 7**, 30–32.

Howard JM, Barker WF, Culbertson WR (1964) Post-operative wound infection: the influence of ultraviolet irradiation of the operating room and various other factors. *Annals of Surgery* **160**(Suppl), 1–192.

Hunt TK (1976) *Fundamentals of Wound Management in Surgery, Wound Healing, Disorders of Repair*. Chirurgeon Inc, South Plainfield.

Hunt TK, Knighton DR, Thakral KK (1984) Studies on inflammation and wound healing: angiogenesis and collagen synthesis stimulated in vivo by resident and activated wound macrophages. *Surgery* **96**, 48–52.

Hunt TK, Halliday B (1980) Inflammation in wounds. From Laudable Pus to Primary Repair and Beyond. In: Hunt TK (ed) *Wound Healing and Wound Infection*. Appleton Century Crofts, New York.

Hunt TK, Linsey M, Grislis G (1975) The effect of differing ambient oxygen tension on wound infection. *Annals of Surgery* **181**, 35–45.

Hunt TK, Zederfeldt B, Godstick TK (1969) Oxygen and healing. *American Journal of Surgery* **118**, 521.

Jaber F (1986) Charting wound healing. *Nursing Times* **Sept 10–16**, 24–27.

Johnson A (1986) Cleansing infected wounds. *Nursing Times* **Sept 10**, 30–34.

Kahan BD (1981) Nutrition and host defence mechanisms. *Surgical Clinics of North America* **61**(3), 557–571.

Kottra CJ (1982) Wound healing in the immunosuppressed host. *AORN Journal* **35**(6), 1142–1148.

Krizek TJ (1979) Difficult wounds: radiation wounds. *Clinics in Plastic Surgery* **6**, 541–543.

Lawrence JC (1982) What materials for dressing. *Injury* **13**, 500–512.

Leaper D (1986a) The wound healing process. In: Turner TD, Schmidt RJ, Harding KG (eds) *Advances in Wound Management*. John Wiley, Chichester.

Leaper D (1986b) Antiseptics and their effect on healing tissue. *Nursing Times* **May 28**, 45–47.

Leaper DJ, Stewart AJ (1986) A comparative trial of Scherisorb Gel and Cadexomner Iodine: Problems of community based trials involving chronic leg ulcers. In: Turner TD, Schmidt RJ, Harding KG (eds) *Advances in Wound Management*. John Wiley, Chichester.

Lock PM (1980) The effect of temperature on the healing of experimental burns. *Nordic Wound Healing Symposium*. Lindgren and Soner, Gothenburg.

Lowthian PT (1978) Pressure sore prevalence. *Nursing Times* **74**(9), 358.

Macklem P (1973) Relationship between lung mechanics and ventilation distribution. *Physiologist* **16**, 580–588.

Mani R, White JE, Creery J (1985) Transcutaneous measurement of oxygen and its significance in the healing of leg ulcers treated with oxygen impermeable dressing. In: Ryan TK (ed) *An Environment for Healing: the role of Occlusion*. Royal Society of Medicine, London.

Mason EE (1981) *Surgical Treatment of Obesity*. WB Saunders, Philadelphia.

Meers PD, Ayliffe GA, Emmerson AM, Leigh DA, Mayon-White R, Mackintosh CA, Stronge JL (1981) National hospital infection study. *Journal of Hospital Infection* **2**(Suppl) 1–11.

Morgan DA (1987) *The Care and Management of Leg Ulcers*. Available from DA Morgan, Pharmacy Department, Whitchurch Hospital, Cardiff.

Morgan D (1987a) *Formulary of Wound Management Products*. Available from DA Morgan, Pharmacy Department, Whitchurch Hospital, Cardiff.

Morrison MJ (1987a) Wound assessment. *Professional Nurse* **July**, 315–317.

Morrison MJ (1987b) Priorities in wound management: part 2. *Professional Nurse* **Sept**, 402–411.

Nichols RL (1981) Surgical bacteriology. *Surgery Annual* **13**, 205–238.

Nielsen ML, Raahave D, Stage J, Justesen T (1975) Anaerobic and aerobic skin bacteria before and after skin disinfection with chlorhexidine: an experimental study. *Journal of Clinical Pathology* **28**, 793–797.

Ninikoski J (1977) Oxygen and wound healing. *Clinics in Plastic Surgery* **4**, 361–368.

Olson M, O'Connor MD, Schwartz ML (1984) A five-year prospective study of 20,193 wounds at Minneapolis V A Medical Center. *Annals of Surgery* **199**, 253–259.

Owens W (1943) Use of pressure dressings in the treatment of burns and other wounds. *Surgical Clinics of North America* **23**, 1354.

Pories WJ, Schear EW, Jordan DR (1966) The measurement of human wound healing. *Surgery* **59**, 821–825.

Rhoads JE, Alexander CE (1955) Nutritional problems of surgical patients. *Annals of the New York Academy of Science* **63**, 268.

Ruberg RL (1984) Role of nutrition in wound healing. *Surgical Clinics of North America* **64**(4), 705–715.

Ryan TJ (ed) (1985) *An Environment for Healing: the Role of Occlusion*. Royal Society of Medicine, London.

Scales JT, Winter GD (1961) The adhesion of wound dressings: an experimental study. In: Slome D (ed) *Wound Healing*. Pergamon, Oxford.

Scales JT, Winter GB (1961) The adhesion of wound dressings: an experimental study. In: Slome D (ed) *Wound Healing*. Pergamon, Oxford.

Schumann D (1979) Pre-operative measures to promote wound healing. *Nursing Clinics of North America* **14**(4), 683–699.

Seropian R, Reynolds BM (1971) Wound infections after pre-operative depilatory versus razor preparation. *American Journal of Surgery* **121**, 251–254.

Shull KC, Nicolaides AN, Fernandes E (1979) Significance of popliteal reflux in relation to ambulatory venous pressure and ulceration. *Archives of Surgery* **114**, 1304–1306.

Siddall S (1983) Wound healing. An assessment tool. *Home Health Care Nurse* **Sept/Oct**, 35–41.

Silver IA (1985) Oxygen and tissue repair. In: Ryan TJ (ed) *An Environment for Healing: the Role of Occlusion*. Royal Society of Medicine, London.

Silver IA (1980) The physiology of wound healing. In: Hope TK (ed) *Wound Healing and Wound Infection*. Appleton Century Crofts, New York.

Stephens FV, Dunphy JE, Hunt TK (1971) The effect of delayed administration of corticosteroids on wound contraction. *Annals of Surgery* **173**, 21–217.

Studley HO (1936) Percentage of weight loss: a basic indication of surgical risk in patients with chronic ulcer. *Journal of American Medical Association* **106**, 458.

Tenorio A, Jindrak K, Weiner M, Bella E, Enquist IF (1976) Accelerated healing in infected wounds. *Surgery, Gynecology and Obstetrics* **142**, 537–543.

Torrance C (1986) The physiology of wound healing. *Nursing* **5**, 162–168.

Turner TD (1986) Hydrogels and hydrocolloids: an overview of the products and their properties. In: Turner TD, Schmidt RJ, Harding KG (eds) *Advances in Wound Management*. John Wiley, Chichester.

Turner TD (1985) Semi-occlusive and occlusive dressings. In: Ryan TK (ed) *An Environment for Healing: the Role of Occlusion*. Royal Society of Medicine, London.

Turner TD (1983) Absorbents and wound dressings. *Nursing Second Series Supplement* **12**, 1–7.

Vaughan R, Englehardt R, Wise L (1974) Post-operative hypoxaemia in obese patients. *Annals of Surgery* **150**, 877–882.

Vaughan R, Englehardt R, Wise L (1976) Intraoperative arterial oxygenations in obese patients. *Annals of Surgery* **184**(1), 35–42.

Westaby S (1985) (ed) *Wound Care*. William Heinemann Medical Books, London.

Westaby S (1981) Wound care healing: the normal mechanism 2. *Nursing Times* **Nov 25**(Supplement).

White H, Cook J, Ward M (1977) Abdominal wound dehiscence. A 10 year survey from a district general hospital. *Annals of the Royal College of Surgeons (Eng)* **59**, 337.

Williams DL, Dykes PJ, Marks R (1985) Effects of a new hydrocolloid dressing on healing of full thickness wounds in normal volunteers. In: Ryan TJ (ed) *An Environment for Healing: the Role of Occlusion*. Royal Society of Medicine, London.

Winter GD (1965) A note on wound healing under dressings with special reference to perforated film dressings. *Journal of Investigative Dermatology* **45**, 299.

Winter GD (1971) Healing of skin wounds and the influence of dressings on the repair process.

In: Harkiss KJ (ed) *Surgical Dressings and Wound Healing*, Bradford University Press and Crosby Lockwood and Sons, London.

Wood RAB, Williams RHP, Hughes LE (1977) Foam elastomer dressing in the management of granulating wounds: experience with 250 patients. *British Journal of Surgery* **64**, 554–558.

Ziegler Cuzzell J (1986) A realistic approach to wound documentation. *American Journal of Nursing* **5**, 600–601.

Chapter 12

Problems with Breathing

INTRODUCTION: THE PROCESS OF VENTILATION AND PERFUSION

Although many metabolic activities take place within the lungs, the respiratory system has two main tasks: ventilation or the movement of air in and out of the airways, and gas exchange or diffusion of oxygen and carbon dioxide into and out of alveolar capillaries (Rokosky, 1985).

Ventilation

Ventilation is the result of pressure changes transmitted from the thoracic cavity to the lungs. The respiratory muscles, activated either by voluntary effort or involuntarily by the brainstem, cause pulmonary ventilation by alternately compressing and distending the lungs, which in turn causes pressure in the alveoli to rise and fall (Guyton, 1981). Inspiration is initiated by contraction of the diaphragm and external intercostal muscles so that the thoracic cavity expands downwards and outwards. The pleural membrane joins the thoracic cavity and lungs, and as a result of this connection the decreased intrathoracic pressure from chest wall expansion is relayed to the intrapleural space and then to the lungs themselves. In response to the drop in alveolar pressure which becomes slightly less negative with respect to atmospheric pressure (normally less than -1 mmHg), air flows into the respiratory passages. During expiration the diaphragm relaxes and the elastic recoil of the lungs, chest wall, and abdominal structures, compress the lungs. During heavy breathing however the elastic forces are not powerful enough to cause rapid expiration, so this is achieved by contraction of the abdominal muscles which forces the abdominal contents upwards against the bottom of the diaphragm (Guyton, 1981).

As a result of several interacting forces the lungs have a continual elastic tendency to collapse and therefore to recoil away from the chest wall. The lung tissue contains many elastic fibres which are straightened by lung inflation and so attempt to shorten. Disruption of the rib-to-pleurae-to-lung relationship causes lung collapse (Rokosky, 1985). A more important factor is the surface tension of the fluid lining the alveoli. This also causes a continual elastic tendency for the alveoli to collapse. This surface tension is reduced by a lipoprotein mixture called surfactant, a detergent-like substance manufactured by alveolar cells.

Compliance

The expansibility of the lungs and thorax is referred to as compliance. This is expressed as the increase in volume that occurs for a given increase in alveolar pressure (Guyton, 1981). Compliance varies according to lung size, but on average every time alveolar pressure is increased by 1 cm water, the lungs expand 130 ml. So inspiration normally requires only a modest effort for a considerable gain in volume. Any condition that destroys lung tissue, causes it to become fibrotic or oedematous, blocks the bronchioles, or in any other way blocks expansion and contraction, causes decreased lung compliance. In addition, problems with expansion of the thoracic cage including deformities such as kyphosis and severe scoliosis; conditions such as paralysed and fibrotic muscles which restrain movement; and conditions which increase mass loading such as obesity, and ascites, can all reduce expansibility of the lungs and thereby reduce the total pulmonary compliance.

Elastance

This is the reverse of compliance and refers to the extent to which the lungs are able to recoil or return to their barely stretched position. During normal breathing respiratory muscle contraction occurs only during inspiration while expiration is an entirely passive process caused by elastic recoil of the lung and thoracic cage structures. Therefore the respiratory muscles normally perform work only to cause inspiration and not at all to cause expiration.

The work of breathing

In order to overcome various resistances and forces the respiratory muscles must perform work. As already mentioned this work is related to inspiration and can be divided into three parts (Guyton, 1981):

1. Compliance work, that required to overcome the elastic forces.
2. Tissue resistance work, that required to overcome the viscosity of the lung and chest wall structures.
3. Airway resistance work, that required to overcome airway resistance during the movement of air into the lungs. The major determinant of resistance is the radius of the airway. Normally resistance is low, so that minimal opposition to airflow occurs.

Physiological measurement shows that during normal quiet breathing most of the work performed by respiratory muscles is used to overcome elastic forces (compliance work); a small amount is used to overcome tissue resistance (Guyton, 1981). During very heavy breathing the greater proportion of the work is used to overcome airway resistance. In pulmonary disease all three types of work may be greatly increased. Compliance and tissue resistance work are especially increased by diseases that cause fibrosis or hardening of the lungs such as alveolar fibrosis and fluid filling of the alveoli. Airway resistance work is especially increased by diseases that obstruct the airway such as asthma, and chronic bronchitis. During normal quiet breathing consumption of oxygen for ventilation purposes accounts for only 2–3% of the total resting consumption of oxygen. However pulmonary disorders that decrease pulmonary compliance, increase airway resistance, or that increase viscosity of the lung or chest wall can at times increase the work of breathing so much that one-third or more of the total energy expended by the body is for breathing alone.

Gas exchange

Following ventilation of the alveoli with fresh air, the next step in the respiratory process is diffusion of oxygen from the alveoli into the pulmonary blood and diffusion of carbon dioxide from the pulmonary blood into the alveoli. Oxygen is continually being absorbed into the blood of the lungs, and new oxygen is continually entering the alveoli from the atmosphere. The more rapidly oxygen is absorbed, the lower becomes the concentration in the alveoli; and the more rapidly new oxygen is brought into the alveoli from the atmosphere the higher becomes its concentration. Therefore oxygen concentration in the alveoli, and its partial pressure as well, is controlled by the rate of absorption of oxygen into the blood, and rate of entry of new oxygen into the lungs by the ventilatory process. Carbon dioxide is continually being formed in the body then discharged into the alveoli from where it is continually removed by the process of ventilation. Therefore the two factors that determine alveolar concentration of carbon dioxide and its partial pressure are the rate of excretion of carbon dioxide from the blood into the alveoli, and the rate at which it is removed from the alveoli by alveolar ventilation.

Ventilation-perfusion ratio

It is the ratio of ventilation to pulmonary capillary blood flow, called the ventilation-perfusion ration (V/Q), that actually determines what the alveolar gas composition will be (Guyton, 1981). There is a normal mismatching of V/Q throughout the lung. Gravity or the weight of the lung causes the difference in ventilation. Differences in blood flow are related to the weight of the blood column or hydrostatic pressure. As there is a greater increase in perfusion than ventilation down the lung, the ratio of ventilation to perfusion decreases from the upper to the lower parts of the lung (West, 1979). Therefore, in the normal person in the upright position, both blood flow and alveolar ventilation are considerably less in the upper part of the lung than in the lower part. However, blood flow is reduced far more than ventilation so at the top of the lung the ventilation-perfusion ratio is as much as three times as great as the ideal value, which causes a moderate degree of physiological dead space in this area. In the bottom of the lung there is ventilation in excess of blood flow with a ventilation-perfusion ratio as low as 0.6 l the ideal value, so in this area some blood fails to become normally oxygenated and this represents a physiological shunt. A change in the distribution of either ventilation or perfusion will alter this ratio and may occur in the presence of diseases such as obstructive airways disease, during exercise, when undergoing mechanical ventilation, or on changing posture (Hough, 1984).

Airway clearance: mucociliary system

The upper airway and trachea transport inspired air and expired gases between the environment and the lungs. In addition the inspired air is warmed, humidified to 100% water vapour, and filtered of most particulate matter before it reaches the trachea. Defensive mechanisms to keep the air clean and free of pollutants include neural reflexes, secretion of mucus, lysozyme, lactoferrin and secretory IgA, and immune responses and reactions at cellular level including macrophages (Jeffery and Corrin, 1984).

The mucociliary system comprises the mucus and cilia, and extends from the posterior two-thirds of the nasal cavity to the terminal bronchioles (Breeze and Wheeldon, 1977). Mucous secretions collect on the interior surface of the airways and organise into two layers. An inner layer of watery periciliary (sol) mucus, and an outer layer of viscous (gel) mucus (Ross and Corrsin, 1974). The cilia are surrounded by watery mucus and islands of gel-type mucus float on top. Cilia move within this watery mucous layer with beating motions which are co-ordinated in waves to propel the layers of mucus and entrapped particles towards the pharynx (Blake, 1975). The normal adult produces about 100 ml of mucus daily, most of which is absorbed through the bronchial lining and about 10–20 ml is cleared and swallowed (Phipps, 1981). Various factors may affect the transport of mucus within the airways. Too much mucus may overwhelm the system, and an absence of mucus would stop the ciliary beating motion (King, 1983). If the mucus is too viscous it will compromise ciliary motion.

When the mucociliary clearance system is impaired or overloaded coughing becomes the primary mechanism of sputum removal (Cosenza and Celentano Norton, 1986).

Two nursing diagnoses to be discussed in this Chapter include:

Ineffective airway clearance

This is defined as a state in which an individual is unable to clear secretions or obstructions from the respiratory tract to maintain a clear airway (Kim and Larson, 1987). Under normal conditions tracheobronchial secretions are dealt with by the muco-ciliary clearance system. However some individuals with airflow limitation related to such conditions as chronic bronchitis, asthma, and emphysema, lower respiratory tract infections, or artificial airway, have a disturbance with the production and clearance of mucus. In these patients when coughing is ineffective in clearing the airways, nursing intervention will be required.

Ineffective breathing patterns

This is defined as states in which the individual's inspiratory and/or expiratory pattern does not provide adequate ventilation (Kim and Larson, 1987). According to Kim and Larson (1987) breathing patterns can be described in terms of respiratory rate, tidal volumes, ratio of inspiration to expiration, and the co-ordinated movements of the respiratory muscles. Normally breathing patterns are effective in meeting the ventilatory needs of the body. However in conditions of airflow limitation such as chronic obstructive airways disease, emphysema and asthma, and restrictive conditions which prevent effective lung expansion such as scoliosis, obesity, ascites, pneumothorax, neuro-muscular disorders affecting respiratory movements, atelectasis, and alveolar fibrosis, breathing patterns are altered in ways which are less efficient and effective in meeting the body's ventilatory needs.

ASSESSMENT AND PROBLEM IDENTIFICATION (Tables 1 and 2)

Rate and depth of respiration

Respiratory rate and tidal volume fluctuate cyclically during quiet breathing but may be affected by a variety of stimuli. For example when the individual is seated during quiet breathing minute ventilation and tidal volume are higher when compared to the supine position (Javaheri et al, 1981). Normal respiratory rates are said to vary from 12 per minute, up to 20 per minute (Ruppel, 1982). Rates in excess of 20 per minute in adults are defined as tachypnoea (Tandberg and Sklar, 1983). Normal tidal volumes range from 400 to 700 ml (Ruppel, 1982). At increased respiratory rates for the same level of ventilation to be present, the total ventilation must increase. This increased ventilation produces smaller tidal volumes, resulting in less effective or wasted venti-lation (Cherniak and Cherniak, 1983). Tidal volume, defined as the volume of gas inspired or expired during the normal breathing cycle, can be measured with a spirometer. As a single measurement tidal volume is most significant when it reflects shallow breathing, as low tidal volumes indicate dead space or waste ventilation (Hunter, 1981).

Patients with chronic airflow limitation, such as those patients with chronic obstruc-tive airways disease, breathe at faster respiratory rates, and with smaller tidal volumes than normal individuals (Gilbert et al, 1972), although the mechanism for this is unclear. Inspection of the chest provides essential information about the rate, rhythm and depth of respiration.

The spirometer can provide information about the patient's tidal volumes. Respiratory rate is typically counted for 15 seconds and multiplied by four. This approach potentially introduces an error of as many as four breaths per minute into a measurement commonly found to be 16–20 per minute (Gravelyn and Wegg, 1980). Gravelyn and Wegg (1980) assessed respiratory rates as an indicator of acute respiratory dysfunction. Defining abnormal rates as those in excess of 24 per minute, elevations in rates without respiratory dysfunction were found in only 4% of all measures. Patients with retention of secretions in airways as evidenced by abnormal breath sounds, cough, or sputum production had abnormal respiratory rates. Following surgery to the abdominal cavity, rapid shallow breaths may be taken because pain prevents deep inspiration.

Accessory muscle use

Patients with chronic airflow limitations tend to have altered patterns of breathing, needing to recruit the external intercostal and accessory muscles to breathe. In the early stages of airflow limitation this is usually confined to situations of high activity. Studies suggest that patients with chronic airflow limitation have a flattened diaphragm which

Table 1. Assessment of Breathing Impairment

Criteria	Methods
Respiratory mechanics—breathing pattern	
Respiratory rate	Inspection
Respiratory depth	Observation
Ratio of inspiration: expiration	Measurement/timing
Accessory muscle use	Dyspnoea Scale (Kinsman et al, 1983)
Ease of breathing	Visual analogue scale (VAS), Borg Scale
	(Burdon et al, 1982)
	Patient self-report
Airway clearance	
Cough	Patient self-report
Breath sounds	Auscultation
Sputum/secretion production	Observation
	Measurement
Body position	
Position adopted for effective breathing	Patient self-report
	Observation
	Spirometry
Activity tolerance	
Self-care, grooming	Patient self-report
Eating	Observation
Walking	12 minute distance walk
Home management	(McGavin et al, 1976)
Occupational, social, recreational activities	
Blood gases	Laboratory analysis
Spirometry	
Volume and flow during specific	Spirometer, peak flow meter
respiratory manoeuvres	

makes it a less effective generator of force during inspiration (Kim et al, 1976) so that intercostal and accessory muscles have to be used to maintain even low levels of ventilation (Stubbing et al, 1982). Inspection of the chest can provide information about the breathing pattern. During normal inspiration the diaphragm moves from its usual domed position, shortens and pushes downwards on the abdomen. If the abdominal muscles are relaxed they are moved outwards. At the same time tension in the diaphragm pushes the lower rib cage upward and outward (Grassino and Goldman, 1986). Therefore during diaphragmatic breathing inspiration is dominated by an outward motion of the rib cage and abdomen. When the diaphragm is impaired and abdominal muscles relaxed, inspiration is achieved by rib cage muscles including external intercostals and accessory muscles of respiration. Then the rib cage is pulled upwards, and the relaxed abdominal muscles are pulled inwards. Therefore when rib cage muscles dominate inspiration the upper chest expands and abdominal muscles move inwards. These patterns reflect extreme conditions, and many patients will display the use of a combination of accessory muscles and diaphragm.

Table 2A. Identification of Different Causes of Breathing Impairment

Criteria	
Respiratory mechanics	
Rate	Normal/tachypnoea (rate >20)
Depth	Normal/shallow
Ratio inspiration: expiration	Normal/prolonged expiration
Accessory muscle use	Not always evident
Ease of breathing	Use VAS, Dyspnoea Scale, Borg Scale
	May be dyspnoeic
Chest expansion	May be restricted
Airway clearance	
Sputum/secretion	Present in excess of 20–30 ml per day
	May be purulent, thick, tenacious
Breath sounds	Abnormal breath sounds present: wheezes, crackles; may be diminished/absent
Cough	Ineffective for expectoration, or absent
Body position	Slumped or supine
Blood gases	Normal/abnormal
Activity tolerance	Limited to some extent
Spirometry	Reduced peak expiratory flow
Diagnosis:	*Ineffective airway clearance*

Table 2B. Identification of Different Causes of Breathing Impairment

Criteria	
Respiratory mechanics	
Rate	Tachypnoea (rate >20/22 per minute)
Depth	Shallow (small tidal volumes)
Ratio inspiration: expiration	Increased, slow expiration
Accessory muscle use	Evident: neck, abdominal, external intercostals recruited
Ease of breathing	Use VAS, Dyspnoea Scale, Borg Scale
	Dyspnoea either at rest or on activity
Chest expansion	Diminished (<2.5–3″ expansion)
Airway clearance	
Sputum	May or may not be present in excess
Breath sounds	Normal/abnormal
Cough	If present usually effective
Body position	Standing or sitting upright, leaning forward, shoulders hunched, arms supported on a surface
Blood gases	Abnormal
Activity tolerance	Usually severely restricted
	Tires quickly
	Feels weak
Spirometry	Decreased peak expiratory flow.
Diagnosis:	*Ineffective breathing pattern*

Ease of breathing

Many states of respiratory dysfunction result in subjective and objective signs of difficulty with breathing. The sensation of dyspnoea is subjective and includes both the perception of laboured breathing by the patient, and the reaction to that sensation (Carrieri et al, 1984). In nursing literature the terms breathlessness, shortness of breath, and dyspnoea are used interchangeably. Their precise definitions have not been established. The word dyspnoea originates from the Greek '*dys*' which means abnormal or disordered, and '*pnoia*' which means breath—disordered breathing. For the purposes of this chapter the terms dyspnoea, breathlessness, and shortness of breath are used interchangeably as is consistent with the published work on dyspnoea (Carrieri et al, 1984).

Dyspnoea refers to a sensory experience that is perceived, interpreted and rated solely by the patient himself (Widinsky, 1979). The sensation involves the interaction of physiological, biochemical and psychological components; however its precise mechanism is unclear. For a review of current theories the reader is referred to various sources (Lancet, 1986; Bass and Gardner, 1985; Carrieri et al, 1984). Both obstructive and restrictive lung dysfunction can lead to intermittent or permanent states of perceived dyspnoea. Patients with airways obstruction experience changes in their breathing pattern which include increased rate, smaller tidal volumes and use of accessory muscles of respiration. In addition airflow obstruction or limitation alters pulmonary mechanisms and impairs inspiratory muscle function. All these factors lead to inadequate ventilation especially during activity. This inadequate ventilation leads to dyspnoea either at rest or during activity (Lareau and Larson, 1987). Restrictive lung conditions also produce dyspnoea by restricting lung expansion. Restrictive disease may occur as a result of disrupted thoracic cage movements (extrapulmonary). For example scoliosis alters the pattern of lung expansion; neuromuscular diseases such as Guillain-Barré syndrome inhibit thoracic expansion by impairing neuromuscular transmission of impulses to the diaphragm and other muscles of inspiration. Increased mass loading which occurs with obesity, ascites, and pregnancy, restricts and alters the pattern of lung expansion. Restrictive disease may also be intrapulmonary involving lung parenchyma. Parenchymal inflammation characteristically causes restriction as in pneumonia. Atelectasis, lung resection and pulmonary fibrosis all have the common features of reduced pulmonary compliance, and increased elastance or elastic recoil. So the lungs are hard to expand but recoil tightly. Therefore it can be seen that restrictive disorders that decrease lung expansion, increase the work of breathing, and produce varying degrees of dyspnoea (Hopp and Williams, 1987), reflecting changes in effort that the patient perceives as the work of breathing increases.

Assessment of dyspnoea

In trying to understand dyspnoea from a nursing perspective it may be useful to place it within a familiar framework (Lareau and Larson, 1987). The pain model is useful, since like pain dyspnoea is a subjective experience of varying intensity. Like pain, individual patients' responses to dyspnoea and tolerance of it varies a great deal. Like pain, dyspnoea is accompanied by related clinical signs including increased rate and decreased depth of breathing. The assessment of dyspnoea can take several different forms:

1. Asking patients to report their usual level of dyspnoea.
2. Asking patients to report the level of dyspnoea with certain activities.

The assessment can be made more objective by using a scale or other measuring instrument. A visual analogue scale (VAS) similar to that used for pain assessment provides a reasonably reliable and valid measure of the severity of breathlessness, and it has proved sensitive enough to be used to detect small changes in the severity of breathlessness over time (Woodcock et al, 1981; Gift et al, 1986). Gift et al (1986) found that a 10 cm vertical line with verbal anchors at each end—'no shortness of breath' at the low end, and 'shortness of breath as bad as it can be' at the high end (Figure 1)— was a reliable measure. Patients rate the intensity of their breathlessness and mark the corresponding point on the line. The VAS can be used to report the usual amount of dyspnoea or the amount of dyspnoea while performing a specific activity. This is a useful and helpful tool for use in the clinical setting to monitor changes over time. The modified Borg Scale (Burdon et al, 1982) is a 10-point category scale for rating perceived breathlessness. Words describing breathlessness are anchored to numbers between 0 and 10. Patients are free to select whole numbers or fractions (Figure 2). As with the VAS the Borg Scale can be used to report the usual amount of dyspnoea or the extent of dyspnoea while performing specific activities. Burdon et al (1982) found that scores on the Borg Scale were validated by physiological measures. It was found that breathlessness as indicated by scores on the Borg Scale increased as the forced expiratory volume in 1 second (FEV_1) decreased in all subjects. Like the VAS this could prove to be a useful and effective clinical tool for nurses to use. A category scale can be used to classify the severity of dyspnoea in relation to activity tolerance or functional impairment (Figure 3). These scales are insensitive to small changes in dyspnoea. This type of scale may be appropriate for use in the patient's home where functional activity could be monitored over time. It has been stated that dyspnoea is a subjective experience and as such each individual's perception of it will be different. It is said that the relationship between pulmonary dysfunction and the severity of dyspnoea is close only within individual disease entities (Widinsky, 1979). It would seem that restrictive lung diseases provide moderate correlations between the perception of dyspnoea and pulmonary function tests, whereas some patients with chronic obstructive disease may have poor pulmonary function tests and not complain of dyspnoea (Fishman and Ledlie, 1979). Psychological and emotional factors may also influence the perception of breathlessness, including anger, anxiety and frustration (Carrieri et al, 1984).

Assessment of airway clearance

Breath sounds

An important characteristic defining the diagnosis of ineffective airway clearance is abnormal breath sounds, since this sign most directly reflects the presence of secretions remaining in the airway. This is especially so in patients with artificial airways such as tracheostomy or endotracheal tube. A small study by Knipper (1984) assessed the effectiveness of abnormal breath sounds in predicting the presence of tracheobronchial

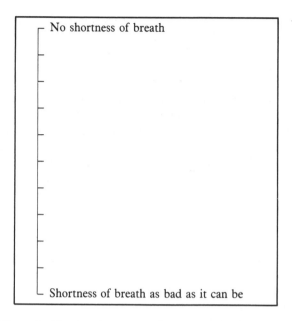

Figure 1. Visual analogue scale for assessment of dyspnoea

0	Nothing at all
0.5	Very, very slight
1	Very slight
2	
3	Moderate
4	
5	Severe
6	
7	Very severe
8	
9	Very, very severe
10	Maximal

Figure 2. Modified Borg scale (Burdon et al, 1982)

Grade 0	No shortness of breath with normal activity. Shortness of breath on exertion comparable to a well person of the same age, height and sex.
Grade 1	More shortness of breath than a person of the same age while walking on the level or climbing stairs.
Grade 2	More short of breath and unable to keep up with persons of the same age and sex while walking on the level.
Grade 3	Short of breath while walking on the level and while carrying out usual tasks.
Grade 4	Short of breath while carrying out usual self-care activities.

Figure 3. Category scale for grading dyspnoea (Morgan, 1982)

secretions and found that over three-quarters of patients with abnormal breath sounds (crackles and crepitations) yielded a significant amount of secretions on suction compared with those patients without crackles present. Abnormal breath sounds such as crackles and wheezes (rhonchi) reflect the presence of mucus in the smaller and larger airways respectively. If obstruction of the airway has occurred the breath sounds will be diminished or absent. Abnormal breath sounds will frequently be found in patients with chronic airflow obstruction and asthma, and also in patients with lower airway infection such as pneumonia, and in patients with artificial airways.

Auscultation is a skill which clinical nurses can acquire. It provides valuable information which can be used for problem identification. Listening to breath sounds without a stethoscope will also reveal the presence of stridor which is a harsh or musical inspiration indicative of upper airway obstruction (Sterling, 1983).

Secretion production and clearance

Evidence of retained secretions includes sputum production. Lung mucociliary clearance has been found to be impaired in chronic bronchitis, bronchiectasis, and cystic fibrosis (Lourenco et al, 1972; Wood et al, 1975). Although the normal adult produces about 100 ml of mucus daily most of this is resorbed through the bronchial lining and about 10–20 ml is cleared and swallowed (Hirsch and Kory, 1967). In patients with chronic bronchitis it was found that the mean daily sputum production was 160 ml confirming the presence of excessive lung secretions (Bateman et al, 1981). In chronic bronchitis goblet cells increase in number and submucosal glands hypertrophy in response to chronic irritation thereby accounting for the increase in mucus production seen in many patients. Acute inflammatory conditions stimulate mucus production which may also be purulent in character. Abnormal conditions also change the physical character of secretions (change the gel or sol layer) in such a way that normal mechanisms of clearance will not work adequately. Severe inflammation increases the rigidity of mucus increasing intramolecular bonds (Cosenza and Celentano Norton, 1986). This change can cause physical damage to cilia, or may cause areas of mucosa to be stripped and produce mucostasis (Hirsch, 1980).

Purulent sputum has decreased elasticity and increased viscosity due to the presence of highly viscous white cell DNA. Sputum in asthmatic patients is more viscous because of changes in the glycoprotein and water content (Johansen and Gould, 1977). In chronic bronchitis secretions are more tenacious probably because there is more mucus than serous fluid. Patients with cystic fibrosis have goblet cell hyperplasia and hypertrophy of bronchial glands with a resultant thick copious secretion. Some infective organisms including influenza A virus and *Mycoplasma pneumoniae* can cause damage to the mucociliary clearance system for several months thus impairing the movement of lung secretions (Camner et al, 1973; Jaarstrand et al, 1975). Secretion clearance rates are also slower in patients with cystic fibrosis, chronic bronchitis, and bronchial asthma (Cosenza and Celentano Norton, 1986). With an artificial airway in place part of the mucociliary system is bypassed. Dry air breathing (loss of normal warming, humidifying, and filtering function) was found to reduce significantly tracheal mucus velocity in intubated dogs (Hirsch et al, 1975). This may be related to the dysfunction of the mucociliary system, or a change in character of the secretions or both. In summary, assessment of sputum production and clearance may involve the following parameters:

1. Amount.
2. Consistency, colour.
3. Ability to clear it.
4. Rate of clearance.

Cough

Cough is a protective mechanism against lung aspiration in the upper airway, and is normally a secondary mechanism for airway clearance in the lower airway (Hanley and Tyler, 1987). A cough is a forced expiratory manoeuvre that is partly reflex and partly voluntary. When the normal mucociliary clearance mechanism is impaired or overloaded, coughing becomes the primary mechanism of sputum removal. Coughing is initiated by stimulation of irritant receptors found in the larynx, trachea, bronchi, or carina. The normal cough sequence comprises a deep inhalation which increases lung volume and airway calibre so allowing air to pass distal to the obstructing secretion; closure of the glottis; contraction of the expiratory muscles; and, after about 0.2–0.4 seconds, the glottis opens suddenly, and expiratory flow begins (Leith et al, 1986). The linear velocity of air generated by coughing produces a shearing force to dislodge particles and mucus so that they may be expelled. The cough is generally effective in clearing secretions in the major airways, but it may also be effective in clearing peripheral or smaller airways in patients with bronchitis (Traver, 1985). Cough can be assessed by asking the individual to cough and observing the outcome. The sound made during coughing should be evaluated. If it is coming from the throat it is a short sharp high-pitched sound, from lower in the airways it is a deeper resonant sound. Hoffman (1987) grades cough according to its ability to generate force and clear secretions:

1. Functional: adequate to clear all secretions. No assistance required.
2. Weak-functional: adequate to clear the throat and small amounts of secretions. Assistance is required if secretions increase in volume, such as with respiratory infection.
3. Non-functional: unable to generate any cough.

For coughing to be effective, propulsive airflow distal to the secretions must be adequate and the mucus must have the proper properties. For example patients with cystic fibrosis or chronic bronchitis can cough so ineffectively that they cause a retrograde movement of mucus, or aspiration from one lung to another (Newhouse et al, 1973). With an artificial airway in place the cough reflex may be less effective. The glottis is bypassed and this eliminates its role in producing an effective cough. Also airway resistance is increased by an artificial airway owing to the smaller tube diameter and decreased distensibility as compared to a normal airway. As a result, the ability to generate the high airflow rate necessary for expulsive force is diminished (Newhouse et al, 1976). Also a complicating muscular or neurological disease may decrease the propulsive force. Patients with painful abdominal wounds may not produce an effective cough because they are unable to take a deep breath that expands the airways enough to ensure that air will flow distal to any secretions that may be present. Although coughing may be a painful nuisance to patients, it is vital when the mucociliary system is overloaded. Presence of a moist but unproductive cough has been prospectively identified as a most important early sign of secretion retention (McMichan et al, 1980).

Assessment of activity intolerance

Patients with both restrictive and obstructive lung pathology experience impaired ventilation and perfusion which may limit their activity. Some patients who cope adequately when at rest, may have inadequate function when undertaking even mild activity. The activity assessment should be comprehensive including information about what patients are capable of doing in relation to self-care, grooming, eating, walking, care of the house and social and recreational activities. A more objective test which provides information about a patient's ability to perform daily activities is the 12 minute distance walk (12MD) (McGavin et al, 1976). This is a simple test which could be carried out in a normal hospital ward, or in the community. It consists of measuring the maximum distance that a patient can walk in 12 minutes at their own rate, taking as many rests as required. It necessitates a prolonged submaximal effort which is similar to that required on a daily basis. Some testing of its validity as a measure of functional ability shows that it is both reliable and valid in patients with chronic airflow limitation. In healthy subjects, when compared to the maximal exercise test, it correlated highly (r= 0.94) with direct measure of maximal oxygen consumption (Wyndham et al, 1971). Among patients with chronic bronchitis the 12MD correlated (r=0.52) with maximal oxygen consumption (McGavin et al, 1976). Further use and testing of this tool could show its potential for clinical use.

Blood gases

This is a complex subject and for a full discussion the reader is referred to texts dealing with the topic (Shapiro et al, 1977). Alterations in respiration are reflected in the arterial partial pressures of oxygen (PaO_2) and carbon dioxide ($PaCO_2$), and fall into four main interdependent categories (Webb and Cochrane, 1981):

1. Change in alveolar ventilation.
2. Venous to arterial shunting.
3. Impaired diffusion.
4. Mismatching of alveolar ventilation and pulmonary blood flow.

Pulmonary disorders which can result in abnormal blood gas values include chronic airways obstruction (ventilation-perfusion mismatching); pulmonary oedema and fibrosing alveolitis (diffusion impairment); and pneumonia and adult respiratory distress syndrome (ARDS) (venous to arterial shunting) (Webb and Cochrane, 1981). Cyanosis is an unreliable and late sign of hypoxaemia. When cyanosis does indicate hypoxaemia it only appears once the haemoglobin is desaturated to the level of venous blood. Mental confusion and tachycardia are more accurate reflections of hypoxaemia (Rokosky, 1985). In some situations cyanosis may not indicate hypoxaemia. Peripherally it may result from vasoconstriction related to cold. When the amount of haemoglobin is significantly increased as in polycythaemia, it can never be fully saturated and cyanosis is characteristic.

The forced expiratory manoeuvre

As most generalised lung disease affects the mechanical properties of the lungs and airways, the main clinical tests of these are based on forced expiratory manoeuvres (Sterling, 1983). An important point to make in these tests is that the main driving pressure for airflow during forced expiration is the elastic recoil of the lungs, and since this is proportional to the degree of lung inflation, the most important aspect of the test is to ensure that the patient has taken a really full inspiration before starting to exhale. Using a spirometer, the measurements taken most commonly during this manoeuvre are the forced vital capacity (FVC), and forced expiratory volume in one second (FEV_1). A useful measurement for frequent use in wards and at home which can be taken using this manoeuvre is the peak expiratory flow (PEF). The peak flow meter and its derivative, the light-weight plastic peak flow gauge, give less detailed information, but are very useful in the assessment of treatment of airflow obstruction. When measuring PEF consistency in technique is extremely important. Assessment should be done with the individual in the same position. Air leak around the lips should be minimised. As with spirometry, an essential part of the technique is maximal inspiration before a forced expiration, which in this case is a short sharp blow. Typically, three measurements are obtained and the best result taken. Significance of the values obtained can be assessed by:

1. Comparing trends in patient effort over time.
2. Comparing values to those predicted for normal individuals.
3. Comparing patient values to those considered minimally acceptable to allow independent spontaneous ventilation without development of atelectasis (Hoffman, 1987).

The basic functional abnormality in airflow limitation is a reduction in FEV_1 and PEF. The monitoring of the peak flow in patients with airflow limitation is now a well-established practice. In diseases which are inherently variable it is of greater value to make a simple measurement such as peak flow on many occasions, rather than more sophisticated measurements on a much smaller number of occasions (Webb and Cochrane, 1981).

Assessment data has been presented to aid in problem identification for the following aetiologies related to the stated diagnoses.

1. Ineffective airway clearance related to airway infection.
2. Ineffective airway clearance related to presence of an artificial airway.
3. Ineffective breathing patterns related to decreased lung expansion.
4. Ineffective breathing patterns related to airflow limitation or obstruction.

These are independent diagnoses, and it is unlikely that a patient with long-term pathology will have only one set of problems. Restrictive and obstructive diseases may result in a combination of problems with airway clearance, and disturbed breathing patterns.

RATIONALE AND INTERVENTIONS

Modification of breathing patterns

Breathing exercises

Whether airway obstruction is related to secretions in the airway, muscle spasm, inflammation in airway walls, or loss of elastic recoil, the obstruction can be reduced with increases in lung volumes (Menkes and Britt, 1980). Increasing lung volume decreases airway resistance and improves ventilation to poorly ventilated lung areas (Macklem and Mead, 1967; Menkes and Britt, 1980).

Diaphragmatic breathing is a technique used to achieve improved lung volumes and distribution of ventilation. Abdominal or diaphragmatic breathing is designed to increase the use of the diaphragm during inspiration. Studies have indicated that active contraction of the diaphragm should result in improved airflow to the base of the lung where perfusion is greater (Froese and Bryan, 1974). Abdominal or diaphragmatic breathing is taught by asking patients to relax the abdominal muscles and push them outwards during inspiration so that the abdominal cavity expands and allows for the unobstructed descent of the diaphragm, and then to slightly tighten the abdominal muscles during expiration to augment the upward movement of the diaphragm. Although diaphragmatic breathing is commonly used as an intervention to reduce dyspnoea, research has not provided significant evidence for its efficacy in changing the distribution of ventilation (Grimby et al, 1975).

Slow deep breathing is another way to redistribute airflow (Menkes and Britt, 1980). Bake et al (1974) have shown that normal individuals have more ventilation to dependent areas of the lungs at low airflows, whereas at high airflows ventilation is distributed more evenly. The distribution of flow at high flows in normal individuals is similar to the pattern seen in patients with chronic airflow limitation related to chronic obstructive airways disease (COAD) at their usual rate of breathing. Therefore if patients with COAD breathe at lower flows whilst maintaining the lung at higher volumes for a longer time during the respiratory cycle, the distribution of ventilation should improve. This can be achieved by slow deep breathing which slows the rate of respiration, increases tidal volume, and improves gas exchange (Thomas et al, 1966).

Pursed lip breathing is a technique often seen adopted naturally by dyspnoeic patients with airflow limitation. This achieves the slow deep pattern described above. By the patient mildly blowing against pursed lips, the expiratory time is prolonged, rate is slowed, and tidal volumes increase. Pursed lip breathing may also be accompanied by a decrease in $PaCO_2$, and an increase in PaO_2. Subjective relief of dyspnoea is felt by patients using this breathing pattern may either be related to added positive airway pressure during expiration, or to change in breathing pattern (Thomas et al, 1966). Post-operative respiratory problems may also be related to a decrease in lung volumes most marked after upper abdominal operations (Peters and Turnier, 1980). Trunk surgery restricts movement of the chest cage and diaphragm which leads to increase in alveolar collapse and lobar atelectasis.

Factors contributing to these complications include decreased number of respiratory 'sighs' (normal intermittent deep breaths); and pain and muscle spasm disrupting chest wall function and reducing lung volumes. Slow deep breathing will act to prevent these complications. Recently the use of incentive spirometry (IS) is gaining wide popularity as a method for inducing deep inspiration, so preventing alveolar collapse. IS devices consist of one or more chambers, each containing a plastic ball. Inspiratory activity causes the ball to be sucked up the chamber, the ball falling if inspiratory flow is not maintained (Jenkins and Soutar, 1986). Use of an IS device duplicates the effect of a deep breath, while at the same time providing objective documentation of increases or decreases in the volume inhaled. Pre-operative teaching of such techniques followed by post-operative supervision is necessary for this to be an effective intervention. Relaxation training and biofeedback have been used to reduce the rate of breathing and increase tidal volumes in patients with obstructive airways disease and asthma (Sitzman et al, 1983, Freedberg et al, 1987). Relaxation training may be useful in reducing dyspnoea in some patients, but further research is needed to clarify its mechanisms and effects.

Therapeutic coughing

Therapeutic coughing is a primary pulmonary defence mechanism in patients with excessive secretions because of chronic inflammation, irritation, or infection. Even with the glottis bypassed when an artificial airway is in place, some patients remain able to cough quite effectively (Leith et al, 1986).

The use of coughing as an intervention has to be directed and evaluated by nurses. Ineffective coughing technique is tiring and will be detrimental to the patient. Huff coughing or forced expiratory technique (FET) is useful for patients who have small airway closure (severe obstructed disease) following multiple coughs (de Boek and Zinman, 1984). These patients usually have difficulty in expectorating secretions lodged in the upper airways. The huff cough is a forced expiratory manoeuvre with open glottis. The glottis is kept open by saying the word 'huff'. Clinically coughing is recommended only when secretions are audible by ear or with stethoscope, to avoid irritation and unnecessary fatigue (Luce et al, 1984). The position for coughing should be sitting upright with the body flexed at the waist; a side-lying position with the knees bent is preferable to the supine recumbent position (Hanley and Tyler, 1987). After any expiratory manoeuvre such as coughing the patient should perform a voluntary maximal inhalation of 3–10 seconds to aid in reinflating the collapsed alveoli. This can help to avoid the complications of pooled mucus, decreased oxygenation and increased risk of infection (Cosenza and Celentano Norton, 1986). The use of incentive spirometers for this manoeuvre is effective. The reinflated alveoli stay inflated for at least one hour, so the patient should be encouraged to perform these exercises hourly and after each cough (Bartlett et al, 1973).

Body positioning

Patients often adopt specific positions in order to relieve the feeling of dyspnoea. This includes standing up with the arms in front while leaning on a table, and leaning forwards with arms supported on a flat surface and hunched shoulders (in the sitting position). Some dyspnoeic patients also appear to breathe easier while lying fairly supine much to the surprise of many nurses. There are good physiological and anatomic mechanisms to support the effectiveness of these positions in patients with airflow limitation. A mechanism proposed by Sharp et al (1980) is that in the supine position the effects of abdominal contents tend to push up the diaphragm lengthening the muscle fibres and increasing its tension generating potential. In the seated leaning forward position the abdomen is compressed which would stretch the diaphragm upwards and improve its tension generating capability. Also, leaning forward may help in the use of accessory muscles of respiration. A study by Crosbie and Myles (1985) examined the effects of different positions on lung function in normal individuals. Results showed that the 'slumped half-lying' position seen in so many post-operative patients and medical patients, appears to cause a decrease in vital capacity and FEV_1 of 12% and 15% respectively from those obtained in the sitting position, and also tends to show lower values compared with prone and supine positions particularly for FEV_1. As has been previously stated the normal uneven ratio of ventilation to perfusion of inspired gases can be disrupted by changes in pulmonary function. A mismatch of perfusion in excess of ventilation (V/Q inequality) is a most common cause of hypoxaemia in patients with pulmonary dysfunction. This hypoxaemia results from the mixing of poorly oxygenated blood from underventilated lung regions with well-oxygenated blood from well-ventilated lung regions, therefore decreasing the overall PaO_2 value. This mismatch may be improved by suitable positioning of the patient.

Lateral position

Positioning patients with unilateral lung disease (lobar pneumonia) so that the 'good' lung is down and the affected lung uppermost may lead to an improvement in PaO_2. This is probably as a result of improved matching of ventilation to perfusion when the unaffected lung is dependent (Remolina et al, 1981). This mechanism may also account for the relief felt by dyspnoeic patients when lying on their side (Hough, 1984). The high-side lying position may be used to relieve dyspnoea if the patient is made comfortable and the trunk is not side-flexed. In the mechanically ventilated patient with unilateral lung disease (with or without low levels of positive end expiratory pressure [PEEP]) the best V/Q appears to occur with the good lung down (Celentano Norton and Conforti, 1985). Side lying is also the optimum position for the administration of fluid or drugs through a nebuliser so as to facilitate the more distal distribution of the droplets (Hough, 1984).

Sitting up

A study by Crosbie and Sim (1986) examined the effects of posture on lung function in patients following abdominal surgery. Positions studied included sitting, lying supine, right and left side lying, and slumped half-lying. Results showed that lung function as measured by FEV_1 and FVC was significantly greater in the sitting position than in any other of the positions. The results would suggest that the sitting position allows less restricted descent of the diaphragm without the need for assistance from the oblique externus abdominus muscle. In the seated position the accessory respiratory muscles in the cervical region and shoulder girdles may be more easily recruited to increase inspiration (Crosbie and Sim, 1986). It would seem that the upright sitting position is advantageous for post-operative patients and should be actively promoted.

Suction

In patients who are unable to cough effectively it is often necessary to perform nasotracheal or endotracheal suctioning. Tracheobronchial suctioning is associated with many risks.

Hypoxaemia has been documented as an adverse effect of suctioning in many studies (see Young, 1984). The mechanism for this effect may include suction induced atelectasis (Rux and Powaser, 1979), and reflex bronchoconstriction caused by mechanical stimulation of the trachea (Naigow and Powaser, 1977). Various techniques to reduce suction-induced hypoxaemia have been assessed including: manual inflation by 'bagging'; preoxygenation by bagging or via change in ventilator rate; insufflation through suction catheter or endotracheal tube adaptor: hyperoxygenation by bagging; hyperinflation by bag or ventilator; and hyperventilation by bagging or increase in ventilator rate (Barnes and Kirchoff, 1986). For a full review of these techniques the reader is referred to Barnes and Kirchoff (1986).

Atelectasis was observed following formation of obstructive crusting in infants who required mechanical ventilation and frequent suctioning for more than 20 days by Nagaraj et al (1980). Failure to re-expand collapsed areas of lung may predispose to infection.

Cardiac arrhythmias: Shim et al (1969) demonstrated that the incidence of transient cardiac arrhythmias during tracheal suction in patients was significant while breathing air. Breathing 100% oxygen before suction resulted in complete abolition of the arrhythmias.

Tracheobronchial trauma to mucosa can occur with the passage of the catheter alone, and ulceration is greater with higher negative pressures (Kusenski, 1978). Decreased ciliary action for up to three hours after suction has been shown by Landa et al (1980).

Given the serious nature of potential consequences of suction, the use of this intervention to clear secretions should be based on clear clinical signs of retained secretions. In non-intubated patients every effort should be made to enhance secretion clearance by less risky methods. The frequency of suctioning should be based on careful assessment. The patient's breath sounds should act as a guide to the need for suctioning (Knipper, 1984). The ideal suction technique ensures maximum removal of secretions with minimum tissue damage and hypoxaemia (Shekleton and Nield, 1987). Damage to tracheal tissue can result if suction pressures above 100–120 mmHg are applied to adults and above 80 mmHg in children (Kusenski, 1978). The duration of suction has been shown to be related to development of hypoxaemia. A cumulative decrease in PaO_2 has been shown to occur with each pass of the suction catheter, and at least 60 seconds are required before PaO_2 returns to baseline levels (Baun and Flones, 1984). Larger catheters increase the risk of mechanical trauma, and can cause airway collapse and atelectasis. Catheter size should be less than half the diameter of the trachea (Young, 1984). Nasotracheal suctioning should also only be carried out if other clearance techniques such as coughing are ineffective.

Upright positioning and neck hyperextension may help catheter passage. Minitracheotomy is a new technique in which a cannula with an internal diameter of 4 mm is inserted into the trachea. Insertion is by a simple puncture technique which does not require general anaesthesia or sedation and once in place the cannula allows tracheal suction to be carried out as often as desired using a 10 FG suction catheter. Because the cannula is small in relation to the trachea the patient breathes normally through the nose or mouth and is able to speak and cough normally (Preston et al, 1986). This can be used in the short- or long-term for management of secretion clearance in patients with various respiratory difficulties.

Oxygen therapy

Oxygen therapy is given to patients suffering from hypoxia or from conditions that may lead to hypoxia including acute respiratory failure caused by respiratory infection, pulmonary embolism, abnormal breathing patterns related to chest wall injury, and for maintenance of acute exacerbations of chronic airways disease, asthma, and emphysema. Hypoxia occurs when the supply of oxygen to the tissues is inadequate to maintain normal tissue respiration. The administration of oxygen-enriched breathing mixtures to acutely ill patients is based on the premise that this form of treatment can overcome the ill effects of tissue hypoxia. Therapeutic practices are based on the knowledge of the physiology of oxygenation in normal and diseased individuals and on knowledge of pulmonary oxygen toxicity rather on demonstrated alterations in disease outcomes (Snider and Rinaldo, 1980). The arterial PO_2 (PaO_2), when markedly decreased, indicates oxygen deprivation of tissues especially in unstable or acute states. Therefore the PaO_2 remains a useful guide for initiating and monitoring oxygen therapy in many circumstances. Clinical symptoms of hypoxia are non-specific and include mental confusion, impaired judgement and agitation. Cyanosis is an unsatisfactory guide to hypoxia because it occurs only with severe hypoxaemia and may be absent in anaemia and polycythaemia. The presence of inadequate oxygenation in the acute situation requires a high index of suspicion in any patient showing non-specific signs such as described above (Snider and Rinaldo, 1980). Even without these signs certain clinical situations are associated with a high incidence of gas-exchange abnormalities that may result in hypoxaemia, and this would include nearly all acute pulmonary disorders, and some chronic pulmonary disorders. Ideally the institution of oxygen therapy should be initiated when hypoxaemia is present as revealed by a PaO_2 value of 8 kPa (60 mmHg) or less (Snider and Rinaldo, 1980), although certain conditions such as pulmonary embolism or pneumonia may require oxygen therapy at PaO_2 values higher than that stated above. In certain conditions such as chronic obstructive airways disease, oxygen therapy should be treated with caution. Hypercapnia (raised $PaCO_2$) after oxygen therapy in patients with acute exacerbation of COAD is well recognised. Various mechanisms are proposed for this process including reduced hypoxic drive due to rise in PaO_2, hypoventilation and deterioration in ventilation perfusion matching (Stradling, 1986). Following a review of research, Stradling (1986) concludes that reduced hypoxic drive and hypoventilation may still be the responsible mechanism. These patients should receive low dose oxygen therapy to give them a small increase in arterial oxygen tensions sufficient to increase significantly the arterial oxygen saturation but not to depress seriously the ventilatory drive (Campbell, 1960). After an adequate level of oxygen therapy has been determined by arterial blood gas analysis, the oxygen therapy device that is used should be capable of delivering consistent, reliable concentrations of oxygen. Low flow oxygen therapy devices (for example the nasal cannula) provide the patient with only a partial amount of the inspired gas by entraining room air to mix with the oxygen. Oxygen concentrations may differ from patient to patient with this type of device with changes in breathing rate and pattern. High flow devices provide the total volume of inspired gas for the patient. Therefore they can deliver precise concentration of oxygen as well as controlled consistent humidification. Small adjustable valves can be fitted so that oxygen concentration will be accurate. Some manufacturers suggest the flow rate to be set at specific levels for optimal functioning of the masks. Humidification is desirable to overcome the drying effects of the inspired gas. Studies show that the percentage of inspired oxygen that is delivered may not be affected by the use of a humidifier (Cohen et al, 1977). Most patients require oxygen to help them over an acute period of illness. However some patients require oxygen therapy in the long term in their home environment. Transtracheal oxygen delivery through microcatheter is a new technique for long-term oxygen therapy in patients with chronic airways disease. A small (16 gauge) catheter inserted percutaneously into the trachea allows oxygen to be delivered directly into the lungs. Patients can achieve adequate oxygenation at lower flow rates and humidification is unnecessary because the nasopharynx is bypassed. This has been found to reduce breathlessness in patients with severe hypoxaemia due to COAD (Banner and Govan, 1986).

Oxygen therapy must be tailored to meet the needs of individual patients. These needs are determined and assessed by evaluating clinical signs and symptoms of hypoxaemia. Understanding the applications and limitations of oxygen therapy devices provides the nurse with guidelines for appropriate oxygen therapy.

Hydration therapy

Purulent secretions are characteristically thick and tenacious. This problem is exacerbated by pyrexia, diuretics, and tachypnoea. A study by Chopra et al (1977) of the effects of dehydration on mucociliary transport rates in dogs found that dehydration significantly decreased mucociliary transport rates, and rehydration returned rates to normal. Rehydration of dehydrated patients has been demonstrated to increase mucociliary clearance rates in persons with rates below their normal baseline (Cosenza and Celentano Norton, 1986). In addition the discovery that hydration with enteral or parenteral fluids did not increase clearance rates above baseline has led to the suggestion that excessive fluid intakes may not be needed to keep secretions from becoming tenacious (Moody, 1977). A normal level of hydration should be the aim, taking account of effects of pyrexia and other adverse factors. Local hydration can be provided by humidifers or nebulisers via a mask or wide-bore mouthpiece. Inhalation of normotonic or hypertonic saline aerosols has been found to stimulate mucociliary clearance rates significantly in patients with chronic bronchitis (Wanner and Rao, 1980). However, the efficiency of such aerosols in humidifying airway secretions has been called into question by studies that show they produce only a slight decrease in viscosity of secretions and in addition the mist was deposited in the upper airways with small amounts only in the lower airways (Wanner and Rao, 1980). In patients with artificial airways, inspired air lacks the humidity provided by the upper airways. Humidity and aerosol generating devices can be used to saturate the air, with the aim of preventing mucosal drying, keeping secretions moist, and maintaining the integrity of the mucociliary clearance system (Shekleton and Nield, 1987). A humidifier frequently used in ventilator circuits is the cascade type of bubble humidifier, which is warmed and provides 100% humidity. Nebulisers will create a vapour mist breathed in via a T-tube connection attached to the tracheostomy or endotracheal tube. Studies on the deposition of particles produced by jet or ultrasonic nebulisers raise doubts of their efficiency in moisturising the lower airways (Asmundsson et al, 1973), and in addition there is evidence that these treatments may cause a fall in blood oxygen levels and an increase in airway resistance (Cheney and Butler, 1968). Adequate systemic hydration is an important contribution to maintaining an adequate mucociliary system.

Energy conservation

There is little research which focuses on interventions to conserve energy in patients with respiratory dysfunction. Interventions previously described to improve breathing patterns (relief of dyspnoea, slowing and increasing depth of respiration, oxygen therapy for long-term maintenance) may help to improve activity tolerance in some patients. Some respiratory rehabilitation programmes are designed to optimise the functional status of patients with a combination of general body exercises, patient education, and nutritional support (Larson and Kim, 1987). Various exercise training regimes and their effects on exercise tolerance in patients with chronic airflow limitation, have been studied by Booker (1984), and Tydeman et al (1984). The results of these studies do not provide clear guidelines for type and length of exercise training that benefits these patients. What may be clear is that the value of group activity in creating confidence and a positive outlook in patients is vital (Tydeman et al, 1984). Some interventions have been studied in an attempt to affect directly respiratory muscle function. This includes exercising respiratory muscles to improve strength and endurance. A review of two techniques to improve inspiratory muscle function includes: (1) isocapnic hyperventilation, which entails patients exercising their respiratory muscles by breathing for 15 minutes at the maximal ventilation they can sustain; and (2) resistive breathing, which is breathing at normal levels of ventilation but the inspiratory muscles are loaded so they must generate more tension with each inspiration (Larson and Kim, 1987). Studies to date appear to show that the effects of these techniques on respiratory muscle function are variable and further research is required.

IMPLICATIONS FOR NURSING

'Breathing' is a familiar activity of daily living to all nurses (Roper et al, 1985), but it is doubtful if nursing assessment and interventions for this activity and its dysfunctions are as comprehensive and effective as they might be.

As can be seen from the contents of this chapter there are some objective assessment methods that could be easily incorporated into routine nursing assessment. This would have the dual purpose of increasing objectivity and providing a firmer basis on which to select interventions, whilst in addition, repeatedly using such tools would highlight their effectiveness or not as clinical tools.

There are also interventions available with a reasonable theoretical and research base. Frequent nursing interventions such as those to help patients breathe and cough with ease and efficiency could be improved upon. The nurse's role as a health educator could be crucial in keeping patients with chronic breathing problems functioning at their optimum level at home. Nursing interventions for these patients would include education concerning medicinal and nutritional needs, and monitoring their activity and rest patterns.

FUTURE RESEARCH

1. Evaluative studies on the effect of more systematic respiratory assessment education on nurses' ability to identify breathing problems.
2. Studies on the clinical efficacy of respiratory assessment tools.
3. Studies to identify psychological and physiological factors related to patients' perceptions of dyspnoea.
4. Studies to identify strategies used by patients to relieve dyspnoea.
5. Studies to explore the mechanisms underlying such strategies.
6. Studies to identify the ability of patients with respiratory impairment to carry out activities of daily living.
7. Studies to explore different modes of exercise and activity to improve activity tolerance of patients with chronic breathing impairment.
8. Studies to evaluate patient education programmes for self-care of chronic breathing impairment.

REFERENCES

Asmundsson T, Johnson RF, Kilburn K (1973) Efficiency of nebulisers for depositing saline in the human lung. *American Review of Respiratory Diseases* **108**, 506.

Bake B, Wood L, Murphy B, Macklem PT, Millic-Emili J (1974) The effect of inspiratory flow rate on the regional distribution of inspired gas. *Journal of Applied Physiology* **37**, 8.

Banner NR, Govan JR (1986) Long-term transtracheal oxygen delivery through microcatheter due to chronic obstructive airways disease. *British Medical Journal* **293**, 111–114.

Barnes CA, Kirchoff KT (1986) Minimising hypoxaemia due to endotracheal suctioning. A review of the literature. *Heart and Lung* **15**(2), 164–176.

Bartlett R, Gazzaniga A, Geraghty T (1973) Respiratory manoeuvres to prevent post operative pulmonary complications. *Journal of the American Medical Association* **224**, 1017–1020.

Bass C, Gardner W (1985) Emotional influences on breathing and breathlessness. *Journal of Psychosomatic Research* **29**(6), 599–609.

Bateman JRM, Newman SP, Daunt KM (1981) Is cough as effective as chest physiotherapy in the removal of excessive tracheobronchial secretions. *Thorax* **36**, 683–687.

Baun MM, Flones MJ (1984) Cumulative effects of three sequential endotracheal suctioning episodes in the dog model. *Heart and Lung* **13**, 148–154.

Blake J (1975) On the movement of mucus in the lung. *Journal of Biomechanics* **8**, 179–190.

deBoek R, Zinman R (1984) Cough versus chest physiotherapy. A comparison of the acute effects on pulmonary function in patients with cystic fibrosis. *American Review of Respiratory Diseases* **129**, 182–184.

Booker HA (1984) Exercise training and breathing control in patients with chronic airflow limitation. *Physiotherapy* **70**(7), 258–260.

Breeze RG, Wheeldon EB (1977) The cells of the pulmonary airways. *American Review of Respiratory Diseases* **116**, 705–777.

Burdon JGW, Juniper EF, Killian KJ (1982) The perception of breathlessness in asthma. *American Review of Respiratory Diseases* **126**, 131–135.

Camner P, Jaarstrand C, Philipson K (1973) Trachiobronchial clearance in patients with influenza. *American Review of Respiratory Diseases* **108**, 131-135.

Campbell EJM (1960) A method of controlled oxygen administration which reduces the risk of carbon dioxide retention. *Lancet* **ii**, 12–14.

Carrieri VK, Janson-Bjerklie S, Jacobs S (1984) The sensation of dyspnoea: a review. *Heart and Lung* **13**(4), 436–446.

Celentano Norton L, Conforti LG (1985) The effects of body position on oxygenation. *Heart and Lung* **14**(1), 45–52.

Cheney FW, Butler J (1968) The effects of ultrasonically produced aerosols on airway resistance in man. *Anaesthesiology* **29**, 1099.

Cherniak RM, Cherniak L (1983) *Respiration in Health and Disease* 3rd Edition. WB Saunders Co, Philadelphia.

Chopra S, Taplin GV, Simmons DH (1977) Effects of hydration and physical therapy on tracheal transport velocity. *American Review of Respiratory Diseases* **115**, 1009–1014.

Cohen JL, Demers RR, Saklad M (1977) Air entrainment oxygen masks: A performance evaluation. *Respiratory Care* **22**, 227–282.

Cosenza JJ, Celentano Norton L (1986) Secretion clearance: State of the art from a nursing perspective. *Critical Care Nurse* **6**(4), 23–36.

Crosbie WJ, Sim DT (1986) The effect of postural modification on some aspects of pulmonary function following surgery of the upper abdomen. *Physiotherapy* **72**(10), 487–491.

Crosbie WJ, Myles S (1985) An investigation into the effect of postural modification on some aspects of normal pulmonary function. *Physiotherapy* **71**(7), 311–314.

Fishman AP, Ledlie JF (1979) Dyspnoea. *Bulletin European Physiopathology and Respiration* **15**, 789.

Freedberg PD, Hoffman LA, Light WC, Kreps MK (1987) Effect of progressive muscle relaxation on the objective symptoms and subjective responses associated with asthma. *Heart and Lung* **16**(1), 24–30.

Froese A, Bryan AC (1974) Effects of anaesthesia and paralysis on diaphragmatic mechanics in man. *Anaesthesiology* **41**, 242.

Gift AG, Plaut H, Jacox A (1986) Psychologic and physiologic factors related to dyspnoea in subjects with chronic obstructive pulmonary disease. *Heart and Lung* **15**(6), 595–601.

Gilbert R, Auchinloss JH, Brodsky J (1972) Changes in tidal volume frequency, and ventilation induced by their measurement. *American Review of Respiratory Diseases* **124**, 685–689.

Grassino AE, Goldman MD (1986) Respiratory muscle coordination. In: Macklem PT, Mead J (eds) *Handbook of Physiology, Section 3 The Respiratory System, Vol 3, Mechanics of Breathing, Part 2.* American Physiological Society, Bethesda, Maryland.

Gravelyn TR, Wegg JG (1980) Respiratory rate as an indicator of acute respiratory dysfunction. *Journal of the American Medical Association* **244**, 1123–1125.

Grimby G, Oxhoj H, Bake B (1975) Effects of abdominal breathing on distribution of ventilation in obstructive lung disease. *Clinics in Science and Molecular Medicine* **48**, 193–199.

Guyton AC (1981) *Textbook of Medical Physiology.* WB Saunders, Philadelphia.

Hanley MV, Tyler ML (1987) Ineffective airway clearance related to airway infection. *Nursing Clinics of North America* **22**(1), 135–149.

Hirsch JA, Tokayer JL, Robinson ML (1975) Effects of dry air and subsequent humidification on tracheal mucous velocity in dogs. *Journal of Applied Physiology* **39**, 242–246.

Hirsch SR (1980) Mucociliary clearance: pathology and clinical features. *Comprehensive Therapy* **6**, 56–61.

Hirsch S, Kory R (1967) An evaluation of the effect of nebulised n-acetylcysteine on sputum consistency. *Journal of Allergy* **39**, 265–273.

Hoffman LA (1987) Ineffective airway clearance related to neuromuscular dysfunction. *Nursing Clinics of North America* **22**(1), 151–165.

Hopp LJ, Williams M (1987) Ineffective breathing pattern related to decreased lung expansion. *Nursing Clinics of North America* **22**(1), 193–205.

Hough A (1984) The effect of posture on lung function. *Physiotherapy* **70**(3), 101–103.

Hunter PM (1981) Bedside monitoring of respiratory function. *Nursing Clinics of North America* **16**(2), 211–224.

Jaarstrand C, Camner P, Philipson K (1975) Mycoplasma pneumoniae and tracheobronchial clearance. *American Review of Respiratory Diseases* **110**, 415–419.

Javaheri S, Blum J, Kazemi H (1981) Pattern of breathing and carbon dioxide retention. *American Journal of Medicine* **71**, 228–234.

Jeffery P, Corrin B (1984) Structural analysis of the respiratory tract. In: Brainstock J (ed) *Immunology of the Lung and Upper Respiratory Tract*. McGraw Hill Book Co, New York.

Jenkins SC, Soutar SA (1986) A survey into the use of incentive spirometry following coronary artery by-pass graft surgery. *Physiotherapy* **72**(10), 492–493.

Johanson WG, Gould KG (1977) Lung defence mechanisms. *Basics of Respiratory Disease* **6**(2), 1–6.

Kim MJ, Larson JL (1987) Ineffective airway clearance and ineffective breathing patterns. *Nursing Clinics of North America* **22**(1), 125–134.

Kim MJ, Druz WS, Dannon J (1976) Mechanics of the canine diaphragm. *Journal of Applied Physiology* **41**, 369–382.

King M (1983) Mucous and mucociliary clearance. *Respiratory Care* **28**, 335–344.

Kinsman RA, Yaroush RA, Fernandez E (1983) Symptoms and experiences in chronic bronchitis and emphysema. *Chest* **83**, 755–761.

Knipper J (1984) Evaluation of adventitious sounds as an indicator of the need for tracheal suction. *Heart and Lung* **13**, 292–293.

Kuzenski BM (1978) Effect of negative pressure on tracheobronchial trauma. *Nursing Research* **27**, 260–263.

Lancet Editorial (1986) The enigma of breathlessness. *Lancet* **i**, 891–892.

Landa J, Kwoka MA, Chopra GA (1980) Effects of suctioning on mucociliary transport. *Chest* **77**, 202–207.

Lareau S, Larson JL (1987) Ineffective breathing pattern related to airflow limitation. *Nursing Clinics of North America* **22**(1), 177–191.

Larson JL, Kim MJ (1987) Ineffective breathing pattern related to respiratory muscle fatigue. *Nursing Clinics of North America* **22**(1), 205–223.

Leith DE, Butler JP, Sneldon SC (1986) Cough. In: Macklem PT, Mead J (eds) *Handbook of Physiology*. American Physiological Society, Bethesda, Maryland.

Lourenco RV, Luddenkemper R, Carton RW (1972) Patterns of distribution and clearance of aerosols in patients with bronchiectasis. *American Review of Respiratory Diseases* **106**, 857–866.

Luce J, Tyler MC, Peirson D (1984) *Intensive Respiratory Care*. WB Saunders Co, Philadelphia.

McGavin CR, Gupta SP, McHardy GJR (1976) Twelve minute walking test for assessing disability in chronic bronchitis. *British Medical Journal* **1**, 822–823.

McMichan JC, Michell C, Westbrook PR (1980) Pulmonary dysfunction following traumatic quadriplegia. *Journal of American Medical Association* **243**, 528–531.

Macklem PT, Mead J (1967) Resistance of central and peripheral airways as measured by a retrograde catheter. *Journal of Applied Physiology* **22**, 395.

Menkes H, Britt J (1980) Rationale for Physical Therapy. *American Review of Respiratory Diseases* **22**(5), 127–131.

Moody LE (1977) Primer for pulmonary hygiene. *American Journal of Nursing* **77**, 104–105.

Morgan WKC (1982) Pulmonary disability and impairment. Can't work? Won't work? *Basics of Respiratory Disease* **10**, 1–6.

Nagaraj HS, Fellows R, Shutt R, Yacoub U (1980) Recurrent lobar atelectasis due to acquired stenosis in neonates. *Journal of Paediatric Surgery* **15**, 411–514.

Naigow D, Powaser MM (1977) The effect of different endotracheal suction procedures on arterial blood gases in a controlled experimental model. *Heart and Lung* **6**, 808–816.

Newhouse M, Sanchis J, Bienstock J (1976) Lung defence mechanisms. *New England Journal of Medicine* **295**, 990–998.

Newhouse MT, Sanchis J, Dolovich M (1973) Mucociliary clearance in children with cystic fibrosis. In: Mangos JA, Talano RC (eds) *Fundamental Problems of Cystic Fibrosis and Related Diseases*. Stratton, New York.

Peters RM, Turnier E (1980) Physical therapy. Indications for and effects in surgical patients. *American Review of Respiratory Diseases* **122**(5), 147–154.

Phipps RJ (1981) The airways mucociliary system. In: Widdicombe JG (ed) *International Review of Physiology: Respiratory Physiology III* Vol 23. University Park Press, Baltimore.

Preston IM, Matthews HR, Ready AR (1986) Minitracheotomy. A new technique for tracheal suction. *Physiotherapy* **72**(10), 494–497.

Remolina C, Khan AJ, Santiago TV, Edelman NH (1981) Positional hypoxaemia in unilateral lung disease. *New England Journal of Medicine* **304**, 523.

Rokosky JS (1985) Assessment of the individual with altered respiratory function. *Nursing Clinics of North America* **20**, 196–209.

Roper W, Logan WW, Tierney AJ (1985) *The Elements of Nursing*. Churchill Livingstone, London.

Ross SM, Corrsin S (1974) Results of an analytical model of mucociliary pumping. *Journal of Applied Physiology* **37**, 333–340.

Ruppel G (1982) *Manual of Pulmonary Function Testing*. CV Mosby, St Louis.

Rux MI, Powaser MM (1979) Effect of apnea and three levels of negative pressure on the fall in arterial oxygen tension produced by endotracheal suctioning in dogs. *American Review of Respiratory Diseases* **119**, 193.

Shapiro B, Harrison R, Walton J (1977) *Clinical Application of Blood Gases*. Year Book Medical Publishers Inc, Chicago.

Sharp JT, Drutz WS, Moisan T, Foster J, Machnach W (1980) Postural relief of dyspnoea in severe chronic obstructive pulmonary disease. *American Review of Respiratory Diseases* **122**, 201–211.

Shekleton ME, Nield M (1987) Ineffective airway clearance related to artificial airway. *Nursing Clinics of North America* **22**(1), 167–177.

Shim C, Fernandez K, Fine M, Williams H (1969) Cardiac arrhythmias resulting from tracheal suctioning. *American International Medicine* **71**, 1147–1153.

Sitzman J, Kamiya J, Johnston J (1983) Biofeedback training for reduced respiratory rate in chronic obstructive pulmonary disease. A preliminary study. *Nursing Research* **32**(4), 212–223.

Snider GL, Rinaldo JE (1980) Oxygen therapy in medical patients hospitalised outside of the intensive care unit. *American Review of Respiratory Diseases* **122**, 29–36.

Sterling GM (1983) *Respiratory Disease*. William Heinemann Medical Books Ltd, London.

Stradling JR (1986) Hypercapnia during oxygen therapy in airways obstruction: a reappraisal. *Thorax* **41**, 897–902.

Stubbing DG, Mattur PN, Roberts RS (1982) Some physical signs in patients with chronic airflow obstruction. *American Review of Respiratory Diseases* **125**, 549–552.

Tandberg D, Sklar D (1983) Effect of tachypnoea on the estimation of body temperature by an oral thermometer. *New England Journal of Medicine* **308**, 945–946.

Thomas RL, Stokes GL, Ross GL (1966) The efficacy of pursed lips breathing in patients with chronic obstructive pulmonary disease. *American Review of Respiratory Diseases* **93**, 100.

Traver GA (1985) Ineffective airway clearance. Physiology and clinical applications. *Dimensions of Critical Care Nursing* **4**, 198–209.

Tydeman DE, Chandler AR, Graveling BM, Culot A, Harrison BDW (1984) An investigation into the effects of exercise tolerance training on patients with chronic airway obstruction. *Physiotherapy* **70**(7), 261–264.

Wanner A, Rao A (1980) Clinical indications for and effects of bland, mucolytic and antimicrobial aerosols. *American Review of Respiratory Diseases* **122**, 79–87.

Webb JR, Cochrane GM (1981) Arterial blood gases and acid-base balance. In: Webb JR (ed) *Assessment of a Patient with Lung Disease*, NTP Press, Lancaster.

West J (1979) *Respiratory Physiology. The Essentials*. 2nd Edn. William and Wilkins Co, Baltimore.

Widinsky J (1979) Dyspnoea. *Cor Vasa* **21**, 128.

Wood RE, Wanner A, Hirsch J, Farrell PM (1975) Tracheal mucociliary transport with cystic fibrosis and its stimulation by terbutaline. *American Review of Respiratory Diseases* **111**, 733–738.

Woodcock AA, Gross ER, Geddes DM (1981) Drug treatment of breathlessness: contrasting effects of diazepam and promethazine in 'pink puffers'. *British Medical Journal* **283**, 343–346.

Wyndham CH, Strydon NB, van Graan CH (1971) Walk or jog for health. *South African Medical Journal* **45**, 53–57.

Young CS (1984) A review of the adverse effects of airway suction. *Physiotherapy* **70**(3), 104–108.

Index

i 133 234 90